Cognitive and Perceptual Dysfunction

A Clinical Reasoning Approach to Evaluation and Intervention

Cognitive and Perceptual Dysfunction

*A Clinical Reasoning Approach
to Evaluation and Intervention*

Carolyn Unsworth, PhD, OTR
School of Occupational Therapy
Faculty of Health Sciences
La Trobe University
Bundoora, Victoria
Australia

 F. A. DAVIS COMPANY • Philadelphia

F. A. Davis Company
1915 Arch Street
Philadelphia, PA 19103

Printed in the United States of America

Last digit indicates print number: 10 9 8 7 6 5 4 3 2 1

Publisher, Health Professions: Jean-François Vilain
Senior Editor: Lynn Borders Caldwell
Developmental Editor: Crystal Spraggins
Production Editor: Stephen D. Johnson
Cover Designer: Louis J. Forgione

As new scientific information becomes available through basic and clinical research, recommended treatments and drug therapies undergo changes. The author and publisher have done everything possible to make this book accurate, up to date, and in accord with accepted standards at the time of publication. The author, editors, and publisher are not responsible for errors or omissions or for consequences from application of the book, and make no warranty, expressed or implied, in regard to the contents of the book. Any practice described in this book should be applied by the reader in accordance with professional standards of care used in regard to the unique circumstances that may apply in each situation. The reader is advised always to check product information (package inserts) for changes and new information regarding dose and contraindications before administering any drug. Caution is especially urged when using new or infrequently ordered drugs.

Library of Congress Cataloging-in-Publication Data
Unsworth, Carolyn, 1966–
    Cognitive and perceptual dysfunction : a clinical reasoning
approach to evaluation and intervention / Carolyn Unsworth.
        p.   cm.
    Includes bibliographical references and index.
    ISBN 0-8036-0399-1 (alk. paper)
    1. Cognitive disorders—Patients—Rehabilitation Case studies.
    2. Cerebrovascular disease—Patients—Rehabilitation Case studies.
    3. Perception, Disorders of—Patients—Rehabilitation Case studies.
    I. Title.
        [DNLM: 1. Brain Injuries—rehabilitation Case Report.
    2. Cognition Disorders—rehabilitation Case Report.   3. Occupational
    Therapy Case Report.   WL 354 U59c 1999]
    RC553.C64U57   1999
    616.8'—dc21
    DNLM/DLC
    for Library of Congress   99-19072
                                                                              CIP

Foreword

Adults with brain injury who struggle with residual cognitive and perceptual deficits know only too well that these problems can sometimes make even the simplest life activity impossible. Occupational therapy practitioners hoping to help these clients need to understand: (1) the functional implications of cognitive and perceptual dysfunction, from the client's perspective; (2) the neurological underpinnings of cognition, perception, and learning; and (3) the range of evaluation and intervention approaches available to address different cognitive and perceptual problems. *Cognitive and Perceptual Dysfunction: A Clinical Reasoning Approach to Evaluation and Intervention* helps practitioners gain these understandings. This book helps students and practitioners work with adults with cognitive and perceptual problems in effective, holistic, and humane ways.

There are several features of this book that distinguish it from other texts currently available on this topic. First, it uses current occupational therapy clinical-reasoning language to explain the thought processes associated with cognitive and perceptual evaluation and intervention. The clinical-reasoning and case-study chapters include firsthand practitioner explanations of the clinicians' thought processes, making them accessible to readers. This is important, because these thought processes are not obvious during practitioner-client interactions and can only be learned when they are made explicit.

Second, the material on specific cognitive and perceptual dysfunctions is organized around case studies (Chapters 4–11). These case studies walk readers through the evaluation and intervention reasoning process associated with the cognitive and perceptual problems most commonly seen with brain injury. This organization makes the material personal and directly relevant to practice. The client-centered focus and emphasis on functional outcomes in the case studies highlight the importance of designing intervention around the goals of clients and their families, to ensure good intervention oucomes.

The case-study chapters also present a diversity of theoretical approaches to evaluation and intervention. This diversity highlights the complexity of cognitive and perceptual practice and the need for practitioners to keep an open, analytic mind in choosing the best evaluation and intervention strategies for any given client in any given practice setting.

Third, contributors are an international group of experts in the areas on which they are writing. This international representation should expand the thinking of students and practitioners who use the book by highlighting the commonalities of occupational therapy practice around the world and by demonstrating differences in practice in varied practice settings.

Taken together, these features make the book a welcome addition to the literature on cognitive and perceptual dysfunction in adults. Students and practitioners alike should be able to use this text to improve the quality of evaluation and intervention for clients with cognitive and perceptual dysfunction around the world.

Maureen E. Neistadt, ScD, OTR/L, FAOTA

FOREWORD

Books and articles in occupational therapy have tended to take one of three approaches: (1) theory (theory and philosophy of the profession), (2) practice (theories and principles of practice), or (3) application (applications of principles and techniques to particular patient populations, diagnostic conditions, or occupational dysfunctions). Another focus, *clinical reasoning*, was added in 1982 when Rogers and Massagatani sparked interest in the thinking strategies used by therapists during the occupational therapy assessment process. Since then there has been considerable interest in studying and explicating the clinical-reasoning processes and skills of therapists in both assessment and treatment (for a comprehensive review of the trends in this literature see Chapter 2). Dr. Unsworth has designed a unique book that blends theory, practice, and clinical reasoning. This strategy makes such good sense that it is sure to become a popular approach with occupational therapy writers.

In the first three chapters, Dr. Unsworth presents an excellent understanding of the theoretical approaches to practice in cognitive perceptual dysfunction, a superb overview of clinical reasoning, and an integration of how both the theoretical knowledge and the reasoning capacity of the therapist are combined in practice.

In the ensuing chapters, Dr. Unsworth, together with well-recognized theoreticians, has organized each chapter around a case study of a patient who illustrates the impairment under discussion. These case-study chapters are organized in two ways. The first is concerned with cognitive and perceptual impairments. Each of the case-study chapters provides details concerning a particular class of cognitive or perceptual dysfunction and an overview of the neuroanatomy/neurophysiology of the problem. A broad view is taken where the problems discussed are not necessarily specific to a particular disease or injury but produce functional limitations in the person's occupational performance. This allows the reader to move away from the restrictions of the medical model view of the patient's disease and helps the therapist frame the questions to be addressed from an occupational therapy perspective. The therapist can then more rapidly select appropriate evaluation and treatment models and methods.

Second, each chapter focuses on the therapeutic journey undertaken by the therapist and client and takes the reader through the entire evaluation and intervention process while explicating the therapist's reasoning. Until now the notion of how to select evaluation and intervention methods has been typically "hitched" to diagnostic categories. Clinical reasoning has been described as an important process but one that is studied more or less as a phenomenon in itself and is located in the mind of the therapist. While many authors use case studies of stories or clinical examples to illustrate the clinical-reasoning process, the structure that Dr. Unsworth has created highlights the importance of multiple perspectives—disease, impairment, disability, theory, technique, and clinical reasoning—and the necessity for them to be highly integrated. The experienced theorists and clinicians who have contributed to this book illustrate for the reader how to do this. Thus, the reader learns not only techniques of evaluation and intervention but how to frame the question initially so that selection of a theoretical model for evaluation and treatment, the particular evaluation tools to be used, and the treatment strategies used will be the best match for the condition presented.

It has been said that the slogan of occupational therapists is "We put it all together." Dr. Unsworth and her colleagues have indeed "put it all to-gether" for those who do or will work with individuals with cognitive and perceptual deficits and the functional problems that result. This book will be especially useful for academic and clinical faculty in teaching students the theory, principles, and techniques of practice within the context of de-veloping the students' reasoning skills. It follows the new intellectual and educational focus on developing analytical skills while maintaining a tra-ditional respect for established theory and valid treatment approaches. Until now individual educators have developed course materials and in-structional methods on their own in an attempt to integrate this material for students. Now, for at least one area of practice, there is a compilation and a guide that will be much appreciated. This text will also be an excel-lent source for the new practitioner and the clinical supervisor responsible for teaching and staff training.

I think this book is destined to become a classroom classic and a clinical handbook that all therapists will find informative, challenging, and inspir-ing. It will also hopefully inspire other talented therapists and teachers to write similar texts in other areas of occupational therapy practice. Just as the authors have provided models of excellent practice and the reasoning behind it, others will find the format of the book a model for their own work.

Maureen Hayes Fleming, EdD, OTR, FAOTA

Preface

". . . the aim of occupational therapy education is to teach students how to think like practitioners, that is, how to engage in clinical reasoning" (Neistadt, 1996, p. 676).

Over recent years, I have been crafting my courses on cognitive and perceptual dysfunction around a clinical reasoning framework. I have found that this approach offers students both a firm grounding in problems of a cognitive or perceptual nature and the freedom to examine and question the reasoning behind the theoretical approaches, evaluations, and interventions adopted. In particular, the use of a clinical-reasoning framework seems to encourage both students and clinicians to reflect on their practice or clinical experiences and to provide a language for further discussion.

The aim of this book is to provide occupational therapy students, novice clinicians, and clinicians who are new to the field with an understanding of how experienced therapists reason during their evaluations of and interventions with clients who have cognitive and/or perceptual problems. Specifically this book aims to provide the reader with:

- An overview of the different theoretical approaches that guide practice when working with clients who have cognitive and perceptual problems,
- An understanding of how theory integrates with practice in this field,
- An overview of the role of clinical reasoning in occupational therapy practice,
- Information on a variety of standardized assessment techniques that can be used to identify a client's cognitive and perceptual problems, or functional problems, which may be due to cognitive and perceptual impairments,
- An understanding of the reasoning behind assessment choice and application and the interpretation of assessment findings,
- Information on a variety of intervention approaches, techniques, and activities that can be used to remediate or compensate for a client's cognitive or perceptual problems,
- An understanding of the reasoning behind treatment choice and implementation, and treatment monitoring and modification, and

- Information on techniques that can be used to evaluate the effectiveness of intervention, and an understanding of the reasoning behind intervention evaluation.

These aims are achieved through the provision of research-based information concerning the neuroanatomical and physiological mechanisms that produce cognitive and perceptual problems, the different theoretical orientations that guide therapy, and the variety of evaluation and intervention procedures that can be adopted. Then, through the presentation of case studies the reader is guided through the clinical reasoning that supports occupational therapy practice in a particular area. Consistently, educators select the case-study method as an approach that retains the richness and complexity of practice and yet provides students and novice clinicians with an entree to the expert reasoning of clinicians (Neistadt, 1996; Dutton, 1995; Robertson, 1996; Higgs & Jones, 1995). The case-study method adopted in this book, combined with the use of the language of clinical reasoning (Mattingly & Fleming, 1994), has provided us with a means of raising tacit knowledge to conscious awareness so it can be examined, discussed, and passed on to students and novice clinicians.

Acquired brain damage rarely produces a single discrete problem. Rather, clients present with a variety of motor, sensory, and cognitive-perceptual problems and subsequent difficulties in carrying out their daily work, self-care, or leisure activities. Because no two clients present with the same kinds of problems, the therapy process will differ with every client. Recognition of the client's unique pattern of strengths and weaknesses is crucial to a successful therapy program. Thus, while the case-study chapters focus on one particular cognitive or perceptual impairment, the client will also experience a range of other problems that will figure more largely in the overall therapy program. However, space limitations require us to remain focused on the reasonings behind our evaluations and interventions. Although this book was written for occupational therapy students and practitioners, a variety of other health professionals may also find it useful.

The book is divided into 11 chapters. In Chapter 1, several of the theoretical approaches are explored, which therapists use to guide their evaluations and interventions while working with clients with cognitive and perceptual problems. A different theoretical orientation is then adopted in each of the case-study chapters (Chapters 4 through 11) to illustrate how this approach guides practice. Chapter 2 examines how clinical reasoning can be better used to understand and improve practice, and to share our practice with student and novice clinicians. The purpose of Chapter 3 is to explore aspects of clinical reasoning specific to evaluation and intervention of clients with cognitive and perceptual problems. The aim of this chapter is to provide the reader with an overview of the therapy process and associated reasoning prior to the case-study chapters. A range of standardized assessments are presented in detail in this chapter, and are discussed by the various expert contributors in the case-study chapters.

Chapters 4 through 11 are arranged to examine cognitive problems and metacognitive problems, as well as the more spatial, or perceptual, problems that can follow acquired brain damage. Chapter 4 examines problems with concentration from a neurodevelopmental approach; Chapter 5 builds on the information in Chapter 4 by exploring memory, using a quadraphonic approach. Chapter 6 examines the metacognitive problem of disorders of executive abilities and functions, using a rehabilitation approach. Praxic problems are the focus of Chapter 7, whereas Chapter 8 examines problems with simple perceptual problems: the agnosias. Using a cognitive retraining approach, Chapter 9 examines the problem of unilateral neglect, and Chapter 10 then tackles the complex perceptual problems, known as spatial-relations disorders. In Chapter 11, the focus is on group work with clients with cognitive and perceptual problems and the challenges often faced by facilitators of these groups. Although the case-study chapters present clients engaged in one-to-one therapy, the majority of clients are also involved in some form of therapeutic or self-help group.

For the most part a similar format has been used throughout. Chapters open with a review of the cognitive or perceptual problem under study, discussing the neuroanatomical-neurophysiological basis for this problem. A case study follows, which provides details of the client and the treating therapist, including the particular theoretical orientation adopted by the therapist. Assessment, intervention, and therapy evaluation procedures are then presented, including clinical reasoning boxes, which detail the therapist's thoughts and rationale. Finally, each chapter concludes with a series of questions for the reader to discuss and complete. These questions enable readers to test their understanding of material presented in the chapter, and can be used for classroom review and for clinic discussions and debates. Finally, a few comments on writing style. The clinical reasoning boxes have been written in the first person because they are personal explanations (narratives) of therapy involving the thoughts of a particular therapist. They have been provided to assist the reader to understand more about what the therapist is thinking and therefore why he or she performs certain actions. Each chapter opens with a list of key terms. An understanding of these terms is essential to working through each chapter, and these terms are all defined in the glossary. Unless otherwise stated, the book has been written with the therapist and client usually referred to in the singular male form, which has been done for ease of reading.

Carolyn Unsworth

Acknowledgments

This book is the product of the expertise of many individuals to whom I express my sincere thanks. My interest in using clinical reasoning as a foundation for teaching students about cognitive and perceptual problems was sparked through teaching master's-level students at The Boston School of Occupational Therapy (BSOT), Tufts University, a program organized around a clinical-reasoning framework. I thank all of my colleagues at BSOT for sharing their ideas on clinical reasoning with me, and Maureen Hayes Fleming, in particular, for developing, along with Cheryl Mattingly, the language of reasoning, which is now used internationally and has been adopted for use in this book. Thanks to all of my students from Tufts University and La Trobe University. Your constant demand for the most up-to-date information and thirst for knowledge motivated me to write this book.

I would like to thank Betty Abreu, Guðrún Árnadóttir, Jenny Butler, Louise Corben, Leslie Duran, Anne Fisher, Alison Laver, and Sharan Schwartzberg, from the United States, Iceland, Canada, England, and Australia, for sharing their knowledge and expertise by contributing chapters to the book. I have found our national and international collaboration to be both stimulating and enriching. Chapter authors also acknowledge those who have assisted in the development of chapters in some specific way.

The book was reviewed by a team of talented occupational therapy educators, who are listed below. In particular, I would like to thank Sandra David, Anne Fisher, Arlene Lorch, Gwendolyn Parker, and Barbara Prudhomme White. The thoughtful and stimulating nature of their feedback challenged us all to improve the quality of the text.

M. Carolyn Baum, PhD, OTR/L, FAOTA
Elias Michael Director
Program in Occupational Therapy
Washington University School of Medicine
St. Louis, Missouri

Sandra K. David, MHE, OTR/L
Senior Staff Therapist
Department of Occupational Therapy
Medical College of Georgia
Augusta, Georgia

Anne G. Fisher, ScD, OTR, FAOTA
Professor
Department of Occupational
   Therapy
and Director
Assessment of Motor and Process
   Skills Project
Colorado State University
Fort Collins, Colorado

Lianne Hewitt, MPH, OTR
Program Director and Assistant
   Professor
Occupational Therapy Assisting
   Department
Loma Linda University
Loma Linda, California

Arlene Lorch, OTR, MS, CHES
Clinical Instructor
Department of Occupational
   Therapy
College of Health Professions
Thomas Jefferson University
Philadelphia, Pennsylvania

**Maureen E. Neistadt, ScD, OTR/L,
   FAOTA**
Assistant Professor
Department of Occupational
   Therapy
University of New Hampshire
Durham, New Hampshire

**Gwendolyn L. Parker, MA, OTR,
   OTC**
Program Director
Department of Occupational
   Therapy
Texas Tech University Health
   Sciences Center
Odessa, Texas

**Barbara Prudhomme White, PhD,
   OTR**
Assistant Professor
Department of Occupational
   Therapy
School of Health and Human
   Services
University of New Hampshire
Durham, New Hampshire

Crystal Spraggins and Lynn Borders Caldwell of F. A. Davis have offered a great deal of assistance and support from a considerable distance. There is very little that cannot be done through e-mail communication and express mail! Thanks to the team at F. A. Davis for making this book possible.

Finally, I would like to thank my husband, David, my parents, Wilma and Warwick, and all of my family for their interest in, enthusiasm for, and support of this project.

Carolyn Unsworth

Contributors

Beatriz C. Abreu, PhD, OTR,
  FAOTA
Clinical Professor, University of
  Galveston
and
Director of Occupational Therapy
Transitional Learning Community
  at Galveston
Galveston, Texas, USA

Guðrún Árnadóttir, MA, BOT
Senior Occupational Therapist
Reykjavík City Hospital
Reykjavík, Iceland

Jennifer A. Butler, BScHons, Dip
  COT, T.Cert (HE), PhD
Senior Lecturer
School of Occupational Therapy
Dorset House
Oxford Brookes University
Oxford, England

Louise Corben, BAppSci (Occ
  Ther), MA Candidate
Senior Clinician
Department of Occupational
  Therapy
Monash Medical Center
Clayton, Victoria, Australia

Leslie Duran, MS, OTR
Research Associate and Assistant
  Director
Assessment of Motor and Process
  Skills Project
Colorado State University
Fort Collins, Colorado, USA

Anne G. Fisher, ScD, OTR, FAOTA
Professor, Department of
  Occupational Therapy and
Director, Assessment of Motor and
  Process Skills Project
Colorado State University
Fort Collins, Colorado, USA

Alison Laver, PhD, OT (L),
  DipCOT, SROT
Assistant Professor
School of Rehabilitation Science
Faculty of Health Sciences
McMaster University
Hamilton, Ontario, Canada

Sharan L. Schwartzberg, EdD,
  OTR, FAOTA
Professor and Chair
The Boston School of Occupational
  Therapy
Tufts University
Medford, Massachusetts, USA

Contents

1

Introduction to Cognitive and Perceptual Dysfunction: Theoretical Approaches to Therapy

CAROLYN UNSWORTH, PhD, OTR

- Ability
- Adaptation
- Agnosia
- Apraxia
- Attention
- Capacity
- Cognition
- Concentration
- Disability
- Executive Functions
- Generalization
- Impairment
- Insight
- Judgment

- Learning
- Memory
- Metacognition
- Neuropsychology
- Perception
- Performance Areas
- Performance Components
- Performance Contexts
- Problem Solving
- Rehabilitation
- Remediation
- Residual
- Taxonomy
- Unilateral Neglect

On completion of the chapter, the reader will be able to:

- Define cognition and perception
- List the main causes of cognitive and perceptual problems in adults
- Describe a range of ways to classify cognitive and perceptual capacities and impairments
- Discuss several different theoretical approaches a therapist might use when working with clients who have cognitive and perceptual problems
- Successfully work through the Review Questions

Cognitive and perceptual problems are some of the most puzzling and disabling difficulties that a person can experience. Thinking, remembering, reasoning, and making sense of the world around us are fundamental to carrying out everyday living activities. Problems with capacities such as thinking or remembering can have a devastating effect on an individual's life and the lives of his or her family members. Although some degree of habilitation or rehabilitation is often possible, many people with cognitive and perceptual problems are not able to live alone, hold down paid employment, or sustain a family life and relationships. The development or acquisition of cognitive and perceptual problems can produce great personal difficulties, hardships, and burdens for family and considerable financial cost to the individual, his or her family, and the community. The purpose of this chapter is to provide the reader with a foundation of knowledge concerning cognition and perception. The chapter opens with a review of some of the causes of cognitive and perceptual problems in adults. From there, attention turns to the different classification systems used to describe normal and abnormal cognition and perception and some of the models and theoretical approaches that occupational therapists use to guide practice in this field. This chapter aims to provide the reader with an overview of what cognition and perception are so he or she can adopt the clinical reasoning framework presented in Chapter 2 to successfully work through the case study chapters (Chapters 4 to 11). This chapter provides many references for further exploration of areas if the reader requires further information.

☰ INTRODUCTION

This book has been written for occupational therapy students who are learning about, and clinicians who work with, adolescent and adult clients who have cognitive and perceptual problems. Many of the approaches outlined in the book may be applied to a pediatric clients who have brain damage at birth, head injury after trauma, or developmental or learning problems. However, the prognoses and therapeutic needs of children with cognitive and perceptual problems are often different from those of adolescents and adults and are not specifically addressed in this text.

In 1980, the World Health Organization (WHO) adopted the classification system of disease, impairment, disability, and handicap to describe the sequelae of a health event. This book is organized around cognitive and perceptual impairments (such as reduced memory or apraxia) but also considers the disabling impact of these problems on daily living activities. Although an understanding of the client's disease or diagnosis provides the therapist with information about expected outcomes and prognosis, clients with quite different diagnoses can present in a similar manner, with similar impairments and disabilities, and respond to treatment in a similar way. Conversely, clients with the same diagnosis can present in therapy with very different problems and needs. **Impairment** and **capacity** are the terms used when describing performance components, and **disability** and **ability** are the terms used when occupational performance areas such as daily living activities are described. After impairments are identified, the emphasis for occupational therapists shifts to assessing and treating the client's disabilities and assisting him to minimize the handicapping aspects of these disabilities.

An example of the WHO model applied to occupational therapy practice in cognition and perception is as follows: A 40-year-old man has cerebrovascular *disease* and as a result of this experiences a cerebral infarct or stroke. As he recovers in the hospital it becomes apparent that he has several impairments, including a left-sided hemiparesis, left **unilateral neglect**, difficulty in **problem solving**, and reduced memory skills. The functional implications of these impairments are classified as *disabilities* and include decreased ability to walk, bumping into things on his left side, inability to manage his financial affairs while in the hospital, and difficulty with dressing. The *handicapping* effects of the stroke may not be fully realized by this man or his family until he returns to live in the community. His handicaps may include not being able to return to work or driving or difficulty in attending his favorite sporting events. The WHO is also considering adding a new classification called *well-being* to the model. Difficulties this man experiences in terms of his personal relationships, mood, and the way he feels about the quality of his life are described under this classification. In this case example, the occupational therapist will obtain information about the client's disease and impairments through discussions with the physician and neuropsychologist. The therapist may confirm the client's impairments through evaluation procedures and will then focus on the client's abilities and disabilities during the intervention program.

CAUSES AND INCIDENCE OF COGNITIVE AND PERCEPTUAL DYSFUNCTION

Although this book is organized around impairments and focuses on disability, it is useful to briefly consider the underlying causes of cognitive and perceptual problems and some of the incidence rates at which these diagnoses occur. The brain may be damaged through several mechanisms. These include:

- Tumors that are benign or malignant
- Trauma resulting from motor vehicle accidents, falls, or violent incidents (e.g., sports or gunshot)
- Infections, such as encephalitis

- Anoxia after near drowning, cardiopulmonary arrest, or carbon monoxide poisoning
- Toxins such as alcohol or substance abuse
- Vascular disease, which may produce an infarct or hemorrhagic stroke

Clients with these specific diagnoses/brain incidents are presented in the case study chapters in the book. Clients with mental health disorders such as schizophrenia or chronic depression, neurological conditions such as Parkinson's disease or multiple sclerosis, and other degenerative diseases, such as Alzheimer's disease, may also experience cognitive and perceptual disorders. The book does not specifically address the cognitive and perceptual problems associated with these chronic or degenerative conditions. However, many of the issues discussed, evaluations used, and interventions described in this book may also be useful for therapists working with these client groups.

The largest two groups of people who acquire cognitive and perceptual problems are those who have experienced stroke and traumatic brain injury. The incidence rates for these two diagnostic groups are briefly reviewed. Traumatic brain injury may be defined as an insult to the brain caused by an external force. Traumatic brain injuries may be described as skull fractures, penetrating head wounds, closed head injuries, or traumatic injury to extracranial blood vessels (Winkler, 1995). Describing the incidence of traumatic brain injuries is difficult because of differences in definitions of brain injury and reporting procedures. In the United States, each year approximately 500,000 persons require hospitalization as a result of brain injury, and 70,000 to 90,000 persons require some form of therapeutic intervention (Goldstein, 1990). Winkler (1995) estimates that the lifetime cost for an individual with a severe head injury exceeds $4 million. He also estimates that head injury costs the community approximately $25 billion annually.

A stroke, or cerebrovascular accident, is a condition of sudden onset caused by an acute vascular lesion in the brain (Thomas, 1997). Stroke is one of the foremost causes of disability among older adults (Kelly-Hayes et al., 1989), and stroke-related disability involves significant use of health and community services. The American Heart Association (1991) estimates that each year approximately 550,000 Americans will have a stroke. It has been documented that at any one time, approximately 3 million people in the United States have a stroke-related disability that requires ongoing management and care (Agency for Health Care Policy and Research, 1995). The costs associated with diagnosis and treatment of stroke and lost productivity are reported to be in excess of $30 billion each year (Matchar et al., 1994). The American Occupational Therapy Association (AOTA) Member Data Survey suggests that approximately 30 percent of occupational therapists work with people after stroke or traumatic brain injury (American Occupational Therapy Association, 1990). Similarly, approximately 21 percent of therapists in Australia are reported to work in **rehabilitation**, mostly with people who have experienced a stroke or head injury (Australian Association of Occupational Therapists, 1991). The significance of cognitive and perceptual problems both in terms of the number of clients who experience such difficulties and the devastating impact these problems have on peoples' lives warrants the profession's continued support of research and practice in this field.

DIFFERENCES BETWEEN COGNITIVE AND PERCEPTUAL FUNCTIONS

Although **cognition** and **perception** have been defined separately for the purposes of this book, some authors believe that the two are indistinguishable. For example, Abreu and Hinojosa (1992) argue that it is almost impossible to differentiate clinically between cognitive and perceptual processing. They put forth the notion that both cognition and perception require sensory recognition, manipulation, and interpretation and that both are subjective processes. At this time, there is insufficient evidence to suggest which approach most accurately reflects the way we think about and perceive information. However, because the majority of work in this field does distinguish between these processes, and because it is probably easier to learn about cognitive and perceptual deficits individually, they are defined separately.

Cognitive processes are generally defined as the abilities that enable us to "think," which includes the ability to **concentrate** (pay **attention**), remember, and learn. Under such a broad definition, many review texts in the field also refer to **executive functions** as cognitive in nature (Banich, 1997; Mapou & Spector, 1995: Mateer, 1997; Zoltan, 1996; Stuss, 1992). Executive functions include the ability to plan, manipulate information, initiate and terminate activities, and recognize errors. These functions are essential for an individual to live independently and adapt to life in the community (Mateer, 1997). However, some researchers more specifically label executive functions as higher-order cognitive functions (Glosser & Goodglass, 1990) or **metacognitive** (Katz & Hartman-Maeir, 1997; Winegardner, 1993). This issue is discussed more fully by Duran and Fisher in Chapter 6. However, for the purpose of this book, executive functions are categorized under metacognitive performance components.

Perception is the ability to transform information from the senses (touch, hearing, vision, smell, taste, and kinesthesia) and then use it to interact appropriately with the environment. Perceptual deficits do not lie in the sensory ability itself but rather with the individual's ability to interpret the sensation accurately and therefore respond appropriately. Lezak (1995) defines perception as the integration of sensory impressions into information that is psychologically meaningful. Disorders of perception presented in this book encompass simple perceptual problems such as the **agnosias**, complex perceptual problems such as difficulties with spatial relations, the **apraxias**, difficulties executing skilled learned movements, and unilateral neglect.

The cognitive and perceptual problems presented in this book are arranged in a somewhat sequential way. In the past, Trexler (1987), among others, postulated that cognitive and higher cognitive subskills are hierarchical in nature, with basic skills such as **memory** and concentration as prerequisites for more advanced skills such as reasoning and planning. Although there is mounting research evidence to suggest that this is not always the case (e.g., Lezak, 1995), this book has retained this approach to organization for convenience of information presentation. Therefore, the first case study chapters describe the cognitive problems of concentration, memory, and **learning** before presenting metacognitive or higher-order cognitive problems such as executive functions and more complex motor and perceptual processing problems.

CLASSIFICATION OF COGNITIVE AND PERCEPTUAL FUNCTION AND DYSFUNCTION

Cognitive and perceptual capacities and impairments have been defined, classified, and grouped in a variety of ways by researchers and writers in this field. Occupational therapists, psychologists, neuropsychologists, speech-language pathologists, and physicians all write about these problems using terminology that has evolved historically in their disciplines. Therefore, reading literature in this field is often complex and challenging. The three main approaches to classifying cognitive and perceptual capacities and impairments are: (1) according to the lobes of the cerebral cortex, (2) relating to the functional systems as proposed by Luria (1966, 1973) (described later in this chapter), and (3) according to major psychological function (Miller & Gil, 1995). Although there are differences in the ways occupational therapists categorize these problems, many of these organizing structures are compatible, and all adopt categorization systems based on psychological function. For example, Árnadóttir's (1990) approach to organizing cognitive and perceptual disorders (including related motor components) adopts the main classification approach of occupational performance areas and components outlined in the AOTA's document on uniform terminology (1994a). However, differences lie in the way each author divides performance components. Several classification systems will be presented to illustrate that occupational therapists and other authors in the field of cognition and perception are not in agreement and that clinicians need to choose an organizing framework that best meets their needs. Clinicians should be directed in their choice of an organizing framework through selection of a theoretical model. These models are discussed later in the chapter.

The AOTA's document on uniform terminology outlines a structure for understanding occupational therapy practice domains (American Occupational Therapy Association, 1994a). Three domains are presented:

1. **Performance areas** that encompass daily living activities, work or productivity, and leisure
2. **Performance components** that are the capacities that are required for successful engagement in performance areas and include cognitive integration and cognitive components, sensorimotor components, and psychosocial skills and psychological components
3. **Performance contexts** that include the temporal or environmental factors that influence an individual's participation in a performance area

Examples of cognitive components within this classification system include perceptual and praxic abilities that are classified as sensorimotor components and memory, which is classified as a cognitive integration/cognitive component.

Árnadóttir (1990) uses the AOTA's broad outline of occupational performance as a background for her work. She presents cognitive and perceptual problems according to area of brain function. As such, damage to the frontal lobe may result in problems such as apraxia, motor perseveration, speech and language dysfunction, disturbed eye movements, reduced problem solving, emotional impairments and affective disorders, reduced **judgment**, decreased arousal, decreased **insight**, problems with memory, and difficulty with organization and sequencing. Damage to the parietal lobes may result in problems such as agnosia, apraxia, spatial-relations syndrome, and topographical disorientation. The occipital lobes are responsible for vision-related tasks; therefore, damage to this lobe may result in homonymous hemianopsia and visual agnosias. Damage to the temporal lobes may result in problems such as aphasia, agnosia (related to audition), agraphia and acalculia, memory problems, and emotional or personality disorders (Árnadóttir, 1990). Although these broad guidelines associating brain regions with various capacities and impairments can be useful, clients with quite similar brain lesions can experience quite different impairments, and vice versa. It is well-established that multiple brain areas are often responsible for a single capacity (Lezak, 1995).

Árnadóttir (1990) divides cognitive and perceptual problems (and related motor components) into neurobehavioral-specific impairments and neurobehavioral-pervasive impairments. A summary of the classification used by Árnadóttir in the Árnadóttir Occupational Therapy Neurobehavioral Evaluation (A-ONE) (1990) (reviewed in Chapter 3), is presented in Table 1–1. Árnadóttir's classification system presents deficits, in contrast to the AOTA self-study series on cognitive rehabilitation, which presents a **taxonomy** of cognitive and perceptual abilities (Mosey, 1993). A summary of Mosey's tax-

---

Table 1–1. Classification of neurobehavioral deficits used in the (A-ONE) (Árnadóttir, 1990)

NEUROBEHAVIORAL SPECIFIC IMPAIRMENTS	NEUROBEHAVIORAL PERVASIVE IMPAIRMENTS
MOTORIC	AGNOSIA
• Perseveration	• Tactile/astereognosis
• Abnormal tone: right side	• Visual object agnosia
• Abnormal tone: left side	• Visual spatial agnosia
APRAXIA	• Associative visual agnosia
• Ideomotor	• Somatoagnosia
• Ideational	• Anosognosia
• Oral	MOTOR COMPONENTS
BODY SCHEME DISTURBANCES	• Motor impersistence
• Unilateral body neglect	BODY SCHEME DISTURBANCES
• Somatoagnosia	• Body part identification
• Anosognosia	• Right/left discrimination
SPATIAL RELATIONS	EMOTIONAL/AFFECTIVE
• Unilateral spatial neglect	DISTURBANCES
• Spatial relations	• Euphoria
• Topographical orientation	• Lability
APHASIA	• Apathy
• Wernicke's aphasia	• Depression
• Jargon aphasia	• Aggression
• Anomia	• Irritability
• Paraphasia	• Restlessness
• Broca's aphasia	• Frustration

(continues)

(continued)

Table 1–1. Classification of neurobehavioral deficits used in the (A-ONE) (Árnadóttir, 1990)

NEUROBEHAVIORAL SPECIFIC IMPAIRMENTS	NEUROBEHAVIORAL PERVASIVE IMPAIRMENTS
OTHER DYSFUNCTIONS • Impaired organization • Perseveration	COGNITIVE DISTURBANCES • Confusion • Impaired judgment • Concrete thinking • Decreased insight MEMORY DISTURBANCES • Short-term memory loss • Long-term memory loss MEMORY DISTURBANCES • Disorientation • Confabulation OTHER DYSFUNCTION • Impaired alertness • Impaired attention • Distractibility • Absent mindedness • Impaired motivation • Performance latency • Impaired initiative

onomy is presented in Table 1–2. Other classification systems adopted by occupational therapists such as Zoltan's (1996) and Grieve's (1993) are presented in Table 1–3. Table 1–3 highlights how Zoltan mixes descriptions of both capacities and impairments. In Grieve's taxonomy, neglect is presented as a disorder of attention, and perceptual problems seem to be divided into visual-perceptual deficits and spatial deficits. Table 1–4 provides an overview of the way Lezak (1995) conceptualizes behavior. In Lezak's approach, three functional systems are described: cognition, emotionality, and executive functions. However, none of these authors provides sound theoretical or empirical rationales for their classification systems.

Table 1–2. Classification of cognition and perception, AOTA self-study series: Cognitive rehabilitation (Mosey, 1993)

COGNITIVE SUBCOMPONENTS

- Alertness
- Orientation
  - time, place, and person
- Learning
  - learning capacity
  - generalization of what has been learned
- Intellectual processes
  - comparing
  - categorizing
  - determining relationships
  - concrete and abstract thinking
  - logical reasoning
  - intellectual flexibility
  - metacognition
  - insight
- Problem solving
  - problem recognition
  - problem identification
  - problem and situation analysis
  - selection of a course of action
  - implementation of the selected course of action
  - execution of the solution chosen
  - evaluation of problem resolution

- Attention
  - concentration
  - selective attention
  - attentional flexibility
- Memory
  - length of retention and recall
  - content relative to time
- Fund of knowledge
  - procedural knowledge
  - factual knowledge
- Task skills
  - considering the consequence of one's actions
  - making judgments
  - assessing task demands
  - determining relevance of information
  - decision making
  - goal setting
  - following directions
  - planning
  - organizing
  - manner of task engagement
  - synchronizing parts of a task
  - monitoring performance
  - detecting and correcting errors

SOCIAL INTERACTION SUBCOMPONENTS

- Quantity of speech
- Self-control
  - impulsivity
  - aggression
  - irritability

- Self-control (*cont.*)
  - agitation
  - social inhibition
  - sexual inhibition/provocation
  - bizarre behavior

(continues)

(continued)

Table 1–2. Classification of cognition and perception, AOTA self-study series: Cognitive rehabilitation (Mosey, 1993)

SENSORY MOTOR SUBCOMPONENTS

- Visual disturbances
  - diplopia
  - homonymous hemianopsia
  - eye movements
- Self and objects in space
  - figure-ground discrimination
  - form consistency
  - spatial relations
  - vertical orientation

- Body Scheme
  - bilateral awareness
  - right/left discrimination
  - finger gnosia
  - position in space
  - topographical orientation
  - gnosia

PERCEPTUAL MOTOR SUBCOMPONENTS

- Praxia
  - ideomotor praxia
  - ideational praxia
  - constructional praxia

- Motor coordination
  - gross motor coordination
  - fine motor coordination/dexterity
- Postural control

RELATED BEHAVIORS

- Thought disorders
  - formal thought disorders
  - delusions
- Cognitive-perceptual disturbances
  - hallucinations
  - depersonalization
  - derealization

- Mood and affect
- Language disorders
  - dysarthria
  - oral apraxia
  - expressive dysphagia
  - receptive aphasia
  - global aphasia

Kielhofner (1992, 1997) wrote that in order for theory development in cognitive and perceptual disorders to proceed, a consistent taxonomy for these problems needs to be developed using a consistent set of criteria. For the purposes of this book, a classification of cognitive and perceptual impairments has been developed that considers the work of Grieve (1993), Hartley (1995), Van Deusen (1993), and Árnadóttir (1990). Also considered is the work on uniform terminology by the AOTA (1994a); the AOTA self-study series, Cognitive Rehabilitation (Royeen, 1993); and the WHO classification system of Impairments, Disability, and Handicap (World Health Organization, 1980). The classification in this book is based on major psychological functions (Miller & Gil, 1995). If we use the terminology of the

Table 1–3. Classification systems used by Zoltan (1996) and Grieve (1993)

CLASSIFICATION USED BY ZOLTAN (1996)	CLASSIFICATION USED BY GRIEVE (1993)
1. Visual processing skills (encompassing visual acuity, ocular alignment and control, visual fixation, visual fields, scanning, and visual spatial inattention),	1. Visual perceptual deficits and agnosias (including deficits in basic visual perception—color/form constancy and figure ground; visual object agnosias—tactile, auditory, and olfactory agnosias, and prosopagnosia)
2. Visual discrimination skills (encompassing spatial relations, figure ground, form discrimination, topographical disorientation, and depth perception)	
3. The agnosias (including visual object, tactile and auditory agnosias, prosopagnosia, simultagnosia, apractognosia, agnosias related to body scheme disorders, and visual spatial agnosia)	
4. The apraxias (including ideomotor, ideational, oral, constructional, and dressing)	2. The apraxias (comprising ideomotor, ideational, constructional, and dressing apraxias)
5. Disorders of body scheme (Including somatoagnosia, anosognosia, unilateral body neglect, right/left discrimination, and finger agnosia)	3. Spatial deficits (including visual field and scanning defects, constructional deficits, disorders of body image and body scheme, and topographical disorientation)
6. Orientation, attention, and memory	4. Disorders of attention (including the neglect syndrome and executive functions syndrome)
7. Executive functions (including initiation, self-monitoring, awareness, planning and organization, problem solving, mental flexibility and abstraction, and generalization and transfer)	5. Memory problems (encompassing short- and long-term memory, visual and verbal memory, and retrieval problems)
8. Acalculia	

Table 1–4. Dimensions of behavior based on the work of Lezak (1995)

COGNITIVE FUNCTIONS

- Receptive functions
- Memory and learning
- Thinking

Sensory reception
The agnosias (perception)
Computation
Reasoning and judgment
Abstracting
Concept formation
Problem solving
Organizing
Planning
Analysis and synthesis

- Expressive functions

Praxia/apraxia
Aphasia
Verbal functions and language skills
Constructional disorders

- Mental activity variables (i.e., behavior characteristics that concern the efficiency of mental processes)

Consciousness
Attention

PERSONALITY/EMOTIONALITY VARIABLES

- Personality

Disinhibition
Emotional distress
Emotional dulling
Depressed moods
Decreased social sensitivity
Lability
Irritability
Changed sexual drive

EXECUTIVE FUNCTIONS

- Volition

Motivation
Self-awareness

- Planning

Identification and organization of steps
Conceptualization of change
Conceptualization of alternatives

- Purposive action

Initiate, maintain, switch, and stop action

- Effective performance

Monitor performance
Self-correction
Behavior regulation

WHO, then the taxonomy in this book classifies impairments. If we use occupational therapy terminology, then we can say that disorders of cognitive integration performance components and sensorimotor performance components are presented in this text. Using the AOTA Uniform terminology (American Occupational Therapy Association, 1994a), sensorimotor performance components incorporates disorders of perception, which are described as having either a sensory or motor basis.

This book examines problems with a cognitive basis before exploring problems that have a sensorimotor basis or are more perceptual in nature. The method of dividing skill deficits within cognitive and sensorimotor performance areas was chosen to represent the deficits that commonly occur in individuals after brain damage. These clients are regularly seen in the clinic. Therefore, this book uses the following classification method:

A. Problems with cognitive or metacognitive performance components
   1. Problems with concentration
   2. Problems with memory and learning
   3. Problems with executive functions

B. Problems with perceptual (sensorimotor) performance components
   4. The apraxias
   5. The agnosias or simple perceptual problems
   6. Spatial relations syndrome or complex perceptual problems
   7. Unilateral neglect

These seven cognitive and perceptual (sensorimotor) performance components and the specific skill deficits they encompass are presented in Table 1–5. Each of the seven case study chapters in this book deals specifically with one of these cognitive or perceptual (sensorimotor) performance component deficits. Speech and language problems are not included in this book because these problems are primarily assessed and treated by speech and language therapists. Visual problems related to perceptual deficits are briefly discussed in the relevant chapters (Chapters 5 to 7). For more detailed information regarding occupational therapy approaches to working with clients with visual deficits, the reader is referred to Scheiman (1996).

BEHAVIORAL PROBLEMS

In addition to cognitive and perceptual problems, many individuals who have a mental health problem such as schizophrenia or those with traumatic brain injuries (and sometimes those who have had strokes) also experience a wide range of emotional and behavioral problems. These include

Table 1–5. An overview of cognitive and perceptual problems used in this book

PERFORMANCE COMPONENT DEFICITS	SPECIFIC PROBLEMS	
COGNITIVE		
Problems with concentration Chapter 4	Decreased or absent • Information processing speed • Sustained concentration	• Focused (selective) concentration • Divided (alternating) concentration
Problems with memory and learning Chapter 5	Decreased or absent • Short-term memory • Long-term memory	• Organize material for storage
METACOGNITIVE		
Problems with executive functions and insight and self-awareness Chapter 6	Decreased or absent • Goal formation • Goal selection • Anticipation of future goals • Planning • Sequencing • Initiation/termination of activity	• Error recognition and correction • Decision making • Empathy • Problem solving • Organizing • Reasoning • Concept formation
PERCEPTUAL (SENSORIMOTOR)		
Motor area: Apraxias Chapter 7	• Ideomotor apraxia	• Ideational apraxia
Perceptual processing area: Simple perceptual problems—the agnosias Chapter 8	• Visual object agnosia • Auditory agnosia • Tactile agnosia	• Face recognition • Perception of color

(continues)

(continued)

Table 1–5. An overview of cognitive and perceptual problems used in this book

PERFORMANCE COMPONENT DEFICITS	SPECIFIC PROBLEMS	
PERCEPTUAL (SENSORIMOTOR)		
Perceptual processing area: Complex perceptual problems—unilateral neglect Chapter 9	• Unilateral neglect - anosognosia - somatoagnosia	
Perceptual processing area: Complex perceptual problems—spatial relationships Chapter 10	Decreased or absent • Spatial relations • Object relationships • Constructional abilities • Form discrimination • Right/left discrimination • Depth perception	• Topographical orientation • Body scheme - anosognosia - somatoagnosia • Figure/ground discrimination Also includes unilateral neglect and apraxia.

(Adapted from Árnadóttir, 1990; Grieve, 1993; Glosser & Goodglass, 1990; Hartley, 1995; Hodges, 1994; Katz & Hartman-Maeir, 1997; Lezak, 1995; Stringer, 1996; and Van Deusen, 1993.)

mood changes, self-centeredness, impulsivity (i.e., difficulty monitoring and checking actions), low frustration tolerance, irritability (e.g., outbursts of temper), physically aggressive behavior, socially inappropriate behavior (e.g., swearing or sexual disinhibition), and a lack of self-awareness (Ponsford, Sloan, & Snow, 1995). Although these behavioral problems are not specifically addressed in the book, problems such as disinhibition, lability, and decreased social sensitivity are briefly discussed in the case study chapters. The role these problems play in a client's rehabilitation and community reintegration cannot be underestimated.

☰ THEORETICAL APPROACHES TO UNDERSTANDING COGNITIVE AND PERCEPTUAL DYSFUNCTION

MECHANISMS OF RECOVERY

Different theoretical approaches to the rehabilitation of patients with cognitive and perceptual problems are based on a variety of assumptions concerning whether or not brain recovery is possible and, if it is possible, how this recovery may occur. The concept of neural plasticity is fundamental to many theories of recovery. *Neural plasticity* is the brain's ability to regenerate and reorganize both in a neurophysiologic, neuroanatomic, and functional sense after damage (Sohlberg & Mateer, 1989). There are also differing beliefs concerning the best timing for intervention after brain damage. Some researchers in this field believe that therapy is most useful in facilitating the brain's own spontaneous recovery, making it most appropriate in the acute phase of recovery. Other researchers suggest that cognitive rehabilitation can assist a person in improving function at any time after injury. As Sohlberg and Mateer (1989) suggest, both views have merit.

Advancement of knowledge in the area of recovery of function has been largely due to work in the fields of neurophysiology, neuropharmacology, neuroimaging, **neuropsychology**, psychology, and neurosurgery. The work of Russian neuropsychologist Alexander Luria (1963; 1966; 1973) has probably had the greatest impact on our understanding of brain function and the problems that result after damage. The knowledge resulting from his research in this field is the foundation for much of our current practice in cognitive and perceptual rehabilitation. Luria (1966) described three functional units of the brain that are functionally integrated: (1) the arousal unit, which is responsible for regulating cortical tone; (2) the sensory-input unit, which is responsible for receiving, analyzing, and storing incoming information; and (3) the organizational and planning unit, which is responsible for activity programs, regulation, and verification.

He also postulated that these three units are hierarchically organized and furthermore that each unit is again hierarchically organized into three cortical zones: (1) primary areas, which receive and send information to the extremities; (2) secondary areas, which process incoming information; and (3) tertiary areas, which integrate information.

Today, the majority of research on mechanisms of brain recovery from a neurophysiological and neuroanatomical perspective refer to Luria's work as a means of demonstrating how our interpretations of brain function have changed yet remained the same. For more detailed discussions on neurophysiological mechanisms of recovery, the reader is referred to Seil (1997); Almli and Finger (1992); and Meier, Strauman, and Thompson (1987).

A client's potential for recovery after brain damage is also determined by multiple factors unrelated to the pathology or injury site. Researchers are only just beginning to realize the impact of these factors. Client-related variables such as age, gender, premorbid health and personality characteristics (including motivation and attitude), and family support all significantly impact on the potential for recovery. For a further discussion of these variables, the reader is referred to Lezak (1995).

REMEDIAL AND ADAPTIVE APPROACHES TO INTERVENTION

Neistadt (1990) suggests that occupational therapy intervention approaches in cognitive and perceptual rehabilitation fall into two main categories: **remedial** and **adaptive**. These approaches may be used separately, concurrently, or sequentially depending on the client's needs and the clinician's theoretical orientation to intervention. Writers and researchers in the field often disagree concerning which approach or combination of approaches achieves the best results with clients. Recently, Neistadt (1994a, 1995a) argued that both of these approaches require the ability to learn and that treatment approaches adopted by the therapist should be guided by the client's learning potential. Further research is required to demonstrate the effectiveness of the adaptive and remedial approaches.

Remedial approaches target intervention at the level of capacity and impairment. In a remedial approach, the therapist and client work toward rectifying problems in the subcomponents of performance. In other words, the emphasis is on restoring cognitive and perceptual capacities. A therapist using this approach assumes that the brain can repair itself by establishing new neural connections or repairing ones that are damaged. The therapist assumes that he or she can work with the client to recover lost capacities or develop alternative functions to replace lost ones. The focus of this approach is on assisting the client to achieve a "correct" performance by using tabletop perceptual drills or specific sequences of sensorimotor exercises to overcome problems experienced. Remedial approaches are also referred to as "bottom-up" approaches because they attempt to recover underlying skills and assume that the client will be able to generalize skills to occupational performance, which is at a higher level (Neistadt, 1990; Trombly, 1995a; Zoltan, 1995). The issue of whether or not skills generalize is discussed further in Chapter 3.

In adaptive approaches, the client's abilities are maximized by providing compensation strategies (Trombly, 1995a; Zoltan, 1995). Compensation strategies include modifications to the environment or the method used to perform a task, provision of adaptive equipment, or activity-specific assistance from another person. The adaptive approach targets intervention at the level of ability and disability. The aim of an adaptive approach is to achieve a "correct" performance by limiting the effects of the deficit through the use of other intact skills. The emphasis is on skills training and reinforcement of successful responses to resolve a problem or complete a task. These approaches place emphasis on facilitating mastery of the tasks that make up occupational performance areas such as dressing, shopping, or using a microwave oven. In an adaptive, or "top-down," approach, the therapist works with the client on specific occupations that are required or those that the client wants to achieve. In other words, the therapist starts at the top, which is the desired occupation, rather than working with the client on the underlying performance components. When using an adaptive approach, the therapist does not assume generalization of compensation strategies from one activity to another.

In the next section, a variety of theories and models that guide occupational therapy practice are explored. Whereas some of these models are top down and promote adaptive approaches in therapy, others are bottom up and favor remedial therapy interventions. The assumptions made by the authors of these models concerning the nature of brain function and dysfunction and the mechanisms for recovery are explored. The ways in which therapists use these models to guide clinical reasoning are briefly explored in Chapter 3 and are examined in more detail in the case studies in Chapters 4 to 11.

THEORIES, MODELS, AND FRAMEWORKS FOR PRACTICE

The importance of adopting and being able to articulate a frame of reference for therapeutic practice cannot be underestimated. This is particularly true when working with clients who have cognitive or perceptual disorders, given that many "recipes" for evaluation and intervention may be thrown together to achieve a program that has no rationale, consistency, or structure. In a study of the clinical decision-making processes of six experienced occupational therapists in Britain, Hagedorn (1996) found that the therapists were not able to articulate which models of practice or frames of reference were guiding their reasoning. However, the researcher observed therapists to be using biomechanical, cognitive/perceptual, and neurodevelopmental approaches in their work. It is suggested that therapists need to be able to articulate the basis for their practice to teach students effectively about applying theory in practice and to provide a better rationale for therapy to clients, colleagues, insurers, and third-party payers.

As outlined by Kielhofner (1992, 1997), theory development in the field of cognition and perception is still in its infancy. The lack of development of empirically based models is probably due to the inability of professions to agree on a theoretical framework for recovery of function, the variety of problems that manifest after damage to different brain structures, and the elusiveness of accurate measures of cognitive and perceptual functioning (Uzzell, 1997). A great deal of work needs to be done to classify and describe the processes underlying normal cognition and perception before work to describe disorders of cognition can proceed (Kielhofner, 1997). Although Kielhofner (1992) originally described a cognitive and perceptual model, he has more recently (1997) acknowledged that instead of a single approach to understanding and treating cognitive and perceptual problems, there are many. However, Kielhofner (1997) suggests that there is a trend toward an increasingly consistent view of cognitive and perceptual problems and intervention. An excellent review of theoretical approaches to practice in the field of cognitive and perceptual rehabilitation may be found in Katz (1992). Katz (1992) and her contributors examine in more detail the quite different models and approaches that are being developed around the world. However, although theoretical development of this field proceeds slowly, clients continue to present to occupational therapy for evaluation and treatment. Therefore, we need to examine what theoretical and model developments have occurred in occupational therapy and determine how we can use these to guide our clinical reasoning in this field of practice. Some of the more popular approaches are briefly presented here. They are (1) the information-processing approach and the quadraphonic approach; (2) the dynamic interaction approach; (3) the retraining approach; (4) the neurofunctional approach; (5) the cognitive disabilities model; (6) the model of human occupation; (7) the rehabilitative/compensatory model; and (8) the group-work model.

Several of these approaches have been used to guide therapy in the case studies described in Chapters 4 to 11. Approaches 1 to 5 have been developed specifically to guide practice with clients who have cognitive and perceptual problems. Approach 6 was developed to describe and understand human occupation; this model can be used with all persons who experience occupational performance limitations, including those who have cognitive and perceptual problems. Approach 7 was developed for persons with physical dysfunction but may also be used to guide therapy with any client group (Fisher, 1997a). Finally, Approach 8 was developed to explain the nature of therapeutic groups and their influence on participants who have psychiatric problems. This model can also be used when working with a wide variety of clients, including those who experience cognitive and perceptual problems. Table 1–6 (beginning on p. 24) provides a summary of the main features of each of these approaches.

Approach 1—The Information-Processing Approach and the Quadraphonic Approach

The information-processing approach as described by Abreu (1981) and Abreu and Toglia (1987) offers a remedial approach to treatment and is therefore a "bottom-up" approach. This model is based on information-processing theory and teaching and learning theories. Abreu and Toglia (1987) state that healthy adults use a variety of strategies to organize and structure information and that after brain injury, information-processing capacity is significantly reduced. Within this model, the perceptual process is thought to involve sensory detection, analysis, hypothesis formation, and response.

Abreu and Toglia (1987) suggest that it is inadequate to assess clients using standardized batteries and neuropsychological tests alone. Rather, the therapist must also assess the quality of the client's performance by engaging him in a series of graded tasks. The therapist must monitor how the client responds to grading and cue use in the task. The goal of treatment is to assist clients in developing strategies to handle, and effectively use, increasing amounts of information (Neistadt, 1990). Three treatment phases are identified in the model. In phase one, the emphasis is placed on the client's ability to detect and respond appropriately to the environment. In phase two, the therapist works with the client to discriminate, organize, and manipulate information from the environment. Phase three emphasizes the client's ability to manipulate and organize internal information such as emotions, ideas, and thoughts (Abreu & Toglia, 1987). Although some remedial approaches assume that treatment should repeat the stages on ontogeny (i.e., normal developmental sequence), Abreu and Toglia believe that the level at which the treatment begins depends on the client's current level of information processing. In the information-processing approach, treatment activities are matched with the client's information-processing capacity. Readers interested in using an information-processing approach should also refer to the work of Diamant and Hakkaart (1989), Mayer (1988), and Sohlberg and Mateer (1989).

More recently, Abreu and Hinojosa (1992) discuss a "process approach" when working with brain-injured adults. In addition to considering a client's cognitive and perceptual problems, this approach also considers the client's postural control dysfunction. This approach seems to build on the information-processing approach outlined above and has been labeled to reflect the therapist's need to continually adjust his assessments and interventions in accordance with the client's fluctuating abilities. The process approach also draws upon information-processing theory and teaching and learning theory but also uses motor learning theories. Although cognition-perception and postural control are two separate units, these authors discuss them as parts of an integrated system (Abreu & Hinojosa, 1992). Similar to the information-processing approach, this approach is based on the assumption that occupational therapy intervention is able to ameliorate dysfunction and that remediation of impaired abilities is possible.

Abreu (1998a) has refined this approach and now refers to it as the "quadraphonic approach." The quadraphonic approach is an interactive rehabilitation program that provides a holistic perspective for the management of stroke, traumatic brain injury, brain tumors, cerebral palsy, and other neurological conditions across the continuum of recovery from coma to community reentry. The quadraphonic approach uses both micro and macro perspectives for evaluation and treatment.

The micro perspective provides guidelines for the management of performance components or subskills: attention, visual perception, memory, motor planning, postural control, and problem solving. Evaluation and treatment of these performance components is based on a frame of reference that incorporates four theories: information processing, teaching/learning, neurodevelopmental, and biomechanical. The quadraphonic approach integrates these theories and uses a team concept (client, therapist, and family group) for rehabilitation.

The macro perspective provides guidelines for the management of functional performance and real-life occupations. Evaluation and treatment are accomplished through the use of narrative, analysis, and synthesis of real-life occupations to explain and predict the behavior of an individual based on four characteristics: lifestyle, lifestage, health, and disadvantage status. Real-life occupations include shopping, cooking, meal preparation, money management, and mobility. The use of this dual perspective provides a holistic basis for the quadraphonic approach. The quadraphonic approach is illustrated in Chapter 5 through the example of a therapist who uses this approach when working with a client who has memory and learning problems.

Approach 2—The Dynamic Interaction Approach

The dynamic interaction approach was developed by Toglia (1989a, 1992a, 1992b) and seems to provide further development of the work she published with Abreu in 1987 (as described previously). Toglia suggests that although traditional approaches have been based on the assumption that cognition and perception can be divided into discrete subskills, the dynamic interaction approach encourages therapists to investigate dynamically the ". . . underlying conditions and processing strategies that influence performance" (Toglia, 1992b, p. 104). One of the fundamental assumptions of the dynamic

Table 1–6. Summary of key features of approaches to working with clients who have cognitive and perceptual problems

APPROACH	KEY READING	POPULATIONS THE APPROACH IS USED WITH	THEORETICAL BASIS OR BASES	EMPHASIS IS REMEDIAL OR ADAPTIVE	ASSESSMENTS ASSOCIATED WITH THE APPROACH
1. The information processing approach and the quadraphonic approach	• Abreu & Toglia (1987) • Abreu & Hinojosa (1992) • Abreu (1998a)	• Traumatic brain injury (TBI) • Stroke • Cerebral palsy	• Information processing theory • Teaching and learning theory • Biomechanical theory • Neurodevelopmental theory	Remedial, and remedial and adaptive	A series of eight assessments developed within the quadraphonic approach are described in Chapter 5.
2. The dynamic interaction approach	• Toglia (1989, 1992a, 1992b)	• Developed for clients with TBI • Can be applied to all populations, including a psychiatric population	• Information-processing theory • Cognitive psychology • Dynamic approach	Remedial and adaptive	• Dynamic visual processing assessment • Toglia Category Assessment (Toglia, 1992b)

(continues)

Table 1–6. Summary of key features of approaches to working with clients who have cognitive and perceptual problems

APPROACH	KEY READING	POPULATIONS THE APPROACH IS USED WITH	THEORETICAL BASIS OR BASES	EMPHASIS IS REMEDIAL OR ADAPTIVE	ASSESSMENTS ASSOCIATED WITH THE APPROACH
3. The retraining approach	• Averbuch & Katz (1992)	• Developed for clients with traumatic brain injury (TBI) • Now applied to all other neuropsychologically impaired clients • Adolescents with learning problems	• Neuropsychological theories • Information-processing theory • Developmental theory	Remedial and then adaptive	• LOTCA (Itzkovich et al., 1990) • RBMT (Wilson et al., 1985) Both these assessments are described in detail in Chapter 3.
4. The neuro-functional approach	• Giles & Wilson (1992) • Giles (1992)	Clients with acquired cognitive impairments resulting from: • TBI	• Learning theory • Neuropsychological theories	Remedial and adaptive	• Behavioral observation • Standardized assessments such as the A-ONE (Árnadóttir, 1990)

(continues)

Table 1–6. Summary of key features of approaches to working with clients who have cognitive and perceptual problems

APPROACH	KEY READING	POPULATIONS THE APPROACH IS USED WITH	THEORETICAL BASIS OR BASES	EMPHASIS IS REMEDIAL OR ADAPTIVE	ASSESSMENTS ASSOCIATED WITH THE APPROACH
4. The neuro-functional approach (*continued*)		• Stroke • Anoxia • Infection			
5. The cognitive disabilities model	• Allen (1985) • Allen, Earhart, & Blue (1992) • Levy (1992) • Stone (1992)	Developed for a psychiatric population but now used with clients who have: • Traumatic brain injury • Dementing illnesses	• Learning theory • Broad-based neurosciences	Adaptive	• RTI • ACL • LCL • CPT (all four in Allen, Kehrberg, & Burns, 1992)

(continues)

(continued)

Table 1–6. Summary of key features of approaches to working with clients who have cognitive and perceptual problems

APPROACH	KEY READING	POPULATIONS THE APPROACH IS USED WITH	THEORETICAL BASIS OR BASES	EMPHASIS IS REMEDIAL OR ADAPTIVE	ASSESSMENTS ASSOCIATED WITH THE APPROACH
6. The model of human occupation	• Kielhofner (1995a) • Kielhofner (1997)	• All client populations This model was developed to broadly describe and understand human occupation	• General systems theory • Biopsychosocial model • Occupational behavior	Can use remedial or adaptive approaches, but the model does not discuss	Not applicable; a number of assessments have been developed related to occupational behavior
7. The rehabilitative/ compensatory model	• Trombly (1989, 1995a, 1995b, 1995c) • Fisher (1997a)	Originally used with clients who have physical dysfunction; now more broadly used with all client populations.	Not fully articulated as yet, but draws upon Learning theory.	Adaptive	A variety of assessments are compatible with this model including AMPS (Fisher, 1997a), and the COPM (Law et al., 1994)

(continues)

(continued)

Table 1–6. Summary of key features of approaches to working with clients who have cognitive and perceptual problems

APPROACH	KEY READING	POPULATIONS THE APPROACH IS USED WITH	THEORETICAL BASIS OR BASES	EMPHASIS IS REMEDIAL OR ADAPTIVE	ASSESSMENTS ASSOCIATED WITH THE APPROACH
8. The group work model	• Howe & Schwartzberg (1995)	Originally developed for use with clients who have psychiatric problems; now more broadly used with all client populations	Based on: • Group dynamics • Social psychology • Motivational theories • Maslow's hierarchy of needs	Can use remedial or adaptive approaches	Not applicable

interaction approach is that cognition is the dynamic interaction between the individual (which includes his learning styles, strategies, and metacognition), the task (including complexity, modality, and familiarity), and the environment (including cultural, social, and physical aspects) (Toglia, 1992b). When using a dynamic interaction approach, the therapist can choose either remediatory or adaptive treatment techniques with the client. The theoretical foundations of this approach are information-processing theory, cognitive psychology, and the dynamic approach to cognitive rehabilitation as described by Trexler (1987).

The assessment and treatment procedures used within this approach reflect the dynamic perspective of cognition. Assessment combines the use of "static" standardized assessments and the dynamic investigative assessments that aim to identify the specific conditions that have the greatest impact on performance (Toglia, 1992b). Assessment includes an estimation of the client's capacity to learn, solve problems, and deal with day-to-day situations. During assessment, the therapist alters cues and components of tasks and observes the client's potential for change. Toglia (1992b) proposes that the use of this approach provides information on how the task and the client's internal processing strategies influence his ability to process information. As the clinician assesses the client, he modifies the task or provides external cues to determine the impact of these on performance. In contrast to the use of standardized assessments, during which the examiner must remain unbiased and neutral, a key feature of dynamic interaction assessment is the relationship between the client and clinician and the dynamic way they interact during the assessment process.

Toglia (1992b) reports that "dynamic interaction" assessment findings directly guide selection of the most appropriate approach to treatment. For example, if assessment reveals that the client's performance is not facilitated through repetition and practice, then adaptive treatment strategies may work well. On the other hand, if such input facilitates performance, then remediation techniques should be used as treatment. Within this approach, treatment may be viewed as reactive, which means that the client's responses determine the kinds of therapy undertaken and there is no predetermined sequence of treatment activities. Treatment involves a number of components, including practice in multiple situations, metacognitive training, and consideration of the learner's characteristics to facilitate transfer of learning. Although transfer of learning is assumed in many treatment approaches, it is explicitly addressed and facilitated in the dynamic interaction approach.

As noted by Toglia (1992b), the limitations of dynamic interaction assessment are that it cannot be used to measure change over time and it requires a high level of expertise from the therapist to successfully use the assessment procedure. Toglia (1992b) also discusses the need for further research to examine the effectiveness of metacognitive treatment techniques and hence determine if clients can develop an awareness of their cognitive capacity and develop self-monitoring skills.

Approach 3—The Retraining Approach

The cognitive retraining approach was described by Averbuch and Katz (1992) and focuses on the remediation of specific skill deficits. Thus, this is predominantly a bottom-up approach. The rationale for this approach is based on neuropsychological, developmental, and information-processing theories and the work of Neistadt (1990) and Toglia (1991). These theories appear to have led the authors of this approach to view the cortical regions as interdependent and finely balanced and to believe that a disruption in one region can have a negative impact on the brain as a whole. In addition, it is thought that there are several different ways to perform cognitive functions; therefore, therapeutic training can create alternative strategies to achieve reorganization of cognitive and perceptual abilities (Averbuch & Katz, 1992). An underlying assumption of this approach is that generalization of skill can occur from practice in one task to other tasks. **Generalization** refers to the ability to use a newly learned strategy or skill in different situations. This is in contrast to the neurofunctional approach (Giles & Wilson, 1992), which assumes that brain-injured clients must practice every activity directly and that generalization of skill cannot be taken for granted.

Client assessment within the retraining approach relies primarily on the administration of two standardized batteries: the Lowenstein Occupational Therapy Cognitive Assessment (LOTCA) (Itzkovich et al., 1990) and the Rivermead Behavioral Memory Test (RBMT) (Wilson, Cockburn, & Baddely, 1991). (Both of these assessments are reviewed in Chapter 3.) Treatment within this framework consists of two phases. In the first phase, the emphasis is on the remediation of specific cognitive and perceptual deficits, and the therapist seeks to ameliorate problem areas. The therapist may also work with the client to strengthen remaining or less-affected abilities. The second phase of treatment is adaptive and aims to generate alternative strategies that the client can use to receive and accumulate information (Averbuch & Katz, 1992). The focus of this second phase is to assist the client in adapting to the environment. The outcome of the retraining approach is measured in the client's real-world environment. Therefore, even though the main part of treatment is the retraining of cognitive and perceptual skills, the approach is said to have been successful only when these skills successfully transfer to the real-life setting (Averbuch & Katz, 1992).

Approach 4—The Neurofunctional Approach

The neurofunctional approach was first described by Giles and Wilson in 1992 and is based on learning theory. This approach was developed specifically for individuals with acquired neurological impairments (Giles, 1992). The focus of this approach is on retraining real-world skills rather than on retraining specific cognitive and perceptual processes (Giles, 1992). Using the guidelines for examining the assumptions of treatment approaches devised by Neistadt (1990), this model may be broadly described as taking an adaptive approach to treatment but incorporating some remedial concepts as well. However, Giles (1992) criticizes both approaches and argues that remediation approaches are largely unproven and thus may result in little functional improvement for the client. He also suggests that compensatory skills or techniques are taught to a client without considering if the gains made in terms of quality of life justify the considerable effort required. He suggests that therapy time may be more profitably spent by working with a client to perform specific functional behaviors in their true contexts (Giles, 1992).

Therapists who use this approach adopt the use of a wide range of standardized and nonstandardized assessment procedures. For example, Giles (1992) suggests that the A-ONE (Árnadóttir, 1990) may be useful but that the therapist's observation skills are most important in identifying the client's problems. By using structured observation, the therapist can gain an understanding of the client's performance in specific functional activities (Giles, 1992), and treatment can focus on retraining these functional activities. Important elements of the treatment process include cognitive overlearning, behavior shaping, control of behavior by antecedents, fading, the opportunity for practicing required behaviors, and client debriefing (in which positive performance is discussed and encouraged) (Giles, 1992). Thus, desirable behaviors are thought to become automatic. However, all members of the therapy team must reinforce this approach, which is thought to work best in a controlled rehabilitation setting (Giles & Wilson, 1992). An example of the use of this model in occupational therapy practice may be found in Yuen (1994).

Approach 5—The Cognitive Disabilities Model

The cognitive disabilities model was developed by Allen (1985) in her work with clients who experienced mental health problems. Her work is now being used by some therapists in the assessment and treatment of clients with brain injury and with clients who have a dementing illness (Levy, 1992; Stone, 1992). The model describes cognitive function on a continuum that is graded on six levels from level 1 (profoundly impaired) to level 6 (normal).

A seventh level of 0 is included for clients in comas. These levels are discussed in detail by Allen (1992) and Allen, Earhart, and Blue (1992). In summary, the levels may be described as follows:

- Level 0—Coma (i.e., a prolonged state of unconsciousness)
- Level 1—Automatic actions (i.e., invariable responses to external stimuli)
- Level 2—Postural actions (i.e., gross body movements that the individual initiates to overcome the effects of gravity and move the body in space)
- Level 3—Manual actions (i.e., using the hands and sometimes other parts of the body to manipulate material objects)
- Level 4—Goal-directed actions (i.e., assist the person to go through the steps required to get to the finished product)
- Level 5—Exploratory actions (i.e., the knowledge that changes in neuromuscular control produces different effects on materials)
- Level 6—Planned action (i.e., the ability to estimate the effects of actions on present, or absent material objects) (Allen, 1992)

Each level describes the extent of a person's disability and the difficulties he has in performing occupations. Allen (1992) has done extensive work to develop three assessments to determine the level of functioning, including the tasks that a person is capable of at each of the six levels (Allen, Earhardt, & Blue, 1992). Several assessments are used within this model, including the Routine Task Inventory (RTI); the Allen Cognitive Level (ACL) screening test; the Lower Cognitive Levels (LCL) test, which was specifically designed to assess clients' functioning at levels 1, 2, or 3; and the Cognitive Performance Test (CPT) (Allen, Kehrberg, & Burns, 1992).

After the client's cognitive level has been identified, crafts and other routine activities the client is capable of performing, or that have been adjusted so the client can engage in the activity, are presented. Treatment activities are guided both by the client's cognitive level and his treatment phase, which is described as either postacute, rehabilitation, or long-term care. Although the model has a neuroscientific base, Allen's work does not focus on neuroplasticity and remediation of function through therapy. Rather, the model assumes that learning and memory are permanently impaired in most clients (with the possible exception of some clients at levels 5 and 6), and the therapeutic focus is placed on adaptive approaches such as environmental modification and strengthening **residual** abilities. Therefore, the model assumes that occupational therapy intervention cannot change the cognitive level of the client. Any change in client ability is assumed to be due to either use of medication or the natural course of healing. The model places a heavy emphasis on educating and informing caregivers and family about safety and possible legal issues related to the client's restricted capacities and abilities. The therapist's role includes providing cautions concerning the kind and amount of supervision the client requires and environmental modifications that are necessary to ensure safety. Additionally, Allen, Earhardt, and Blue (1992) suggest that the occupational therapist must take action to ensure the client does not drive if he or she is not capable and that other legal actions are taken to prevent hazardous situations from arising.

Sharrott (1985, 1986) suggests that this approach is not widely accepted because it classifies or labels clients and assumes that changes in clients' level of function are not due to occupational therapy intervention. However, Kielhofner (1997) states that although the view that clients' performances may not improve because of occupation is controversial, it is important to recognize real limitations in clients' performance and not always attribute poor performances to lack of motivation. Kielhofner (1997) suggests that although it is useful to acknowledge that some functional limitations will be permanent, the therapist should be wary of limiting the client's opportunities to learn or change. Occupational therapists who have discussed the theory or studied the use of this model in a variety of practice settings include Levy (1992), Mayer (1988), and Stone (1992).

Approach 6—The Model of Human Occupation

The model of human occupation (MOHO) was first developed by Kielhofner and Burke (1980) as a conceptual framework for occupational therapy practice. Since that time, a number of people have contributed to its development, and a new refined version of the model has been presented in the second edition of *A Model of Human Occupation: Theory and Application* (Kielhofner, 1995a). The model seeks "to account for the motivation, performance, and organization of occupational behavior in everyday life" (Kielhofner, 1997, p. 188). The model is used with clients who are experiencing occupational performance limitations, and unlike many other models, it can be used with clients of any age and diagnosis (DePoy & Burke, 1992). Therefore, this model has not been specifically developed for use with clients who have cognitive and perceptual problems. The model draws on a number of theories and models, including general systems theory and Engel's biopsychosocial model (Kielhofner, 1992, 1995a).

The model is based on the premise that the human system is composed of three subsystems: a volitional subsystem, a habituation subsystem, and a mind-brain-body performance subsystem. The volitional subsystem is concerned with a person's motives for occupations. This subsystem is made up of dispositions (i.e., cognitive/emotive orientations toward occupations) and self-knowledge (i.e., an awareness of self as an actor in the world). This subsystem enables a person to anticipate, choose, experience, and interpret occupational behavior (Kielhofner et al., 1995). The volition subsystem comprises three areas: (1) personal causation (i.e., a person's knowledge of his abilities and perception of control over his own behavior), (2) values (i.e., personal convictions and sense of obligation), and (3) interests (i.e., the preference for and attraction of some occupations over others). The volitional process is concerned with experiencing, choosing, and interpreting occupational behavior.

The habituation subsystem deals with organizing routines that provide structure in our lives. This subsystem is concerned with habit maps, which guide habitual behavior, and role scripts, which guide role behavior—that is, the habit maps and role scripts guide organized routines and everyday behaviors and are involved in the changes in roles and habits over time (Kielhofner, 1995b). Finally, the mind-brain-body performance subsystem has been described as the system that provides the capacity for performance. Whereas the volition subsystem provides the desire to perform and the habituation subsystem organizes behavior into recognizable routines, the mind-brain-body performance subsystem provides the capacity for performance. This subsystem includes the physical and mental constituents (including musculoskeletal, neurological, cardiopulmonary, and symbolic constituents) of occupational performance (Fisher & Kielhofner, 1995).

A number of observational measures, checklists, and interviews have been designed for use with this model (e.g., refer to The Role Checklist, The Volitional Questionnaire, and the Occupational Performance History Interview reported in Kielhofner [1995a]). These tools are used to gather information concerning a client's volition, interests, roles and habits, and occupational functioning. Within the MOHO, the Assessment of Motor and Process Skills (Fisher, 1997a) and the Assessment of Communication and Interactions Skills (Salamy, Simon, & Kielhofner, 1993) can be used to provide information on clients' performance skills. Principles for therapeutic intervention focusing on change are provided in the model (Kielhofner, 1995a). Although the aim of this model is not to provide specific approaches for intervention, the model emphasizes the importance of selecting therapeutic occupations that relate to the client's life circumstances and the need for future occupational behavior. A number of case examples in Kielhofner's book (1995a) illustrate different approaches to intervention.

When working with clients who have cognitive and perceptual problems, the MOHO provides a generalist perspective that can assist therapists to organize their approach to evaluation and intervention (Kielhofner, 1995a). To illustrate the MOHO perspective, let us use the case of a woman experiencing learning and memory difficulties resulting from a mild head injury sustained in a car accident in which her partner was killed. Whereas an information-processing approach may be taken to specifically address memory difficulties, the MOHO provides a way to conceptualize the occupational problems this woman may experience because of decreased motivation, altered routines, and a reorganization of her life roles. DePoy and Burke (1992) have also outlined two case studies supporting the use of the MOHO to guide their approach to therapy when working with clients who have cognitive and perceptual problems.

In summary, although the MOHO has not been widely adopted for use with adults with neurological dysfunction (Okkema, 1993), it undoubtedly has a place with other models of practice that have more specific application to clients with acquired brain damage. Therefore, the MOHO may be applied broadly as an "umbrella model" to ensure that an occupational approach is taken by therapists.

Approach 7—The Rehabilitative/Compensatory Model

A rehabilitative/compensatory model is commonly adopted by occupational therapists in a wide range of practice settings, including physical dysfunction (Trombly, 1995b, 1995c, 1995d) and cognitive disabilities (Allen, 1992; Allen, Earhart, & Blue, 1992). Although the exact origins of the rehabilitative/compensatory approach are unclear (Kielhofner, 1992), Trombly (1989, 1995c, 1995d) was the first to articulate and develop the rehabilitative/compensatory model into an occupational therapy model of practice. More recently, Fisher (1997b) extended the work of Trombly by (1) articulating more explicitly assumptions made about people within the rehabilitative/compensatory model; (2) generalizing this model beyond persons with physical disabilities to those with developmental, cognitive, or psychosocial disabilities; and (3) adding collaborative consultation to education and adaptation as strategies used to effect change.

The rehabilitative/compensatory model emphasizes the use of an adaptive approach to intervention. Trombly (1995c) asserted that the focus of the rehabilitative/compensatory model of practice is on adaptation or compensation and that it does not address change through remediation of impairments. Therefore, the rehabilitative/compensatory model is applicable at the disability and handicap levels of the WHO classification system (1980). It is important to point out, however, that through the process of providing adaptations that promote competence in occupational performance, Fisher (1997b; in press) believes that the person's resultant increased competence in occupational performance can indirectly lead to some degree of remediation of impairments, including restoration of not only cognitive, perceptual, and motor impairments, but also self-esteem, interests, and values. Nevertheless, the emphasis of the rehabilitative/compensatory model is to teach the client to be as independent as possible by using adapted equipment, using new methods to accomplish functional goals, and/or by adapting the environment (Trombly, 1995b).

The rehabilitative/compensatory model has been confused with the rehabilitation movement (Dutton, 1995) and the biomechanical model (Kielhofner, 1992, 1997). Moreover, because of Trombly's (1989, 1995d) focus, it has been linked almost exclusively to physical rehabilitation. The rehabilitative/compensatory model should not be limited to physical rehabilitation because many occupational therapists working with persons with cognitive or perceptual disabilities and other areas of practice often use the rehabilitative/compensatory model to guide their interventions (Fisher, 1997b). In fact, the cognitive disabilities model discussed earlier can be considered a special version of the rehabilitative/compensatory model.

The rehabilitative/compensatory approach is often chosen by a therapist when further recovery (remediation) of impairments with the client is not expected. Interventions within the rehabilitative/compensatory approach are adaptive or compensatory and focus on teaching the client alternate or compensatory techniques (i.e., adapted methods of doing), designing and providing adaptive equipment, and modifying or adapting the physical or social environment.

> When we teach the client new alternative or compensatory techniques, our aim is to help the client adapt to an existing environment. When we provide adapted equipment or modify the environment, we adapt the environment to better fit the abilities of the client (Fisher, 1997b, p. 20).

Based on the work of Trombly (1989, 1995c, 1995d), Fisher (1997b) articulated the following assumptions made about people when using the rehabilitative/compensatory model:

1. Occupational performance occurs within a multidimensional client-centered performance context that includes a person's motivation, underlying capacities, physical and social environment, and culture, as well as the characteristics of the tasks the person needs and wants to perform.
2. The ability to perform daily life tasks is dependent on the person's basic underlying capacities or motivational characteristics.
3. A minimum level of motivation, as well as neuromuscular, biomechanical, cognitive, and psychosocial capacities are needed for both learning and efficient, effective, and safe daily life task performance.
4. Whenever possible, the person is viewed as one who can become an effective problem-solver, capable of designing new adaptations as the need arises.
5. Loss of competence in occupational performance can occur as a result of a change in a person's personal characteristics, "loss of motivation,

drastic changes in environment, or cultural inaccessibility" (Trombly, 1995c, p. 23). Occupational dysfunction can also occur when the individual fails to develop competence in occupational performance.

6. The person with persistent disability, whose impairments do not respond to remediation, is viewed as a learner who needs to regain competence in occupational performance.
7. People can regain the ability to perform daily life tasks through compensation or adaptation.
8. When a basic underlying capacity is impaired, the occupational therapist teaches the person to adapt his or her methods, tools, and environments to enable the ability to perform daily life tasks.
9. When no adaptations can compensate for the person's residual disability, the person will need to eliminate the task from his or her daily life, manage the task by directing others, or accept the assistance of another person.
10. When caregiver training is provided as part of the intervention, the caregiver becomes the learner.

Evaluation and intervention using the rehabilitative/compensatory model incorporates a top-down approach and involves the following steps (Fisher, 1997b, in press):

1. Establish the client-centered performance context within which occupational performance occurs.
2. Develop therapeutic rapport, a collaborative partnership between the client and the therapist that continues to develop throughout the time they work together.
3. Identify strengths and problems of occupational performance in terms of tasks (not goal-directed actions or impairments) that are currently supporting or hindering the client's role behavior or that the client wants to perform upon discharge.
4. Implement a performance analysis. "Performance analysis is defined as the observational evaluation of a person's task performance to identify discrepancies between the demands of a task and the skill of the person. The person's problems and strengths are described in terms of the quality of the goal-directed actions that comprise the occupational performance, not the client's underlying capacities and impairments" (Fisher, in press). The therapist uses either informal observation of a person's occupational performance or the Assessment of Motor and Process Skills (AMPS) (Fisher, 1997a), a standardized performance analysis, to accomplish the performance analysis.
5. Define the goal-directed actions of performance the client can and cannot perform effectively. These are the client's functional problems or limita-

tions in occupational performance, and they should not be confused with impairments that may impact function.

6. Clarify or interpret the underlying cause for the ineffective performance, which may be the client's impairments or may be caused by environmental factors. Note that in a true top-down approach, the client's impairments are not identified until after the tasks and goal-oriented actions of performance that are causing the client problems are identified.

7. Plan and implement adaptive or compensatory occupation according to the following steps:

• Expand consultative partnerships to include not only the client and his or her family but also persons who have access to needed information or who will be impacted by the proposed changes.
• Implement methods of collaborative consultation (Fisher, 1997b), education (Trombly, 1995d), and adaptation (Fisher, 1997b; Trombly, 1995d) to develop adaptive occupation and enhance the client's occupational performance.

8. Reevaluate the client's occupational performance, again using performance analyses.

Approach 8—The Group-Work Model

Howe and Schwartzberg (1995) proposed the group-work model for occupational therapy in 1986. The model is based on group dynamics as articulated in psychiatry, motivational theories, social psychology, and Maslow's needs hierarchy (Howe & Schwartzberg, 1995; Kielhofner, 1997). Although this model is most often used with clients who have mental health problems, it can be used with a variety of other client groups, including those who have cognitive or perceptual problems. The authors of this model acknowledge that it is still in formation and that it lacks well-developed technology for application and sufficient empirical data to support it (Kielhofner, 1992). The model provides an approach to explain the nature of therapeutic groups and their influence on participants (Howe & Schwartzberg, 1995). A central concern of this model is the ways an individual may achieve satisfaction and growth through occupational behaviors within groups. Using a group-work model approach, group members engage in functional activities, participate in discussions concerning activities, or join in group-centered social action. There are four types of action in the functional group: (1) purposeful; (2) self-initiated; (3) spontaneous, or here-and-now; and (4) group-centered (Howe & Schwartzberg, 1995). The actions can be easily graded in a manner suitable for the individual and group functional level. This is very important given the range of differences in the cognitive, psychological, and social capacities of individuals after head injury or stroke. For more information concerning the use of this model in occupational therapy, the reader is referred to Howe and Schwartzberg (1995).

Ideas and programs for conducting groups with head-injured clients have been presented by Okkema (1993), Prichard and Bernard (1995), and Sohlberg and Mateer (1989). These programs could be strengthened by placing them within the group-work model as proposed by Howe and Schwartzberg (1995). Sohlberg and Mateer (1989) outline a variety of groups for use with head-injured clients, including orientation, communication, and psychosocial and cognitive skill groups. It is suggested that although there are many difficulties associated with conducting groups with head-injured clients (including the heterogeneity of members, involuntary nature of membership, and varying intellectual functioning), there are also many advantages. The aim of cognitive and perceptual rehabilitation is to help clients return to community living. Forming a "community" or group within the rehabilitation setting can help clients to work together toward reinforcing socially appropriate behaviors and interactions because groups require members to respond to environmental expectations. Groups can offer individuals a sense of identity and self-worth. Groups also motivate members to action and encourage members to take responsibility for meeting their own needs while considering those of others. Carefully monitored group work fosters a sharing and acknowledgment of difficulties and promotes occupational skill acquisition or redevelopment (Kielhofner, 1992; Sohlberg & Mateer, 1989). In summary, therapeutic group work can facilitate change, particularly change related to occupational skills and the social aspects of occupational behavior. In Chapter 11, Schwartzberg explores in more detail the use of groups for persons who have cognitive and perceptual problems.

SUMMARY

Cognitive and perceptual dysfunction can have a profound effect on the lives of individuals who experience these problems and their families. This chapter reviewed the definitions of cognition and perception and some of the disease and accident processes that create problems with these capacities. In order to guide practice, therapists who treat clients with cognitive and perceptual problems work within theoretical models or frames of reference. The final section of this chapter presented a series of eight theoretical approaches that therapists can use when working with clients who have cognitive and perceptual problems. However, within these theoretical frameworks, many other factors inform the practice of experienced clinicians.

Competent practice requires skilled *clinical reasoning,* a skill that evolves over time. The ways in which clinicians reason in their practice often reflects their level of expertise. Mattingly and Fleming (1994) describe clinical reasoning as a complex phenomenon involving several different kinds of thinking and perceiving. By examining and exploring expert clinical reasoning and making this tacit information as explicit as possible, students and novice clinicians can improve their practice. As outlined by Neistadt (1996), knowledge of clinical reasoning and its language can help therapists to consciously reflect on their decisions; improve their abilities to explain the rationale behind their treatments to clients, their families, and other health professionals; and improve job satisfaction by making therapists more aware of the complexities of their practice. Chapter 2 examines clinical reasoning in more detail, describing some of the theories behind clinical reasoning and how the study of expert clinical reasoning can offer students and novice clinicians insights to improve their practice. Chapters 4 to 11 provide examples of expert clinicians' reasoning in order to explicate expert practice when conducting evaluations and interventions with clients who have cognitive and perceptual dysfunction.

≣ REVIEW QUESTIONS

1. Describe the six main causes of acquired cognitive and perceptual problems. Which other client groups experience cognitive and perceptual problems?
2. Define *cognition* and *perception.* Discuss whether you believe these are two separate entities or one.
3. The two main therapeutic approaches to working with clients who have cognitive and perceptual problems are remedial and adaptive/compensatory. What are these and what does each entail? Which approach do you favor and why?
4. Eight theoretical approaches/models have been described that can be used to guide practice when working with clients who have cognitive and perceptual problems. Summarize two of these, including the researchers/theorists who have developed the approach; the theories they draw upon; main assumptions; and assessment/evaluation and treatment/intervention techniques used. Discuss an advantage and disadvantage of each approach.

≡ ACKNOWLEDGMENTS

I would like to thank Betty Abreu and Sharan Schwartzberg for reviewing sections of the "Theories, Models, and Frameworks for Practice" component of this chapter. I would also like to thank Anne Fisher for assisting to write the section on the Rehabilitative/Compensatory Model. Sue Sloan, a neuropsychologist and occupational therapist, provided timely and thoughtful discussions surrounding the conceptualization of cognitive and perceptual problems and ways such problems can be categorized.

2

Clinical Reasoning in Occupational Therapy

CAROLYN UNSWORTH, PhD, OTR

- Clinical Reasoning
- Conditional Reasoning
- Cue
- Decision Making
- Diagnostic Reasoning
- Expert Therapist
- Interactive Reasoning
- Narrative Reasoning

- Novice Therapist
- Pattern Recognition
- Phenomenological
- Pragmatic Reasoning
- Procedural Reasoning
- Scientific Reasoning
- Tacit Knowledge
- Theoretical Reasoning

On completion of this chapter, the reader will be able to:

- Define clinical reasoning in broad terms and identify and define at least five different kinds of clinical reasoning
- Discuss the value of learning about clinical reasoning and name at least three approaches to enhancing the development of expert clinical reasoning
- Provide examples of situations in which a clinician might use procedural, interactive, and conditional reasoning
- List the five stages in the development of expertise and the key features of each phase
- Successfully work through the Review Questions in this chapter
- Demonstrate sufficient knowledge of clinical reasoning to successfully work through the case study chapters in this book

The purpose of this chapter is to define and explore clinical reasoning and to examine how students and novice clinicians can gain and improve these skills. By giving a language to the tacit thought processes of expert clinicians, the reader will be able to recognize and discuss how expert clinicians reason in their practice with clients, as discussed in the case study chapters. By understanding clinical reasoning, it is hoped that students will be better prepared for their fieldwork and ultimately for practice as occupational therapists. The chapter opens with a discussion of clinical reasoning and the differences between scientific and narrative forms of reasoning. The different types of clinical reasoning are then presented, focusing on procedural, interactive, and conditional reasoning. The final section examines how clinical reasoning skills develop as students, or new graduates, progress over time from novice to expert. Approaches that can be used to assist students in enhancing their clinical reasoning skills are also presented.

☰ INTRODUCTION

It has been argued that an occupational therapist's reasoning and decision-making processes are different from those of other professionals (Kielhofner, 1997). **Clinical reasoning** is the guiding force in our practice as occupational therapists, but what *is* clinical reasoning? What is the nature of reasoning and reflection in occupational therapy, and how and why are clinical decisions made? Although clinical reasoning is not new, research in this field has been conducted only in the past 15 years and a language to describe this previously **tacit knowledge** has since developed. This chapter presents the language of clinical reasoning and discusses some of the research in this field. Occupational therapists can use this information to make expert clinical reasoning more explicit and therefore easier for students and novice clinicians to learn about and incorporate into their practice. As pointed out by Cohen (1991), clinicians have voiced concerns for years that although students and novice or inexperienced clinicians are well-prepared to apply "standard theories to straightforward cases" (p. 969), they are not able to critically reflect on their practice or employ creative responses. Many academics and clinicians agree that the use of case studies that illustrate expert reasoning provide excellent opportunities for students to develop their own reasoning skills. Therefore, this chapter lays the groundwork for each of the case study chapters in the book by providing the reader with the language of, and theory behind, clinical reasoning in occupational therapy. The case study chapters in this book are aimed at helping students and novice clinicians to look beyond recipes of practice in cognitive and perceptual dysfunction and to use clinical reasoning to reflect on and improve their practice.

☰ WHAT IS CLINICAL REASONING?

DEFINITION OF CLINICAL REASONING

Mattingly and Fleming (1994) make the distinction between theoretical and clinical reasoning. They describe **theoretical reasoning** as being concerned with generalities, or what we can reliably predict or hold to be true. Theoretical reasoning is learned from textbooks. In contrast, they define clinical reasoning as:

- A practical know-how that puts theoretical knowledge into practice
- Concerned with deliberating over appropriate action and then putting this in place
- A complex practical reasoning to find what's best for each client (Mattingly & Fleming, 1994)

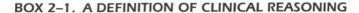

BOX 2–1. A DEFINITION OF CLINICAL REASONING

To me, clinical reasoning is how I think and make decisions when I'm planning to be with a client; when I'm with a client; and afterwards, when I reflect on therapy. It involves intuition, judgment, empathy, and common sense. . . .

- It's how I think about what the client is telling me and what I observe.
- It's what I pay attention to and ignore.
- It's what I respond to immediately or note for future reference.
- It's the way I try to understand my client as a human being.
- It's how I draw on my knowledge of previous clients, their difficulties, and successful and unsuccessful solutions.
- It's the way I draw on my theoretical knowledge and apply it in practice.
- It's the stories I share with other therapists about our clients, the therapy we provide, and how we feel about it.
- It's the way I consider the total picture, including how much therapy time I can spend with the client, financial reimbursement issues, and the support available from the client's family.
- It's the process of deciding what course of action to take with the client, and how I modify or change this over time.

The way I reason has changed over time due to greater experience and mentoring from expert occupational therapists and other health professionals. The way I reason in my occupational therapy practice makes me different from other health professionals.

Clinical reasoning is the thinking or cognitive processes and decision-making that therapists use to guide their work. Although the reader is referred to Mattingly (1991) for a more in-depth discussion of clinical reasoning, an overview of clinical reasoning is presented in Box 2–1.

RESEARCH ON CLINICAL REASONING IN OCCUPATIONAL THERAPY

The first empirical study of clinical reasoning in occupational therapy was conducted by Rogers and Masagatani in 1982. Their pilot study focused on the thinking processes employed by therapists when assessing their clients. The following year, Rogers's Eleanor Clarke Slagle lectureship heightened therapists' awareness of clinical reasoning as a way of understanding and explicating practice (Rogers, 1983). This lectureship, coupled with a presentation by Donald Schön (an expert in the analysis of professional practice) to the American Occupational Therapy Association Commission on Education, stimulated the American Occupational Therapy Research Foundation to set up the Clinical Reasoning Study. This study was designed by an anthropologist (Mattingly) and several occupational therapists, including Fleming, Gillette, and Cohen, and was heavily influenced by Schön as the project's consultant (Mattingly & Gillette, 1991). The study commenced in 1986, was completed in 1990, and was extensively reported in the American Journal of Occupational Therapy's special issue (November, 1991) on clinical reasoning. In 1994, this information was published in a book by Mattingly and Fleming. Articles on clinical reasoning are now a regular feature in international occupational therapy journals. Although ideas and information from several of these articles are presented below, this chapter as well as the thrust of this book has been greatly influenced by Mattingly and Fleming's work in this field.

TYPES OF CLINICAL REASONING

The main forms of clinical reasoning are scientific, narrative, and pragmatic reasoning (Schell and Cervero, 1993; and Strong et al., 1995), and narrative, procedural, interactive, and conditional reasoning (Mattingly, 1991; Mattingly & Gillette, 1991; Fleming, 1991; and Mattingly & Fleming, 1994).

Scientific Reasoning

Medical educators such as Elstein, Shulman, and Sprafka (1978); Dowie and Elstein (1988); and Schön (1983, 1988) have conducted many studies and written extensively on professional judgment in medicine. This knowledge has contributed significantly to our understanding of reasoning in occupational therapy. Medical **decision making** relies almost exclusively on scientific reasoning. **Scientific reasoning** is the process of hypothesis generation and testing that is generally referred to as *hypothetico-deductive reasoning*. This form of reasoning is most often used when making a diagnosis of the client's medical condition. Scientific reasoning assists the clinician in thinking about the medical aspects of the client's condition and the implications even though very little may actually be known about the client as an individual. Schell and Cervero (1993) suggest that from a scientific reasoning perspective, occupational therapists can improve practice by following the scientific model more effectively. This includes:

1. Selection of a frame of reference
2. Development of a systematic approach to data collection and synthesis
3. Hypothesis generation
4. Hypothesis testing

Several occupational therapy writers and researchers use this scientific form of reasoning to assist therapists in improving their practice. Examples include the work of Cubie and Kaplan (1982), Pelland (1987), and Rogers and Holm (1991).

However, the medical model of decision making and the scientific approach to reasoning do not seem to fully explain occupational therapy reasoning. For example, medical decision making:

- Revolves around determining a diagnosis, which is not usual in occupational therapy
- Pays little attention to the interaction of the client with the practitioner
- Whereas medical decision making appears to be largely sequential, clinical reasoning may be circular, with several steps examined and evaluated simultaneously

Rather than subscribing to the medical model and scientific forms of reasoning, Mattingly (1991, p. 979) describes occupational therapy clinical reasoning as being "... largely tacit, highly imagistic, and a deeply phenomenological mode of thinking." Mattingly (1991) suggested that **narrative reasoning** is a better basis for clinical reasoning in occupational therapy. Narrative reasoning uses storymaking and storytelling to assist the therapist in understanding the meaning of the disability or disease to the client. Mattingly distances occupational therapy clinical reasoning from scientific reasoning and prefers using a **phenomenological** framework (Schell & Cervero, 1993).

Pragmatic Reasoning

Schell and Cervero (1993) suggested another form of reasoning, which they describe as **pragmatic reasoning**. These authors define pragmatic reasoning as the reasoning processes associated with the clinician's practice setting and his or her personal context. For example, Schell and Cervero (1993) suggest that organizational, political, and economic constraints and opportunities all impact on a clinician's ability to provide an occupational therapy service, as do personal motivation, values, and beliefs. Undoubtedly, all of these factors influence a clinician's thinking and the way he engages in the therapeutic process; therefore, it appears to be most likely that clinical reasoning in occupational therapy is multifaceted and involves narrative, scientific, and pragmatic forms of reasoning.

Narrative Reasoning and Chart Talk

Given that clinical reasoning is a mental process, it is difficult to access what is going on in a clinician's mind. One of the ways to do this is to ask therapists to tell some stories about working with clients. The use of narratives or stories provides a means of conveying one's reasoning to other professionals and a medium through which practice can be shared with students and novice therapists. Viewed in this light, narrative reasoning is a way of reporting or giving words to the other forms of clinical reasoning, such as procedural, interactive, and conditional reasoning, which are discussed later in this section (Strong et al., 1995). Narrative reasoning is also a form of phenomenological understanding. Narratives reveal how the therapist treated and interacted with the client and also his or her understanding of how the client was managing his disability. Story creation, on the other hand, involves creating a picture of the future with the client. This includes sharing ideas about achievements that can be worked toward in therapy.

Mattingly and Fleming (1994) report that clinicians tend to use a narrative mode of discourse when talking about the meaning of a medical condition with the client. However, they found that when therapists were discussing procedural aspects of the client's physical condition and evaluations or assessments and interventions, they were more likely to use "chart talk" and scientific forms of reasoning. The researchers described that these two distinct forms of language, "story talk" and "chart talk," provided clinicians with different ways of making sense of the client. Mattingly (1994b) stated that therapists in the Clinical Reasoning Study spent about one third to one half of their time in meetings with colleagues or in writing notes in clients' medical records. During this time, the therapists would discuss the client's clinical problems, treatments, and justification for treatments and they would share treatment goals. In addition, therapists talked to their clients about how the therapy was progressing. During these discussions, therapists tended to use a biomechanical way of understanding the client's problems and therefore used "chart talk." This was particularly the case with therapists working with clients who had physical problems. This typically involved therapists' describing a list of problems and the various treatments that are used to address each problem, with little attention paid to the experience of the client (Mattingly, 1994a).

As indicated previously, when therapists consider the meaning of the disability for the client's life, they begin to tell stories about the client and thus use the narrative mode. Mattingly (1994a) describes how clinical problems and treatment activities are transformed from "chart talk" into an unfolding drama in which the cast (including the client, significant people in his life, and the therapist) all have roles to play. Motives, emotions, feelings, and aspirations are all explored in these stories, which is in sharp contrast to the factual, scientific accounts recorded in clients' medical charts. It is suggested that therapists consider the similarities between the current stories they are engaged in with clients and past stories so they can draw ideas from their experience.

However, Mattingly (1994c) points out that not only do therapists need to be adept at telling and creating stories, they also need to be able to change the story in response to a whole range of factors that arise unexpectedly. Changing the story requires the therapist to be flexible and adaptive. As therapy unfolds, the planned interventions may no longer work or may work more quickly than anticipated; or the client may react in an unexpectedly good or bad way to a particular intervention; or the therapist may find the client no longer shares the story and is creating a new one. No matter how well-planned the therapy, revisions will inevitably be required. The therapist must be able to quickly assess the situation and change the direction of the story.

In summary, narratives are used by therapists when they want to better understand the client's illness and the ways his disability or disease affects his life. Storytelling is most predominant when clinicians are carrying out the day-to-day procedures of evaluating and treating clients and trying to understand the client as a person and the things that are happening in therapy (Alnervik & Sviden, 1996). Story creation is more common when clinicians envision a future for the client or engage in "conditional reasoning." The story created for therapy doesn't usually proceed without the need for revision, and experienced therapists are adept in changing the therapeutic story midstream (Mattingly, 1994c).

The Therapist with the Three-Track Mind

In addition to narrative reasoning, during the Clinical Reasoning Study, Mattingly and Fleming (1994) identified three other main forms of thinking used by clinicians: **procedural reasoning** (which may involve scientific reasoning), **interactive reasoning**, and **conditional reasoning** (which may include pragmatic reasoning). These forms of reasoning are discussed in detail in the remainder of this section. Fleming described that in the Clinical Reasoning Study, the investigators found that not only were there three forms of reasoning, but therapists seemed to be thinking along these reasoning "tracks" simultaneously. Therefore, the researchers began to describe therapists as having "three-track minds." Therapists seemed to monitor the procedural aspects of the treatment, such as what was being done with the client and how the client was performing, while interacting with the client to ". . . elicit their cooperation and understand the person's response to the treatment" (Fleming, 1994a, p. 131). Therapists also seemed to be engaged in casting visions of the client's future and predicting how it would be facilitated by the treatments. Mattingly and Fleming (1994) contend that experienced therapists shift smoothly from one form of reasoning to another or use different forms simultaneously. In more junior therapists and students, the shift between the forms of reasoning can appear more halting.

Whereas Mattingly and Fleming (1994) have separated these different forms of clinical reasoning, Strong et al. (1995) contend that procedural, interactive, and conditional reasoning are not separate forms of reasoning but are parts of the reasoning process itself or aspects of content. They suggest that there is, in fact, a complex, universal process of reasoning based on problem solving. Although further research may in fact uphold this view, labeling and examining different forms of reasoning assists us in exploring therapy in a logical manner, and in teaching clinical reasoning to students and novice clinicians. The following excerpt outlines the three "tracks" of clinical reasoning as described by Mattingly and Fleming (1994). Each form of reasoning, together with an example from practice in cognition and perception, is presented in more detail below.

> Early in the Clinical Reasoning Study, we began to realise that occupational therapists were using several reasoning strategies. Different modes of thinking were employed for different purposes or in response to particular features of a problem. One reasoning strategy that therapists frequently employed was very similar to the hypothetical reasoning typically discussed in the medical problem-solving literature. We called this "procedural reasoning." Therapists tended to rely upon a hypothetical, a procedural, style of thinking when considering the person's physical ailment. This is probably because therapists' knowledge of clinical conditions is frequently acquired through medical lecture courses—which may or may not be taught by physicians, but are almost always presented within the philosophical framework of the medical model. This type of reasoning was similar, but not exactly like medical problem solving. The focus of occupational therapy treatment is different from medical treatment. For physicians, the problem to be solved is the clinical condition. For occupational therapists, the problem is to help the person solve problems of daily functioning incurred as consequences of the clinical condition. In a procedural mode of reasoning therapists search for techniques and procedures that can be brought to bear on the physical problem.
>
> A second type of reasoning was employed when therapists interacted with the patient as a person, a social being. We called this "interactive reasoning." When the therapists were interacting with their patients as people, their interactive style would change. Their interactions were clearly guided by some sort of reasoning. As one therapist said:
>
> > When we interact with patients we are honest and real, but we think about how we are acting and why. It's not just some enthusiastic, but unguided interaction like . . . like say—a hairdresser. You know how

> they are, they just talk about anything. There's no purpose behind what they are talking to you about, or how they react to what you say, except to make the time to pass more pleasantly. When therapists talk to patients there is a reason behind what they say that is more than just conversation. When we interact with patients we think about what we are going to say and why.

We could see that the therapists interacted with their patients in a way that was purposeful and structured by some sort of tacit plans and guidelines. We knew that some parts of occupational therapy education are focused on developing therapists' interactive skills. Lectures and assignments are designed to develop various aspects of interaction such as interviewing skills or group process techniques. The tradition of "therapeutic use of self" (Fidler & Fidler, 1963, p. 40) probably also influences occupational therapy practice. Perhaps the primary place where interactive reasoning is acquired is clinical education. The clinical education of occupational therapists includes objectives and experiences aimed at improving students' interactive skills; and part of the evaluation of the affiliating students' clinical performance considers interactive skills. The notion that interaction is guided by a different type of reasoning than hypothetical reasoning is supported by a growing body of literature in psychology and philosophy. Although we developed the idea that interaction was guided by a particular form of reasoning ourselves, it was not difficult to find similar concepts in the current literature. Many authors have postulated the idea that there are several forms of reasoning. . . .

Both procedural and interactive reasoning were employed to address difference aspects of the whole problem. The procedural reasoning strategy was used when the therapist thought about the person's physical and emotional limitations and what procedures were appropriate to improve function. Interactive reasoning was used to help the therapists interact with and understand the person better. Although these reasoning strategies are distinctly different, therapists shifted rapidly from one form of reasoning to another. Reasoning styles changed as the therapist's attention was drawn from the clinical condition to another feature of the problem, and to how the person feels about the problem, almost simultaneously, using different thinking styles; and they did not "lose track of" their thoughts about aspects of a problem as those components were temporarily shifted to be the background while another aspect was brought into the foreground.

Later we realised that there was a third type of reasoning that therapists employed when they thought of the whole problem within the context of the person's past, present and future; and within personal, social and cultural contexts. This was an especially useful form of reasoning, which therapists used when they wanted to, as they say, "individualise" the treatment for the particular person. We called this "conditional reasoning" because it took the whole condition into account.

Extract reprinted with permission from the authors, Mattingly and Fleming, 1994, pp. 119–121.

Procedural Reasoning

Therapists employ procedural reasoning when they think about which evaluation approaches they will use to identify the client's functional problems, set goals, and plan intervention (Fleming, 1994a). Although terms such as *problem identification* and *goal setting* are used in the occupational therapy literature, terms such as *diagnosis, prognosis and prescription, cue identification, hypothesis generation, cue interpretation,* and *hypothesis evaluation* are more common in the medical decision-making literature (Elstein, Shuman, & Sprafka, 1978).

Both the medical and occupational therapy literatures use the term *problem solving*, yet they mean different things (Fleming, 1994b). In the occupational therapy literature, problem solving refers to the invention of unique solutions for the complex problems and issues that the client faces. In contrast, in the medical literature problem solving generally refers to problem identification or diagnosis. Some occupational therapy researchers do use the term **diagnostic reasoning** when referring to the component of procedural reasoning that involves the evaluation and identification of a client's problems from an occupational therapist's viewpoint (Rogers & Holm, 1991; Neistadt & Atkins, 1996). Others may use the term scientific reasoning when discussing the ways an occupational therapist uses cue identification, hypothesis generation, cue interpretation, and hypothesis evaluation to determine the nature of a client's problems. However, the generation of competing hypotheses as possible cause for the client's presenting problems seems common to most of the health personnel studied by Elstein et al. (1978) and Mattingly and Fleming (1994). (The reader is referred to Chapter 3 for a description of hypothesis testing in occupational therapy.) In the Clinical Reasoning Study, Mattingly and Fleming (1994) reported that experienced occupational therapists typically generated two to four possible hypotheses regarding the cause and nature of the client's problems. In contrast, newer therapists seek the right answer immediately and only consider one or two competing hypotheses as the cause of a problem.

Fleming (1994b) identified that when determining what the client's problems might be and selecting appropriate treatments, the therapist is involved in a variety of reasoning strategies and methods of thinking. These include goal-oriented problem solving, task environment and problem space, pattern recognition, and the four-stage model of problem solving. (All these features are discussed later.) All problem solving in occupational therapy is goal-directed; that is, therapists work with clients to help them maximize their ability to participate in everyday activities. The task environment and problem space are often in the medical facility or the client's home, but therapists must look beyond this controlled environment to the client's longer term residence. The most relevant therapy considers not only the problems in the immediate environment but future environments as well. **Pattern rec-**

ognition refers to a therapist's ability to identify the kinds of client **cues** and features that occur together. For example a therapist who observes a client brushing his hair with a toothbrush may wonder if the client has a psychiatric problem or a problem with ideational apraxia. However, knowing that the client has been admitted for rehabilitation after stroke may prompt the therapist to recognize a typical pattern of cognitive problems after this kind of brain incident (Fleming, 1994b). The ability to recognize patterns of cues and behaviors becomes part of the therapist's tacit knowledge (Fleming, 1994b). Procedural reasoning generally begins with problem identification, and Elstein, Shulman, and Sprafka (1978) developed a four-stage model of problem solving that focuses on problem identification. The four stages in this model are:

1. Cue acquisition: the therapist gathers cues or bits of information about the client and his difficulties
2. Hypothesis generation: several plausible explanations for the observed cues are generated
3. Cue interpretation: each hypothesis is compared with the cue set, and the most logical or best hypotheses to explain the cues are selected
4. Hypothesis evaluation: finally, the clinician determines which is the best hypothesis by evaluating which cues are generally thought to be necessary for selecting each hypothesis and for the presence of critical cues for selecting each hypothesis. In this way, one hypothesis should be identified as the best.

Fleming suggests that therapists may use this model when determining the client's occupational problems.

In summary, *procedural reasoning* seems to be a useful umbrella term that describes a therapist's thinking when working out what a client's problems are and what procedures may be used to reduce the effect of those problems. A clinical description of a therapist using procedural reasoning may be found in Box 2–2. In addition, in the case study concentration (Chapter 4), the clinician uses a hypothesis testing approach as part of his procedural reasoning to determine the nature of the client's problems.

Interactive Reasoning

Interactive reasoning occurs as the clinician engages in therapy with the client. It takes place during face-to-face encounters between clinicians and their clients (Fleming, 1994a). In the Clinical Reasoning Study, Mattingly and Fleming (1994) found that although clinicians reported their procedural practices, they did not report their interactions with the client; therefore, these researchers referred to this interactive reasoning as the "underground practice." Although at first the researchers in the Clinical Reasoning Study

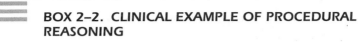

BOX 2–2. CLINICAL EXAMPLE OF PROCEDURAL REASONING

Choosing Assessments to Use with Paul: Therapist Narrative

Paul had been referred for inpatient occupational therapy after his transfer to rehabilitation after 6 days in acute care. Paul is 20 years old and was working as an office clerk (computer operator) for a transport company before his involvement in a motor vehicle accident. The transfer letter from the occupational therapist at the acute facility indicated that Paul had some behavioral problems, reduced concentration, and memory problems. No physical problems were evident. After briefly reviewing Paul's medical history, I met with him for the first time.

I introduced myself to Paul and told him about occupational therapy (OT). I explained that for the first few times he was in OT, we would look at areas he was doing well in and areas that he had trouble with and how together we would decide what we would work on in therapy. Already I had begun to make many observations about Paul, such as the fact that he was dressed neatly and that his expressive language skills seemed good. I decided to assess Paul in two ways. First, I wanted to do a more thorough assessment of Paul's cognitive and perceptual abilities because he had experienced a head injury and the referring therapist had noted some cognitive problems. I wanted to use a standardized assessment for recording purposes and as a means of measuring change. For this purpose I selected the Lowenstein Occupational Therapy Cognitive Assessment (LOTCA) (Itzkovich et al., 1990). I selected this assessment because it's easy to administer and will assist me in screening for a wide variety of cognitive and perceptual problems. Since it takes about 45 minutes to administer the whole test, I decided to use only a few of the 20 subtests during the first session (I thought Paul would tire easily and did not want to push him too hard during his first session). I commenced the assessment with Paul. After about 15 minutes, Paul seemed to get really agitated with the task he was doing, and he swore loudly. I had heard that the nurses had also complained about this behavior. Almost immediately after this outburst, Paul calmed down. There are many therapeutic strategies for dealing with this behavior and for assisting Paul to build his frustration tolerance for activities. However, I wanted to wait and share my preliminary assessment findings with the other team members so we could agree on a consistent strategy to use with Paul. I suggested to Paul that we finish the task he was working on, take a break, and then plan our next therapy session. After a short break, I talked with Paul about his total therapy program and reinforced the information in his memory book (which the speech-language therapist had organized in the morning).

(continues)

BOX 2–2. CLINICAL EXAMPLE OF PROCEDURAL REASONING (CONT.)

The second assessment approach I use with clients is more functional because I want to get an idea of the impact of the client's cognitive and perceptual problems on his or her daily living activities. In Paul's second therapy session, I wanted to do a functional task and use the hypothesis-testing approach to confirm earlier assessment findings. I offered Paul the choice of making a wood-and-pipe windchime or doing a computer activity for this functional assessment. I wanted Paul to have some choice over what he did in therapy, but I also wanted activities that I knew could provide valuable information about his problems. I selected these activities because:

● they offered me scope to generate some hypotheses about the nature of Paul's problems that I could then test out,

● they are age appropriate and culturally attractive,

● I thought that computer literacy would continue to be important for Paul in the future (given that his job at the transport company is computer based) and it would be useful to incorporate a few computer based activities in therapy, and

● I thought Paul might be interested in doing some more therapy in the woodwork room (he mentioned that one of his hobbies in the past had been woodwork) and wanted to introduce him to our woodwork room in a simple way.

Paul chose the windchime activity. I recorded this in his memory workbook and we agreed to meet the next morning.

were puzzled over the use and purpose of the clinicians' interactions with their clients, these interactions were later identified as an important form of reasoning. Rather than being a distraction from therapy, interactive reasoning appears to be a legitimate and necessary therapy mode (Fleming, 1994a).

Therapists use interactive reasoning to describe the client as a person who has interests, needs, and values as well as problems, so that the therapist can understand the disability from the client's perspective. Interactive reasoning stems from the way clinicians value the client as an individual and their deeply held humanistic beliefs. The therapist is also using this form of reasoning when verifying information, asking clients about themselves, and sharing information with clients. Clinicians require great skill to simultaneously monitor both the treatment and the client's feelings about the treatment (Fleming, 1994a). From a variety of authors, Fleming (1994a) put together the following list of purposes for which interactive reasoning is used. Interactive reasoning is used to:

1. Engage the client in therapy (Mattingly, 1989)
2. Know the client as a person (Cohen, 1989)
3. Understand the client's disability from his own point of view (Mattingly, 1989)
4. Individualize the therapy for the client; that is, match the treatment goals with the person, his disability, and his experience of the disability (Fleming, 1989)
5. Convey a sense of acceptance, trust, and hope (Langthaler, 1990)
6. Break tension through the use of humor (Siegler, 1987)
7. Build a shared language of actions and meanings (Crepeau, 1991)
8. Monitor how the treatment session is going (Fleming, 1990)
9. Demonstrate interest in the client and his concerns without indicating disapproval or distaste of the condition (Bradburn, 1992)

A clinical description of a therapist's engaging in interactive reasoning with a client may be found in Box 2–3.

Whereas procedural reasoning is often factually based, interactive reasoning is intuitive. Hammond (1988) described how intuitive reasoning can be more effective than other forms of reasoning when a great deal of information from a variety of sources must be integrated. This occurs in therapy when working with clients who have multifaceted problems or problems that are not well-defined. However, the use of intuitive reasoning seems to develop only with experience, and this is discussed later in the section on expert practice.

Interactive reasoning is concerned with getting the client to collaborate in therapy. This is not always easy when the client is undergoing a frightening experience of readjusting after an accident or illness. In addition, many clients who experience cognitive and perceptual problems also have a clinical lack of insight into their problems. This means the clinician faces the additional difficulty of collaborating with and having meaningful therapy sessions with clients who may not have any understanding of their problems. However, with patience and persistence, the therapist can usually help clients to establish the meaning of their disabilities and their aspirations for the future (Mattingly & Fleming, 1994). Therapists often build rapport with clients not only to be pleasant and make therapy pleasurable but to gain the client's cooperation in the therapy process. Therapists use a number of strategies to engage the client in therapy; this often means recalling the success and failure of past strategies as well as sharing ideas and stories with other therapists about what approach may work best. Mat-

BOX 2–3. CLINICAL EXAMPLE OF INTERACTIVE REASONING

Engaging Shelby in Therapy: Therapist Narrative

I wasn't sure why Shelby was so distracted in therapy today. We had both agreed to bake cookie dough cookies for this session to work on her upper limb movements. Shelby is 38 years old and was admitted to rehabilitation following an aneurysm that burst and was clipped 3 weeks ago. Shelby's main problem is moderate bilateral apraxia in her upper limbs, which means that she requires some assistance to complete all personal activities of daily living.

I knew her husband and children had visited last night and that having her two young children see her in this dependent state sometimes distressed her. Therefore, I decided to try to find out more about what was going on by asking Shelby how the family visit went last night. Shelby's face crumpled and she cried softly. My suspicions were confirmed when she told me how hard it was to have her children see her in the hospital. She said they really didn't understand why she couldn't walk properly and couldn't play with them anymore, and that this upset them. I asked her how her husband was managing at home with them. Shelby replied that he would have to go back to work next week and that her mom would come over and stay each day with the children. Clearly Shelby had a lot of support from family, and it seemed that she was more concerned about the children's perceptions of their mom rather than their well-being. I wanted to make sure I had understood this, so I asked Shelby if this was the problem, and she agreed it was.

Shelby knew I also had a small child, and in many previous sessions we had talked about the trials and joys of raising children and all the tasks this involved. Having this in common had certainly helped us progress in therapy. Shelby had identified that her main aim was to be able to return home and care for herself and her family again, and together we had drawn up a prioritized list of the activities this involved. Although Shelby was making good progress in therapy, she was often angry at herself for not progressing more quickly. I thought it might be a good time to remind Shelby of all the things she could do now that were not possible 2 weeks ago, such as drinking steadily from a cup and using a fork to eat pre-cut food. Shelby nodded agreement that she had made gains.

I began to wonder if we could bring Shelby's children to join in one or two therapy sessions each week. I thought this might be good for several reasons:

● to allow Shelby and her children more time together,

● for the children to get used to what Shelby could do and what she was having trouble with, in a supported environment, and

(continues)

BOX 2–3. CLINICAL EXAMPLE OF INTERACTIVE REASONING (CONT.)

● for Shelby and the children to be involved in fun activities together that would make Shelby's problems seem less frightening and give them a chance to laugh and have fun together.

I suggested to Shelby that we involve the children some more in her therapy. Although I thought she would like this idea, I was concerned that she might want to protect the children from her problems and therefore not want to include them in her therapy. However, she thought it was a great idea. Shelby said how much she missed not having the children with her every day. She asked if they could come in the next day and make cookies together. I was really pleased at how well Shelby had responded to the idea and how much brighter she seemed. I suggested that for the rest of this session we practice rolling dough so she would be able to do this part of the task tomorrow, and the children could do the cutting. I thought that practicing rolling the dough for tomorrow would be a significant motivator for Shelby. We both wanted Shelby to be able to complete this part of the activity successfully in front of her children. For the remainder of the session we planned ways in which we could include the children in the session tomorrow, and yet still make sure Shelby had a lot of opportunity for therapy. Shelby seemed much more motivated toward participating in tomorrow's session than she had in today's!

---

tingly and Fleming (1994) identified the following six strategies that therapists commonly employed in their interactions with clients to facilitate their engagement in therapy:

1. Creating choices. Therapists try to engage clients in therapy by providing choices in relation to problem areas the client wants to work on and the specific occupations or activities they might use in therapy.
2. Individualizing treatment. A therapy program that is uniquely tailored for the client, through both the ingenuity of the therapist and the involvement of the client, generally keeps the client engaged in therapy. Although the goals of therapy may be quite similar for different clients with memory problems, the way the therapy programs are structured and the activities the clients and therapists choose are usually different for each client.
3. Structuring success. Therapists often structure, or manipulate, therapy to provide the client with opportunities for success and thus promote their alliance. Therapists often reveal problems and then work with the client to reduce their impact. Unless the client has some successes along

the way, it is very hard to keep the client motivated or to maintain a positive relationship with the client. Therapists often talk about keeping the client optimally challenged. This includes pushing the client to achieve but not so far that he fails. This has been described as the "just-right challenge" (Berlyne, 1969; Csikszentmihayli, 1975).

4. Joint problem solving. Another approach therapists use to facilitate client engagement in therapy is to ask the client to help them in the problem-solving process. For example, if the therapist has difficulty in using a piece of equipment or in devising a strategy for a transfer, calling on the client for his input enables the client to take a strong and active role in therapy, if only for a short time.

5. Gift exchange. The final two strategies that Mattingly and Fleming (1994) found that therapists use to build an alliance with their clients were more personal in nature. The researchers found that therapists would go out of their way, or outside of their formal roles to do something nice for the client such as bake a cake for a client's birthday. In this way the therapist shows a willingness to care for the client in a more personal way. In exchange, clients often feel more committed to cooperate in therapy. Clients may also give gifts to the therapist. These may be as simple as a flower, a few words of thanks, or a hug, all of which demonstrate their personal thanks for the therapist's involvement in their treatment.

6. Exchanging personal stories. Exchanging personal experiences is another powerful way to develop a bond with a client. Mattingly and Fleming (1994) found this was commonly used by clinicians to engage the clients in therapy and that clinicians were usually aware of the value of this strategy.

Conditional Reasoning

Fleming (1994a) describes the third form of reasoning, conditional reasoning, as the most elusive. Conditional reasoning is not always conscious; therefore, it is more difficult to "get at," understand, and describe. Fleming (1994c) proposed that this form of reasoning is based in the cultural and social processes of understanding one's self and others and is used when the therapist wishes to understand the client from a phenomenological perspective. That is, a clinician uses this form of reasoning when she tries to understand what is meaningful to a client by imagining what his life was like before his illness or disability and imagining what his life could be like in the future.

Conditional reasoning takes the whole of the client's condition into account as the therapist considers the client's temporal contexts (i.e., past, present, and future), and his personal, cultural, and social contexts. Fleming (1994a) states that conditional reasoning requires more than a simple knowledge of the client's condition; it also calls for an understanding of how the condition has affected the individual's work, social situation, leisure, and view of self. Therapists use conditional reasoning to integrate procedural and interactive reasoning to create an image of the client's future. Fleming writes that ". . . in using conditional reasoning, the therapist appears to reflect on the success or failure of the clinical encounter from both the procedural and interactive standpoints and attempts to integrate the two" (Fleming, 1991, p. 1012).

The term *conditional* is used by Mattingly and Fleming (1994) in three different ways:

1. The therapist thinks about the whole condition, including the client's illness, the meaning attached to it, and the client's whole context.
2. The therapist thinks about how the condition could change and what this might mean (this state is conditional and may or may not be achieved).
3. The therapist thinks about whether or not the imagined life will be achieved and realizes that this is conditional on both the client's participation in the therapy program and the shared construction of the future image.

In the Clinical Reasoning Study, conditional reasoning was the term used to describe what clinicians referred to as "putting it all together" and "treating the whole person." Given that conditional reasoning involves considering the total therapy context, this may also cover the pragmatic form of reasoning as described by Schell and Cervero (1993).

Experienced clinicians appear to have a relatively clear image of the person and what his future can be like given appropriate therapy. Clinicians expressed that therapy was on track when the client was moving toward becoming that imagined person. Mattingly and Fleming (1994) described the two forms of thinking that are required to bring about this imagined future as being *imagination* and *interpretation*.

To convey a sense of the client's past, present, and future and to map out how therapy is progressing, the therapist may remind the client (and herself) of a time when he could not do a task or activity (Fleming, 1994c). This may be particularly useful when therapy is progressing slowly or some of the routine aspects have become boring. Importantly, these reminders show both the client and therapist how the condition is progressing and that together they may yet reach their shared vision of the future (Fleming, 1994c).

Fleming (1994c) described how "meaning-making" is central to the concept of conditional reasoning. Therapists are often interested in the client's ability to make new meanings for himself given his current situation. Fleming (1994c) discussed three aspects of meaning-making: intentionality, habit, and symbolic meaning. In essence, intentionality is a ". . . life force through

BOX 2–4. CLINICAL EXAMPLE OF CONDITIONAL REASONING

Discharging Mr. D from Rehabilitation: Therapist Narrative

My 78-year-old client Mr. D is really eager to get home to his wife. He was doing all the cooking and cleaning, as well as helping his wife with her personal care, before his stroke. Mrs. D has been in a skilled nursing facility while her husband has been in rehabilitation. Mr. D has been in rehabilitation for 4 weeks now and we've been working toward his discharge for the past week. Although his physical recovery has been very good, Mr. D persistently neglects visual information on his left side, and he experiences reduced short-term memory. The worst part is that he doesn't seem to have any insight into these problems. Mrs. D seems quite frail, and I really think that if they don't make it at home together, they could end up being moved to a nursing home because there is no family to help them out.

I can imagine that with just a bit of extra support they might be okay at home. I've been working with them both toward an arrangement at home in which Mr. D cares for the house and Mrs. D acts as an "overseer." They seem so eager to be together again that they readily agreed to work toward this plan, but the fact that Mr. D doesn't really understand his problems has me worried. I can imagine that there may be many parts of tasks or activities such as cleaning the house that he just doesn't do, but the Ds say it's OK if they don't live in a perfectly clean house. The Ds have said that their neighbor will help them heat a pre-packaged meal in the oven for their evening meal each day. I've explained to Mrs. D that I'm worried that Mr. D will leave the oven on because the button is on the left side, but I know Mrs. D is good about getting her husband to check things like locking the doors and checking that the gas is off. I asked the Ds if they wanted me to call their neighbor to arrange for her to drop by late each afternoon to help with getting the meal in and out of the oven, but they said they'd already arranged for this. Together we organized for the local church volunteer group to help them by doing the weekly shopping.

I have a pretty clear image of their home from the home evaluation we did last week. When we went out to the house, Mrs. D agreed that it was okay for me to rearrange the furniture to prompt Mr. D to take left turns and to remove some of the smaller tables that he might trip over. Luckily, the kitchen and bathroom doorways were both on the right side of the main room, so I think he won't have too much trouble finding his way around the house.

I think that in the next year or so, the Ds will probably need to move to some other form of housing, particularly if Mrs. D gets any sicker or Mr. D has any other health problems. Although I'm a bit worried about how they'll manage, I think they'll be okay at home for now, and it's definitely their choice to try to manage at home.

which the individual focuses his or her energy for being in the world" (Fleming, 1994c, p. 198). Experienced therapists seem to have an intuitive sense of the importance of intentionality to their clients. Therapists facilitate intentionality by providing opportunities for choice (e.g., in activities) and in motivating clients to have meaningful experiences in their lives. Habits are daily routines, and people form a connection with the world and create meaning through habits. Habits are essential in the building and rebuilding of self after an illness experience. Finally, symbolic meaning is an "understanding'"that is captured through some symbol, which could be as abstract as a concept or as concrete as an object. Therapists offer clients the opportunity to participate in occupations that can be interpreted at different levels of meaning. Clients may derive symbolic meanings from their engagement in these activities. Fleming (1994c, p. 198) suggests that "we think that conditional reasoning revolves around the ways that therapists think about which of the actions that the patient takes have potential for meaning-making." A simple example of a clinician's recounting a story that demonstrates conditional reasoning is shown in Box 2–4. In this narrative, the therapist considers the different kinds of future lives open to her client and his wife. The therapist is aware of the importance attached to, and the meaning associated with, being at home together for this couple.

Fleming (1994a) reported that therapists who were more interested than the clients themselves in clients' medical conditions or occupational therapy treatment procedures did not seem to use conditional reasoning. This is often the case with less experienced therapists who are still grappling with the clients' medical conditions and are still learning about putting an occupational therapy treatment program together. The next section of this chapter explores some of the other differences between students, novice clinicians, and experienced therapists. Through identifying and examining these differences, it is anticipated that students and newer therapists will gain insights into how experts think and work and how they can model their practice on these experts.

≡ FROM NOVICE TO EXPERT

> Expert clinicians are those who are competent in action and, simultaneously, reflect on this action to learn from it (Rogers, 1983, p. 614).

A great deal has been written in the occupational therapy literature about the differences between novice and expert clinicians (Robertson, 1996; Strong et al., 1995; Collins & Affeldt, 1996), and how students can improve their reasoning skills and thereby facilitate the development of expertise

(Cohen, 1991; Neistadt, 1987, 1992a, 1996; Neistadt & Atkins, 1996). The purpose of this section is to review some of the literature concerned with novice and expert differences to provide the reader with insights concerning how a clinician's clinical reasoning changes over time. Although the transition from novice to expert differs for every therapist both in time frame and style, it is anticipated that greater insight into this transition will facilitate a novice's transition from the classroom to the clinic and then on through the stages of proficiency that lead to expertise.

STAGES IN THE DEVELOPMENT OF EXPERTISE

Expert clinical reasoning seems to develop over time along a continuum. Dreyfus and Dreyfus (1980, 1986) presented a five-stage model of skill acquisition based on their study of chess players and airline pilots. They suggested that as a student develops a skill, he passes through five stages of proficiency: novice, advanced beginner, competent, proficient, and expert. Benner (1984) and Benner and Tanner (1987) incorporated this work into their studies of the acquisition of skill in nursing. Benner (1984) suggested that these levels reflect changes in three aspects of skilled performance:

1. A shift in reliance from abstract principles to past experiences
2. A change in perception of the situation, in which there is a shift from perceiving all parts of the picture equally to viewing the whole situation in which only parts are relevant
3. A change from detached observer to involved performer

Table 2–1 outlines Dreyfus and Dreyfus's (1986) stages in the development of expertise and some of the characteristics of clinicians at each stage based on the work of Benner (1984) and Benner and Tanner (1987).

CHARACTERISTICS OF EXPERTISE

Benner and Tanner (1987) proposed that one of the most elusive characteristics of expertise is intuition. *Intuition* may be defined as "understanding without rationale" (Benner & Tanner, 1987, p. 22). These researchers argue that rather than being the basis for irrational acts, intuition and intuitive judgments are the hallmarks of expertise. Although the decision making of **novice therapists** is generally analytical, the expert uses intuition as a basis for judgment. In occupational therapy, Fleming (1994a) described therapists as using intuitive reasoning when they suddenly perceived a problem to be more complex than they had originally assumed. It appears that ex-

Table 2–1. Stages and characteristics in the development of expertise

STAGE	CLINICIAN CHARACTERISTICS
1. Novice	Novices don't have experience of the situations they will be involved in. In order to enter the clinic and gain experience in these areas, students are taught about theories, principles, and specific patient attributes. A novice is usually rigid in the application of these rules, principles and theories. However, rules can't guide the clinician to do all the things she needs to in the multitude of situations and contexts in which she works (Benner, 1984). A clinician can only acquire "context dependent judgment" through participation in real situations.
2. Advanced beginner	Advanced beginners have been involved in enough clinical situations to realize, or have pointed out to them, the recurring themes and information on which reasoning is based. An advanced beginner may begin to modify rules, principles, and theories so that they are adapted to the specific situation. Advanced beginners will do what they are told or what the text dictates as the correct procedure but may have difficulty prioritizing in more unusual circumstances which parts of the procedure are least important or which aspects are vital. Advanced beginners have to concentrate on remembering the rules and therefore have less ability to apply them flexibly. Dreyfus and Dreyfus (1986) suggest that an awareness of the client as a person beyond the technical concerns does not usually develop until the student has advanced to this stage.
3. Competent	Competent therapists are able to adjust the therapy to the specific needs of the client and the situation, but it may be difficult to alter initial treatment plans. Benner (1984) suggests that a clinician is competent once he is consciously aware of the outcome of his actions. This is typical of a clinician who has been in the job for 2 or 3 years. However, a competent clinician is said to lack the speed and flexibility of the proficient clinician. Efficiency and organization

(continues)

(continued)

Table 2–1. Stages and characteristics in the development of expertise	
STAGE	**CLINICIAN CHARACTERISTICS**
	are achieved at this stage through conscious or deliberate planning (Benner, 1984).
4. Proficient	Proficient therapists are flexible and able to alter treatment plans as needed. Proficient therapists have a clear understanding of the client's whole situation rather than an understanding of the components alone. Proficient practitioners have a "perception" of the situation based on experience rather than deliberation. Given that the proficient clinician has a perspective of the overall situation, components that are more or less important stand out, and the clinician can home in on the problem areas.
5. Expert	Expert therapists approach therapy from client-generated cues rather than preconceived therapeutic plans. Experts anticipate and recognize client strengths and weaknesses quickly based on their experience of other clients. The expert clinician does not need to rely on rules and guidelines to take appropriate action but rather has an intuitive grasp of the situation. Experts often find it difficult to explain this intuition.

Adapted from Benner, 1984; Dreyfus & Dreyfus, 1986; Neistadt & Atkins, 1996.

perts rely on intuition to assist them in problem solving when problems are ill-defined and have a large number of facets.

Mattingly (1994b) described differences between novice and **expert therapists** in terms of the way they used narratives in therapy. She suggested that expert therapists had a greater capacity to make revisions to the therapy story as therapy progressed. She suggested that expert therapists were more attentive to the mismatches that occurred between their prospective stories of how the therapy should progress and what was actually happening in therapy. Experts were also reported to be more flexible in changing the narrative when it ran into trouble so that the main story could be preserved, although reached by new paths.

Table 2–2. Comparison of expert and novice clinician reasoning

SUPERVISOR'S CLINICAL REASONING	NEW PRACTITIONER'S CLINICAL REASONING
1. Focuses on many aspects of situation	1. Focuses on one aspect of situation
2. One observation triggers many associations	2. One observation triggers one association
3. Reacts quickly to problem with total solution	3. Reacts slowly to problem with partial solution
4. Reasoning is holistic	4. Reasoning is step by step
5. Reasoning is tacit or unconscious	5. Reasoning requires conscious effort

From *Bridging the clinical reasoning gap*, by Collins & Affeldt, p. 34. Copyright 1996 by the American Occupational Therapy Association, Inc. Reprinted with permission.

Another hallmark of expertise is the way experienced clinicians interact with their clients. Fleming (1994a) suggests that a great deal of a clinician's interactive skill is an intrinsic part of herself and that this is difficult to influence. For example, the degree to which therapists are able to use the different forms of clinical reasoning and make smooth transitions between the different styles of reasoning also seem to depend on the clinician's personality, beliefs, and views. Several of the characteristics of an expert practitioner's reasoning are presented by Collins and Affeldt (1996) in Table 2–2, and these are contrasted with the reasoning approaches of newer graduates.

ENHANCING STUDENTS' CLINICAL REASONING SKILLS

This section presents some of the occupational therapy literature that examines how students and novice clinicians can improve their clinical reasoning and thus hasten their journey from novice to expert. More specific details of teaching strategies to enhance students' development of clinical reasoning skills may be found in Higgs (1992) and Neistadt (1996).

Collins and Affeldt (1996) listed two main ways of assisting novice clinicians to improve their clinical reasoning skills: (1) noting significant similarities and differences between their clients and reflecting on how this can influence treatment and (2) exploring probable consequences of treatments before their enactment. Table 2–3 outlines Collins and Affeldt's suggestions for ways novice clinicians can improve their reasoning. Examples relating to the practice of cognitive and perceptual dysfunction are provided for illustration.

In a study exploring novice and expert differences, Robertson (1996) sought to examine the thinking patterns of students and clinicians in terms of their internal problem representations. She proposed two hypotheses that were supported by the findings of the study: (1) that clinicians would have more integrated problem representations (i.e., a well-organized body of knowledge) and (2) that they would be more likely to take a client-centered approach. Educational implications from Robertson's study (1996) include the need to assist students to:

- Develop relationships between data so that treatment planning is guided by a thorough understanding of the problem situation.
- List the causative factors involved in the situation, a description of the environment and context and the problems, client-specific factors, and therapy goals.
- Use case scenarios from experts to make expert clinician reasoning and hypothesis generation more explicit. In this way, students can learn to "model" their practice on an expert's.

In addition, learning about clinical reasoning through case studies provides the occupational therapy student or novice clinician with:

- An idea of how much attention the clinician pays to client issues in addition to focusing on the clinical problems, such as apraxia or memory problems. As can be seen in several of the case study chapters in this book, the use of a client-centered assessment such as the Canadian Occupational Performance Measure (COPM) (Law, Baptiste, Carswell, McColl, Polatajko & Pollock, 1994), ensures attention is paid to the client's perspective.
- The opportunity to develop more precise thought processes sooner.
- A language to facilitate self-evaluation and improvement in clinical reasoning skills (Neistadt, 1996).

In another study examining the difference between expert therapist and students' clinical reasoning, Strong et al. (1995) reported that experts seemed to use a wider range of information than the students did. Experts also seemed to view it as more important to gain an understanding of their clients both in terms of their illness and disability as well as the client's perceptions of the impact of these on his life. Whereas expert clinicians placed a higher value on good communication skills, students placed more emphasis on knowledge and understanding of the client's problems. Although students are still in the process of consolidating their knowledge of the disability itself, this research

---

Table 2–3. Approaches to improving clinical reasoning skills

PRACTICE COMPONENTS   THERAPIST REASONING

Example Case Study:
After a stroke, Mrs. E has entered rehabilitation. She experiences memory problems and has a right hemiplegia. She is not yet able to walk.

NOTE SIGNIFICANT SIMILARITIES AND DIFFERENCES

I can draw on information about this client and past clients to guide my reasoning.

1. Narrow the focus: the client's cognitive/ perceptual skills and weaknesses are important because they affect the client's function	Through assessment, observation, and hypothesis-testing approaches, I need to identify and then focus on the skill deficits experienced by my client because they will affect his ability to perform self-care, work, and leisure activities. Example: focus on Mrs. E's memory because this will affect her ability to learn the one-handed dressing technique she now needs to use after her stroke. I need to focus on Mrs. E's intact memory of how to get dressed, break down the components of using the new one-handed technique, and then teach it to her and see if it improves her ability to dress.
2. Identify a client/problem area for comparison to reason how this client's skills and weaknesses and functional performance are similar to and different from past clients	I remember that Mrs. T also had problems learning the new dressing technique after her stroke. In addition to not remembering to put on her shirt by dressing her hemiplegic arm first, Mrs. T also had an ideomotor apraxia. Her inability to manipulate her shirt to dress her affected side first seemed to compound the problem. Guided movement and a chart of the steps for dressing seemed to help her . . . perhaps this will also help Mrs. E.

REFLECT ON PROBABLE CONSEQUENCES

Given my knowledge of Mrs. E and her strengths and weaknesses together with my theoretical knowledge and knowledge of other clients such as Mrs. T, I can begin to reason about what other issues may arise in therapy. In this

(continues)

(continued)

Table 2–3. Approaches to improving clinical reasoning skills	
PRACTICE COMPONENTS	THERAPIST REASONING
	way, I can anticipate possible problems and minimize their impact.
1. Reflect on effect of the deficit on function and cause-and-effect links	The particular cognitive and perceptual problems that Mrs. E has are likely to affect other aspects of her functioning. Mrs. E's problem with memory may also affect her ability to learn the new wheelchair transfer techniques and manage her therapy routine.
2. Reflect on what happened in the therapy session	When I taught Mrs. E to follow the memory chart for the steps to get dressed, her performance seemed to improve. Guided movement seemed to help a little but was probably more useful for Mrs. T because of her ideomotor apraxia.

Adapted from Tables 2 and 3 in Collins and Affeldt (1996).

suggests that students also need to pay attention to the client's perceptions of his disability. One way to do this may be to get students to ask the client questions about what the disability means to him after they have explored the more "scientific facts" of the condition.

Finally, another way to enhance student development of clinical reasoning skills is to provide them with structured ways to reflect on their clinical encounters. A key aspect of clinical reasoning is the ability to reflect on what has been experienced in therapy and to go forward in response to this reflection. Having told stories, we need time to reflect on their meaning and significance. Expert reasoning relies on the ability to reflect on, and learn from, therapeutic encounters both as an individual and from sharing experiences with other therapists. A great deal has been written in the medical and education literature on training doctors and teachers to be reflective (Schön, 1983; Valli, 1992; and Witherell and Noddings, 1991). Perhaps there is also a need to teach occupational therapy students and novice clinicians to become more reflective by writing diary entries after therapy sessions and providing opportunities to reflect on their therapy encounters with more experienced clinicians.

☰ CLINICIAN REASONING IN EVALUATION AND INTERVENTION WITH CLIENTS WHO HAVE COGNITIVE AND PERCEPTUAL DYSFUNCTION

There are several occupational therapy textbooks available on the theoretical aspects of evaluation and intervention with clients who have cognitive and perceptual problems (Árnadóttir, 1990; Grieve, 1993; Okkema, 1993; and Zoltan, 1996). In addition to this, a wealth of knowledge is available in neuropsychology texts concerning the nature and assessment of cognitive and perceptual problems (Leon-Carrion, 1997; Lezak, 1995; Walsh, 1994). However, theoretical information from texts and formal education cannot possibly provide us with sufficient information to examine and improve clinical practice or to develop creative solutions to problems that are not mentioned in texts (Cohen, 1991; Schön, 1988). When problems or obstacles arise in therapy, occupational therapists need to be able to reason in order to reach a solution. For example, theoretical knowledge directs us to rule out sensory problems in a client before the assessment of unilateral neglect. But what if the client has insufficient or unreliable language, making sensory testing impossible? What if the client is depressed and refuses to undergo sensory testing? How can students and novice clinicians learn to deal with these situations and the myriad of others that arise in our complex everyday practice?

It is suggested that the complex practice of evaluating and conducting interventions with clients who have cognitive and perceptual problems can be better taught to students and novice clinicians by:

1. Teaching students about clinical reasoning and using teaching strategies that enable students to integrate this knowledge into their cognitive and perceptual dysfunction coursework (Neistadt, 1996). Neistadt and Atkins (1996) suggest that it is particularly important that students learning procedurally oriented courses (e.g., cognitive and perceptual dysfunction) learn to integrate narrative reasoning concepts into their classes, fieldwork, and ultimately their practice. In these courses, scientific and procedural forms of reasoning can dominate to the extent that insufficient attention is paid to the client's experience of the disability, his priorities, and life story.
2. Exposing students to the reasoning of expert therapists through written or video case studies and clinical fieldwork. As Mattingly and Fleming's study revealed (1994), mentoring from an expert therapist is just as influential as formal education to a clinician's practice.

≡ SUMMARY

The clinical reasoning approach presented by Mattingly and Fleming (1994) is based on the assumption that a great deal of knowledge in occupational therapy is tacit; that is, more is known than can be articulated. This chapter has examined a clinical reasoning model of practice that occupational therapists can use when working with clients who have cognitive and perceptual problems.

Having worked through the chapter, the reader will have an understanding of the different kinds of clinical reasoning and how expertise and expert reasoning develop over time. Differences between novice and expert clinician reasoning were explored so students and new graduates can gain insights concerning how to speed their own journey from novice to expert. The next chapter presents an overview of the clinical reasoning used by therapists when evaluating and treating clients. The case study chapters, which make up the remainder of the book, reveal the expert reasoning of several clinicians as they evaluate and conduct interventions with clients who experience a variety of cognitive and perceptual problems.

≡ REVIEW QUESTIONS

1. What is clinical reasoning in occupational therapy?
2. Name and define the three forms of clinical reasoning identified by Mattingly and Fleming (1994).
3. Why is important for all occupational therapists to understand how expert clinicians reason in their practice?
4. Using first-person writing style, write a short narrative about one of your clinical encounters with a client. Reflect on this encounter and identify in the margins what kinds of reasoning you were using at different times during the session.
5. In the case example of Mr. D, the therapist envisioned that he would be able to return home. Imagine the situation in which Mr. D is to be discharged to a retirement home with his wife (i.e., meals and some nursing care are provided, but residents have their own rooms and are able to come and go as they please). What kind of future would you predict for him and what kind of activities would you plan for him in therapy in order to prepare for this new environment?
6. In the case example of Shelby, the therapist hopes to engage Shelby more fully in therapy by introducing her children into treatment ses-

sions. Write the interaction that may take place between the therapist, Shelby, and her children when they meet to make cookies.

☰ ACKNOWLEDGMENTS

I would like to thank Ellie Fossey for reviewing the procedural, interactive, and conditional reasoning narratives presented in this chapter. I would also like to thank my colleagues at The Boston School of Occupational Therapy, Medford, Massachusetts, for sharing their approaches to understanding and teaching clinical reasoning with me.

3

Reflections on the Process of Therapy in Cognitive and Perceptual Dysfunction

CAROLYN UNSWORTH, PHD, OTR

- Activity
- Activity Analysis
- Activity Grading
- Behavioral Goal
- Behavioral Objective
- Generalization

- Hypothesis Testing
- Motivation
- Reliability
- Standardized Assessment
- Unilateral Neglect
- Validity

On completion of the chapter, the reader will be able to:

- Outline the broad steps involved in an occupational therapy approach to working with clients who have cognitive and perceptual problems
- Describe the key characteristics of several standardized assessments used when working with clients who have cognitive and perceptual problems
- Discuss the differences between goals and objectives and outline the approach to writing behavioral goals and objectives
- Discuss the advantages and disadvantages of both remedial and adaptive approaches to therapy
- Describe how an activity can be graded
- Detail factors that need to be considered before a client's discharge
- Successfully work through the Review Questions

In Chapter 1, several of the theoretical approaches that therapists use to guide their assessments and interventions when working with clients who have cognitive and perceptual problems were explored. In Chapter 2, we examined the ways clinical reasoning can be used to better understand and improve practice and share our practice with student and novice clinicians. The purpose of this chapter is to build on the first two by globally examining the therapy process and some of the reasoning associated with practice with clients who have cognitive and perceptual problems.

≡ INTRODUCTION

This chapter is broad in scope, and the reader will need to consult more detailed texts for additional information on the therapeutic process (e.g., see Christiansen & Baum, 1997; Hopkins & Smith, 1993; Trombly, 1995). Rather than duplicate these texts, the purpose of this chapter is to draw out aspects of clinical reasoning specific to assessing and treating clients who have cognitive and perceptual problems. Therefore, the aim of this chapter is to provide the reader with an overview of the therapy process and associated reasoning before the case study chapter (Chapters 4 to 11), which present detailed assessment and treatment information and clinical reasoning related to specific cognitive and perceptual problems.

This chapter provides the reader with an overview of the usual procedures of therapy: evaluation, formation of a problem list and goals and objectives, development of an intervention strategy, and discharge planning. Although information about these procedures can be obtained in many occupational therapy texts, this chapter attempts to highlight issues the therapist should consider when working with clients who have cognitive and perceptual problems. In addition, some of the clinical reasoning associated with these processes is highlighted, and readers are encouraged to reflect on their own views to therapy and examine the reasoning that guides you as you work through this chapter.

≡ INFORMATION GATHERING AND EVALUATION

Information gathering and evaluation are the processes whereby clinicians gain an understanding of their clients' strengths and limitations, their backgrounds, and who they are as people. Whereas some of this information is gained through reviewing the medical record or conducting informal interviews, other data are collected through the administration of tests. Although *testing* refers to the measurement of a client's capacities or abilities, *evaluation* refers to the meaningful interpretation of these findings (Kaplan, 1996). The goal of evaluation is usually for the client and clinician to write a prioritized problem list and a series of long-term behavioral goals and short-term objectives that will guide treatment. It is important for therapists to identify client strengths so these can be maximized and built upon to ensure that the client achieves some success in carrying out his everyday living activities.

More specifically, therapists use some or all of the following approaches to gather information about and evaluate their clients:

- Review the client's medical chart
- Conduct an initial interview with the client (and/or his family)
- Administer standardized assessments
- Administer nonstandardized assessments, make behavioral observations, and conduct hypothesis testing using functional activities
- Conduct site visits at the client's home, workplace, or both

BOX 3–1. THERAPIST REASONING—MEDICAL CHART INFORMATION

Information from the medical chart helps me form an initial sketch in my mind of who the client is and his medical background. This sketch is only temporary, and a more complete picture will form after I actually meet the client and carry out my own evaluations. Knowledge of the client's diagnosis and details of his medical problems direct my thinking about his prognosis and possible functional problems. I look at what medication the client is taking and consider if this may make him drowsy or produce other side effects that impair performance. I draw on my knowledge of clients I have treated in the past with similar medical conditions and think about the outcomes of their therapy. I also use the information from the client's chart to plan my initial interview or first meeting with the client.

Each of these approaches, and some of the accompanying clinical reasoning, is discussed.

MEDICAL CHART REVIEW

Information relating to the client's diagnosis, results from medical tests, precautions, medical history, concomitant medical problems and medication can be gathered from the client's medical chart (Box 3–1). The chart may also reveal details related to the client's employment status, leisure interests, and educational background. More experienced therapists often consider clients they have previously treated with similar medical problems and reflect on how their therapy progressed. In the clinical reasoning literature, this is referred to as *pattern recognition*; it provides some guidance for the clinician.

INITIAL INTERVIEW WITH THE CLIENT

A therapist may use the first meeting with the client as a means of establishing rapport and gaining some initial information (Box 3–2). The therapist can confirm information contained in the medical record with the client (i.e., confirm facts and learn more about the client's recall and perceptions of events). The therapist begins informal assessment at this time through observations of the client's behavior during the interview. In addition, the therapist may explore the client's roles and habits and begin to

> ## BOX 3-2. THERAPIST REASONING—INITIAL INTERVIEW
>
> When I first meet a client, it's very important to establish rapport. I will be working closely with the client for a number of weeks, so it's important that he or she trusts me and feels comfortable. The initial meeting is really a time for information exchange. I tell the client about occupational therapy and what it can offer them, and I try to confirm information in the client's medical record and begin informal assessment. Of course, the degree to which the client may be able to participate in this initial interview varies enormously. If the client has memory problems or is experiencing posttraumatic amnesia (as commonly occurs after head injury), then I know that he won't be able to retain very much from the meeting. In most cases, I find it useful to talk with the client's relatives or family as well so I can fill in any missing information from my session with the client and get to know the family and how much support they are willing to provide.

examine values. Information about the client's typical day before his hospitalization may be gained. Speaking with relatives over the phone or in person can establish the client's previous functional abilities, type of residence and with whom he lived, and what sort of discharge placement may be possible.

STANDARDIZED ASSESSMENTS

Administering standardized assessments is an important method of information gathering for therapists. This section of the chapter reviews what standardized assessments are and describes factors that may adversely affect the results from an assessment. It also presents summaries of nine assessments widely used by therapists who work with clients who have cognitive and perceptual problems. Some of the clinical reasoning associated with assessment selection and use is provided.

What Is a Standardized Assessment?

A **standardized assessment** possesses two key features. First, a standardized assessment has a uniform procedure to administer and score the assessment. This includes a description of the set of assessment materials to be used and operational definitions for all procedures (Anastasi, 1988; de Clive-Lowe, 1996). In this way, the tester can be confident that every time the assessment is administered, it is done in the same way. This approach ensures that differences between clients' scores reflect their differing abilities, not differences in the way the assessor administered or scored the assessment. Although an assessment may provide information about how the client scores, how do these scores compare with those of other people or criteria that we expect people to meet?

There are two approaches to assist us in determining how well or how badly the client has performed. The first requires that his results be compared with the scores obtained by representative groups from the population, which are called *normative data* (i.e., a norm-referenced assessment) (de Clive-Lowe, 1996). A standardized assessment with normative data has been administered to a large group of people from the general population and from the population of people for whom the test is intended. The assessment manual details the resulting tables of normative data, which provide the distribution or spread of the scores. These norms provide information about how well the client performed when compared with a particular group of people (de Clive-Lowe, 1996; Law, 1987). The second approach involves comparing the client's scores with predetermined criteria (i.e., criterion-referenced assessment). Assessments that interpret data by reference to certain criteria have the advantage that the developer can specify the functional significance of a score (Kielhofner, 1995a). For example, if a keyboard operator must type 90 words per minute to manage his job, then if he scores only 50 after a hand injury, his score can be more easily interpreted. Therefore, the second feature of a standardized assessment is that it has some formal basis for interpreting the data (Anastasi, 1988).

However, assessments that are standardized provide more than uniform administration and scoring procedures and a formal basis for interpreting the data. The manuals of these assessments also contain information concerning their **reliability** and **validity,** which are essential for correct interpretation of results (de Clive-Lowe, 1996). There are many different forms of reliability and validity; the main kinds are described in this chapter. A *reliable assessment* is one in which the scores obtained are stable over time (i.e., test-retest), and between different examiners (i.e., inter-rater). The validity of an assessment refers to the degree to which it actually measures what it purports to measure. Several kinds of validity are discussed in the literature. These include content validity (i.e., the content of the assessment represents the domain of characteristics it purports to measure), criterion-related validity (includes predictive validity, which is the ability of the assessment to predict future performance and concurrent validity, which is agreement between results obtained on the assessment and another well-known measures of the same characteristic), and construct validity (i.e., the degree to which an assessment measures the theoretical construct and its ability to distinguish between normal and impaired or disabled subjects). For further information on the reliability and validity of assessments, the reader is referred to Anastasi (1988), Law (1987), and Kaplan (1996).

Results from standardized assessments can be communicated to other therapists who share an understanding of the client's capacities or abilities. Sometimes standardized assessments can be administered both at admission and discharge. The purpose of administering an assessment on admission may include one or more of the following: identifying the client's problem areas; establishing a baseline for treatment; providing information for treatment planning; or predicting performance in activities of daily living. Reassessment on discharge serves two purposes: (1) it assists referral agents to understand the client's capacities or abilities on discharge and (2) it serves as a point of comparison to determine the extent of improvement made by the client during therapy. This is also referred to as "measuring client outcomes" and is one way therapists can determine the effectiveness and efficiency of their therapy programs (de Clive-Lowe, 1996; Kaplan, 1996). This issue is examined at the end of the chapter.

When selecting a standardized assessment, the therapist must consider many factors. In subsequent chapters, we will examine the reasoning of experienced therapists as they determine which assessments to administer to a particular client. Some of the questions a therapist may ask to guide his selection of a standardized assessment are included in Table 3–1. Essentially, the selection of a standardized assessment depends on what the therapist wants to learn about the client and what the assessment can potentially reveal. In many cases, a single assessment will not provide all the information required by a therapist to plan treatment, so several assessments may be administered. Although this is a good idea, in order to maintain its reliability and validity, each assessment must be administered in exactly the way intended by the authors. This usually means administering the entire assessment, not just the parts that the therapist believes are relevant with a particular client. The only exception to this rule is when a test contains subtests that can be administered independently.

Therapists should be aware of their responsibilities to the client and the professional community when using standardized assessments.

> A lot of published tests look very convincing, highly objective and very straightforward to administer and score. That may be so, but the skill (and responsibility) in using such an instrument is in the clinical interpretation of results. This requires a thorough grounding in the technical aspects of test construction as well as clinical expertise. To use a test effectively, you need to understand how it has been constructed and to identify its limitations (for example, in terms of normative sampling, validation and reliability) for the particular context in which you will be using it (de Clive-Lowe, 1996, p. 362).

Table 3–1. Therapist considerations when selecting a standardized assessment

CLIENT-RELATED QUESTIONS	THERAPIST REASONING
1. Is the client ready to participate in formal assessment?	My client requires sufficient behavioral and sensory skills, such as vision and audition, to be able to engage in the assessment. I need to know that my client will be able to work with me on the assessment for the amount of time required.
2. What is the age and diagnosis of my client?	I want to choose an assessment relevant to my client, an assessment developed for a similar population, or an assessment that is not diagnosis specific.
3. What further information do I want to know about this client?	Now that I have some background information, I know some of the areas that the client is experiencing difficulty with, and I want to investigate these further. I need to choose an assessment that will provide me with more information about client performance in these areas.

ASSESSMENT-RELATED QUESTIONS	THERAPIST REASONING
1. What model guides my practice, and does it favor a remedial or adaptive orientation?	Before selecting an assessment, I need to consider the model that guides my practice and its orientation as either remedial or adaptive. The assessment I choose needs to be compatible with this approach.
2. What population was this assessment developed for?	The content domain must be suitable for my client given his or her age, diagnosis, and problems.
3. Am I qualified to use this assessment?	I need to have the necessary skills, experience, and qualifications if I am to use this assessment properly and obtain valid and reliable results.
4. Am I satisfied that I can interpret the data and that the assessment has acceptable reliability and validity?	If there is normative data, I can compare my client's results with someone from a similar background and determine if my client's skills are above or below average. Alternatively, if the assessment is criterion-referenced, I can compare the client's assessment data with functionally significant scores. I want to administer an assessment that will give me reliable and valid information so I can accurately record client status and measure the outcomes of my therapy.

(continues)

(continued)

Table 3–1. Therapist considerations when selecting a standardized assessment

ASSESSMENT-RELATED QUESTIONS	THERAPIST REASONING
5. What domains or cognitive and perceptual areas does this assessment cover? Do I want to target these domains?	If I am working from a bottom-up approach, I want to choose an assessment that contains items that will assess my client in the areas in which I hypothesize he is having difficulties. If I am working from a top-down perspective, I may not want to identify the specific cognitive and perceptual difficulties my client is having. Instead, I may want to use an assessment that identifies what functional tasks my client is having difficulties with.
6. Is the assessment sensitive to change in client status?	The scoring system used in the assessment needs to possess enough levels to detect changes in client status when they arise. If an assessment only has two scoring levels, such as "competent" and "incompetent," then I might not use this assessment if I am looking to record small improvements or deteriorations in my client's abilities.
7. Can the assessment be used before and after intervention to measure change?	I need to check the test manual to determine whether the assessment can be administered on more than one occasion, and that I can compare pre- and postintervention scores to determine whether client performance has changed.

It is necessary to have a thorough understanding of an assessment before contemplating its use. Reviews of some of the standardized assessments used in this book are described in the next section.

Factors Influencing Assessment

In addition to the client's cognitive and perceptual abilities, a variety of factors may influence assessment outcomes. It is important to minimize the effects of these factors during evaluation so that the client's best potential performance is obtained and the therapist does not erroneously attribute poor performance to cognitive or perceptual difficulties. Table 3–2 contains a list of factors that may adversely affect assessment performance and sug-

Table 3–2. Factors that may adversely affect a cognitive and perceptual assessment and ways to minimize their influence

FACTORS INFLUENCING ASSESSMENT PERFORMANCE IN AN ADVERSE WAY	THERAPIST REASONING: WAYS TO MINIMIZE THE IMPACT OF THESE FACTORS
Client may have reduced receptive and expressive communication skills	Before assessment, I find it useful to reflect on the client's receptive and expressive communication skills (and possibly discuss these with the speech-language pathologist) and determine whether the client's communication is reliable.
Client may have sensory disturbances	If I conduct a sensory assessment, I can establish if the client has sufficient sensory abilities to proceed with the cognitive/perceptual assessment (this includes visual screening as well as tactile sensory testing).
Client may tire easily	I consider when the client will be well-rested (possibly in the morning) and administer the assessment at that time.
Client may be emotionally unsettled	I avoid conducting assessments when the client is emotionally distressed.
Client may be taking medication	Before assessment, I establish what medications the client is taking and consider how side effects may affect performance.
Client may have problems with motor, postural, or balance skills	During assessment, I try to ensure the client's postural stability and monitor motor abilities.

gestions of ways to minimize these problems. The presence of these factors may threaten both the validity and reliability of a standardized assessment.

Review of Standardized Assessments

The following review details nine assessments commonly used by occupational therapists when working with clients who have cognitive and perceptual problems. These assessments are reviewed here because there are very few other sources that provide a global summary of all these assessments and their features. Several of these assessments are discussed in more detail in the case study chapters of the book. Therapist reasoning associated with the selection, use, and interpretation of results using these standardized assessments is presented in the case study chapters. Whereas some of these assessments target identification of specific cognitive or perceptual impairments (i.e., a "bottom-up" approach), others are designed to assess an individual's disabilities (i.e., a "top-down" approach) that may be caused by cognitive or perceptual impairments. In some of these assessments (e.g., see AMPS [Assessment of Motor and Process Skills]), no attempt is made to identify the underlying cognitive and perceptual impairments. Although a few of these assessments use daily living contexts or tasks (e.g., see SOTOF [Structured Observational Test Of Function], AMPS, and A-ONE [Árnadóttir Occupational Therapy Neurobehavioral Evaluation]), the majority of the assessments reported rely on specific tabletop activities and pen and paper tasks. For reviews of other standardized assessments of cognitive and perceptual capacities, the reader is referred to Lezak (1995), Zoltan (1996), and Okkema (1993). A summary of the key features of the nine assessments reviewed below is presented in Table 3–3.

1. The Árnadóttir Occupational Therapy Neurobehavioral Evaluation (A-ONE) (Árnadóttir, 1990)

The A-ONE was developed by Árnadóttir for occupational therapists to measure their clients' neurobehavior through five daily living tasks: dressing, grooming and hygiene, transfer and mobility, feeding, and communication. A manual (Árnadóttir, 1990) and scoring forms are used to guide the assessment. No other special equipment is required. The assessment consists of two parts. The first part includes the Functional Independence Scale, which is scored with the Neurobehavioral Specific Impairment Subscale, and the Neurobehavioral Pervasive Impairment Subscale. The Functional Independence Scale measures the client's level of independence in activities of daily living (ADLs) on a four-point scale from 0 (unable to perform) to 4 (independent for the domains of feeding, dressing, grooming and hygiene, transfers and mobility, and communication). The Neurobehavioral Specific Impairment Subscale is used to rate the severity of any impairments noted during the five ADLs (including communication activities) and is scored from 4 (unable to perform due to neurobehavioral impairment) to 0 (no neurobehavioral impairments observed). The Neurobehavioral Pervasive Impairment Subscale examines for the presence (scored as 1) or the absence (scored as 0) of a range of impairments noted during any ADL. This part of the assessment is completed on the Neurobehavioral Scale Summary score sheet and is optional. Part II of the assessment guides clinicians to list the client's impairments and then use the chart and processing figures in the manual to identify associated sites of disrupted neuronal processing. In this way, the problems the client experi-

Table 3–3. Summary of standardized assessments

ASSESSMENT	AUTHORS	DEVELOPED FOR OR BY OCCUPATIONAL THERAPISTS	USED WITH REMEDIAL, ADAPTIVE, OR BOTH APPROACHES	TRAINING COURSE REQUIRED	USES ADL	IS PARTIAL ADMINI- STRATION RECOM- MENDED	NORM OR CRITERION REFER- ENCED
A-ONE	Árnadóttir, 1990	Yes	Remedial (both)	Yes	Yes	Yes	Yes
SOTOF	Laver & Powell, 1995	Yes	Remedial (both)	No	Yes	No	Yes
AMPS	Fisher, 1997a	Yes	Adaptive (both)	Yes	Yes	No	Yes
ACL	Allen, 1990	Yes	Adaptive	No	Yes	No	Partial
COTNAB	Tyerman et al., 1986	Yes	Remedial (both)	No	No	No	Yes
RPAB	Whiting et al., 1985	Yes	Remedial (both)	No	No	No	Yes
BIT	Wilson, Cock- burn, & Halligan, 1987a	Yes	Remedial (both)	No	No	Yes	Yes
LOTCA	Itzkovich et al., 1990	Yes	Remedial (both)	No	No	No	Yes
RBMT	Wilson, Cock- burn, & Badde- ley, 1991	Yes	Remedial (both)	No	No	No	Yes

EVIDENCE OF TEST-RETEST RELIABILITY	EVIDENCE OF INTER-RATER RELIABILITY	EVIDENCE OF CONTENT VALIDITY	EVIDENCE OF CRITERION VALIDITY	EVIDENCE OF CONSTRUCT VALIDITY	TIME TO ADMINISTER (MIN)	APPROXIMATE COSTS
Preliminary data	Yes	Yes	No	Yes	30–40	The book and 20 scoring forms are $50. The 5-day training course and certification are $500.
Yes	Yes	Yes	Yes	Preliminary data	45	Manuals and a set of 20 scoring forms are $110. Further packs of scoring forms are $50.
Yes	Yes	Yes	Yes	Yes	30–60	AMPS manual, computer software, 5-day training course, and calibration cost $650.
Yes	Yes	Preliminary data	Yes	Preliminary data	20	Cost of the lacing kit $10.
No	Preliminary data	No	No	Preliminary data	60–80	Test kit and set of four manuals $2000
Yes	Yes	Yes	Yes	Yes	60	Test kit is $1400. 25 score sheets cost $36.
Yes	Yes	Preliminary data	Yes	No	60	Test kit, manual, and score sheets cost $360.
No	Yes	Yes	Yes	Yes	30–45	Test kit costs $400.
Yes	Yes	Yes	Yes	Yes	30	Test kit costs $290; revised manual costs $30; 25 score sheets cost $30.

ences are related to specific brain regions. The assessment manual contains detailed instructions to guide scoring, and the assessment forms provide room for related comments and spaces for summaries.

Although A-ONE courses have been taught around the world, the main English publication supporting the use of this assessment is Árnadóttir's book (1990). However, the A-ONE and the Behavioral Inattention Test (presented in detail below) have been recommended as the two tools most suitable to measure perceptual and body image dysfunction (Rubio & Van Deusen, 1995). Árnadóttir (1990) cites a few studies supporting the reliability and validity of the tool. For example, content validity was achieved through literature review and canvassing expert opinion. Concurrent validity was established by comparing the average scores from 50 clients with stroke with those of 79 normal subjects. Scores on the A-ONE were found to discriminate between persons with and without brain dysfunction. Inter-rater reliability (using Kappa) between four therapists rating 20 clients was reported to be K = 0.84. A pilot study of test-retest reliability has been performed showing agreement (using Spearman rank-order correlation coefficient) of 0.85 or higher. Very few studies have been published in journals to support the reliability, validity, or use of this tool in practice. Data supporting the use of this tool with a variety of clients in a variety of settings are urgently required. Therapists who wish to administer the A-ONE to their clients are required to undertake a 5-day training course and certification examination.

How to obtain this assessment. Árnadóttir's book (1990) details the assessment. Further information can be obtained from A. Arnason, PO Box 3171, 123 Reykjavik, Iceland.

2. The Structured Observational Test Of Function (SOTOF) (Laver & Powell, 1995)

The SOTOF was designed for occupational therapists to assess older persons' level of occupational performance and neuropsychological functioning after neurological damage of cortical origin (Laver, 1994a). The assessment provides therapists with information on four levels of function: occupational performance, performance components, behavioral skill components, and neuropsychological deficits (Laver, 1994a). The assessment requires the therapist to administer a screening assessment, complete a neuropsychological checklist, and complete four ADL scales with the client. The ADL scales are eating from a bowl, pouring a drink and drinking, putting on an upper body garment, and washing and drying the hands. After analyzing observational data, neuropsychological deficits are extrapolated and recorded on the assessment forms (Laver & Powell, 1995).

The content validity of the SOTOF was established through peer and expert review with 44 occupational therapists. Face validity was established using three sample groups of occupational therapists and students. Survey results indicated that the tool was relevant for the client group for whom it was designed and measured dysfunction in occupational performance and specific neuropsychological deficits. Therapists also reported the test to be easy to use, carry, and clean and quick to administer (Laver, 1994a). To examine criterion-related validity, the performance of a sample of 22 clients with stroke on the SOTOF was compared with their performance on the Rivermead Perceptual Assessment Battery and the Chessington Occupational Therapy Neurological Assessment Battery (both described below), as well as the Middlesex Elderly Assessment of Mental State (Golding, 1989). All assessments were found to reflect a similar level of dysfunction as identified through the use of the SOTOF.

The SOTOF is reported to have acceptable test-retest, inter-rater, and internal consistency reliability as demonstrated through studies with 32 occupational therapists and 37 clients. The average test-retest reliability for the screening assessment was reported to be $K = 0.92$, and inter-rater reliability was found to be an average of $K = 0.94$. The average test-retest reliability for the four ADL scales was found to be between $K = 0.37$ and 0.67, and the average inter-rater reliability was found to be between $K = 0.50$ and 0.77. Average test-retest reliability for the neuropsychological checklist was reported to be $K = 0.55$, and average inter-rater reliability was found to be $K = 0.54$. Kappa statistics could not be calculated for all variables because of the lack of variability in the data; therefore, percent agreement was also calculated for all items. Normative data are available for the SOTOF for clients aged between 60 and 97 years (Laver, 1994a).

How to obtain this assessment. Marketing Services Department NFER-Nelson Publishing Company Ltd., Darville House, 2 Oxford Road East, Windsor, Berkshire SL4 1DF, UK. Phone: 01753-858961. Or obtain through: Western Psychological Services, 12031 Wilshire Boulevard, Los Angeles, CA 90025. Phone: 1-800-648-8857.

3. The Assessment of Motor and Process Skills (AMPS) (Fisher, 1997a)

The AMPS (1997a), developed by Fisher, is a structured, observational evaluation of clients' performances of ADLs. This assessment can be administered to persons over 3 years of age regardless of diagnosis. The assessment examines clients' functional competence in two or three familiar personal or instrumental ADLs of their choice. Hence, the assessment is client-centered. Examples of possible assessment tasks (there are over 60 of these) include meal preparation, re-potting a plant, making a bed, getting dressed, or folding laundry. The ADLs selected should reflect the client's interests and present an appropriate challenge.

When using AMPS, the therapist observes the client's performance and then rates the quality of this performance in terms of how effortless, efficient, safe, or independent the person's ADL motor and ADL process skills are in the context of the task performance (i.e., the dynamic interaction of the person with the environment). ADL motor skills are observable actions related to moving the body or the task objects to complete the assessment task (Fisher, 1997a). Examples of ADL motor skills assessed by the AMPS include Reaches, Manipulates, Lifts, and Endures. ADL process skills refer to the ". . . observable actions of performance that reflect the person's ability to logically sequence the actions of the ADL task performance over time, select and use appropriate tools and materials, and adapt his or her performance when problems are encountered" (Fisher, 1997a, p. 4). Examples of ADL process skills assessed by the AMPS include Initiates, Chooses, Gathers, and Accommodates. Each action is a goal-directed unit (e.g., reaches for the glass, gathers the juice to the table) of the total task performance.

The client is scored in relation to 16 motor and 20 process skills for each of the two or three ADL tasks performed. The scoring is criterion-referenced on a scale of 1 (deficit) to 4 (competent). A score of 4 is given if the quality of performance of that skill item is competent; a score of 3 is given if the quality of performance of the skill is questionable; a score of 2 is given if the quality of performance of that skill item is ineffective so that it disrupts or interferes with task progression; and a score of 1 is given if the quality of performance of the skill is so deficient that it stops the task performance, brings about imminent danger to the person or damage to the task objects, or results in a need for assistance. The client's final ADL motor and ADL process ability measures take into account the degree of task difficulty. Many-faceted Rasch analysis has led to the development of ADL motor and ADL process scales of ability that consider skill item difficulty, task challenge, and rater severity (Fisher, 1993, 1997a, 1997b).

Advantages of this assessment are that the client is engaged in assessment tasks that are familiar, culturally relevant, and that he or she chooses. AMPS is a practical, life-relevant assessment that can be undertaken without special equipment in the client's residence or other relevant setting such as the occupational therapy clinic (Fisher, 1997a). Therapists are required to undergo a 5-day training course and to become a calibrated (i.e., reliable) AMPS rater to use this assessment. The AMPS is reported to be both a reliable and valid assessment (Fisher, 1997a). A number of articles have been published examining the reliability and validity of the AMPS across cultures (Bernspång & Fisher, 1995b; Dickerson & Fisher, 1995; Fisher et al., 1992; Goldman & Fisher, 1997; Goto, Fisher, & Mayberry, 1996; Magalhães et al., 1996), across genders (Duran & Fisher, 1996), across age groups (Dickerson & Fisher, 1993, 1997), with a variety of diagnoses (Bernspång & Fisher, 1995a; Doble et al., 1994; Doble et al., 1997; Kottorp et al., 1995; Pan & Fisher, 1994), between clinic and home environments (Nygård et al., 1994; Park, Fisher, & Velozo, 1994; Darragh, Sample, & Fisher, in press) and as a sensitive outcome measure (Oakley & Sunderland, 1997).

Unlike most of the assessments reviewed in this chapter, the AMPS is not a test of impairments nor was it designed to identify the specific cognitive or perceptual impairments that limit ADL performance. Rather, AMPS is a test of disability and focuses on clients' ADL skills; however, this does not mean that AMPS cannot be used with persons who have cognitive and perceptual problems. The therapist needs to be clear about the information they will gain from the assessment. When assessing a client using AMPS, the therapist gains knowledge about how effortlessly, efficiently, safely, and independently the client compiles the ADL motor and ADL process actions that comprise the task performance and whether or not the person has ineffective overall ADL task performance. On the other hand, when using an assessment such as the Chessington Occupational Therapy Neurological Assessment Battery (COTNAB) (Tyerman et al., 1986) or Rivermead Perceptual Assessment Battery (RPAB) (Whiting et al., 1985), the therapist is assessing at the level of impairment and gains information about the client's cognitive or perceptual capacities.

The AMPS is an assessment of the quality of a person's ADL performance; it is not a neuropsychological assessment. The AMPS is appropriate for use in top-down occupational therapy assessment to more clearly define specific strengths and problems with ADL task performance. Cognitive and perceptual tests may then be given to clarify the specific reason for the problem.

In summary, the AMPS provides clinicians with an opportunity to assess clients based on their occupational performances and identify ADL performance skill deficits. The assessment provides therapists with clinically useful information concerning the problems a client has with an occupation and the level of complexity of ADL tasks that the client is able to perform (Fisher, 1997a).

How to obtain this assessment. More information can be obtained by writing to AMPS Project, Occupational Therapy Building, Colorado State University, Fort Collins, CO 80523.

4. Allen Cognitive Level Test (ACL) (Allen, 1990)

The ACL is frequently used as a screening tool to estimate a person's cognitive level (Allen, 1992). The *cognitive levels* are described as ". . . a functional classification system, hierarchically arranged with the levels representing increasing ability to attend to and use the available task environment" (Mayer, 1988, p. 177). However, the ACL is most appropriate for use with clients who are thought to be functioning at level 3 (manual actions), 4 (goal-directed actions), or 5 (exploratory actions) on Allen's six-level scale of cognitive function (Allen, Earhardt, & Blue, 1992). Although originally developed for use with clients who have psychiatric problems, this assessment is also used with people who have acquired brain damage or experience a dementing illness such as Alzheimer's disease. After an interview to gain information concerning the client's educational and work background, the client is observed performing the visuomotor task of leather lacing. It is assumed that the client's cognitive functioning is reflected through their motor actions.

The assessment has been in use since 1973, and five versions have been trialed and reported: (1) the ACL-Original (Allen, 1982, 1985); (2) the ACL-Expanded (Earhart & Allen, 1992); (3) the ACL-Problem Solving (Josman & Katz, 1991); (4) the ACL-Large (Allen, Kehrberg, & Burns, 1992; Kehrberg, 1993); and (5) the ACL-90 (Allen, 1990, 1992).

The ACL-90 test kit contains leather laces, needles, and pieces of prepunched leather to be laced together. The assessment consists of asking the client to do three different leather lacing stitches in order of complexity: a running stitch, whip stitch, and single cordovan. First the task is demonstrated, and then the client is asked to attempt the lacing task. The client is scored according to the stitch undertaken, his accuracy, and his ability to correct mistakes. Detailed instructions for administration and scoring are provided by Allen, Earhardt, and Blue (1992). Allen (1992) reports that assessment findings assist to identify the client's ability to perform actions, indicate the client's readiness for discharge, suggest the level of assistance the client will require on discharge, and indicate cautions and warnings concerning the client's safety.

Reliability and validity information for several versions of the ACL are presented in Allen, Earhardt, & Blue (1992). In summary, the test is reported to be both reliable and valid. Inter-rater reliability studies have demonstrated good to excellent reliability with Pearson's r (r = 0.75 to 0.99). A variety of validity studies have been conducted to demonstrate concurrent and predictive validity (Katz & Heimann, 1990). Josman and Katz (1991) reported a study comparing the performance of normal subjects and those with mental illness using the ACL-Problem Solving. This study provides some normative data and preliminary evidence of construct validity. The tool can be used with people who have impairments that sometimes limit assessment opportunities. For example, Allen claims that if the client is deaf or has difficulty understanding the instructions, pantomiming the instructions is possible. It is difficult to administer this assessment to clients with visual impairments. However, the large version (the ACL-Large) (Allen,

Kehrberg, & Burns, 1992) assists some clients in overcoming visual deficits. Clients who cannot use their hands may be given a verbal form of the assessment. When administering the test using modified instructions, Allen notes that the therapist must be more cautious in interpreting the results (Allen, Earhardt, & Blue, 1992).

As described in Chapter 1, the Cognitive Disabilities Model incorporates the use of several assessments. Although the ACL was reviewed here in detail, it is interesting to note the other assessments used with this model. These include the Routine Task Inventory (RTI); the Lower Cognitive Levels test (LCL), which was specifically designed to assess clients functioning at levels 1, 2, or 3; and the Cognitive Performance Test (CPT), which was developed for use with clients who have Alzheimer's disease (Allen, Kehrberg, & Burns, 1992). In particular, the CPT is becoming popular with therapists who work with a variety of clients who have cognitive and perceptual deficits. This assessment uses ADL-based tasks (labeled "Dress," "Toast," "Shop," "Telephone," "Travel," and "Wash") to determine a client's functional level. Administration procedures, reliability and validity data, and scoring forms for the CPT, and all the assessments used with the Cognitive Disabilities Model, are provided by Allen, Kehrberg, and Burns (1992).

How to obtain this assessment. Allen, Earhardt, & Blue's book (1992) details the assessment. The ACL lacing test kit (item number HC98) can be obtained from: S & S Arts and Crafts, PO Box 513, Colchester, CT 06415-9232. Phone: 1-800-243-9232.

5. Chessington Occupational Therapy Neurological Assessment Battery (COTNAB) (Tyerman et al., 1986)

The COTNAB was designed to assess cognitive and perceptual deficits in clients age 16 years and older after stroke or head injury. The authors claim that the assessment aims to identify areas of functional difficulty and guide treatment planning (Tyerman et al., 1986). The battery consists of 12 tests divided into four sections assessing visual perception, constructional ability, sensory-motor ability, and ability to follow instructions. The assessment is contained in a large wooden box on wheels with all equipment included. Four manuals are also included: the introductory manual containing information on assessment development, normative data, patterns of functional impairment in head-injured clients, and sample scoring forms; two files providing comprehensive descriptions of each assessment and how it should be administered and scored; and a detailed treatment resource file. Because of the time required to complete the whole assessment, the authors suggest that it can be administered over more than one session.

An overall performance score (graded from 0 [unable or unwilling to attempt] to 5 [normal limits]) is generated from scores for each COTNAB item in relation to the client's ability to complete the task and the time taken. Ability to complete the task usually represents the number of items correctly completed. Clients' scores can be compared with the normative data. Originally, normative data were collected from 150 persons (75 men and 75 women) in three age groups from 16 to 65 years (Tyerman et al., 1986). More recently, Laver and Huchison (1994) collected normative data from 47 clients aged 65 to 87 years. In another study with an older population, Stanley et al. (1995) compared the scores of normal subjects aged 50 to 65 years with scores of those aged 66 years and older. Differences were found between these two groups, and normative data for persons aged 66 years and older were provided.

Although the COTNAB manual reports that this assessment is both reliable and valid, no information is provided to support this claim. In addition, a journal search revealed no refereed articles supporting the psychometric properties of this assessment. A study by Sloan et al. (1991) compared the use of the Rivermead Perceptual Assessment Battery and the COTNAB with 16 clients after head injury. These authors concluded that although the COTNAB took considerably longer to administer, the results of the assessment were clinically very useful. Although the results of this study infer that COTNAB possesses criterion-related validity, further empirical studies are required to support the use of this assessment.

How to obtain this assessment. Nottingham Rehab Limited, 17 Ludlow Hill Road, West Bridgford, Nottingham NG2 6HD, UK. Phone: +44 602 452345.

6. Rivermead Perceptual Assessment Battery (RPAB) (Whiting et al., 1985)

The RPAB was designed for occupational therapists to assess visual perceptual deficits in clients after head injury or stroke and is suitable to administer to clients aged 16 years and older. Although the majority of test instructions are visual, English language skills are required to understand the initial instructions, which are provided verbally. All materials required for the assessment are contained in the test kit, and therapists do not require special training to use this evaluation. The RPAB is a battery consisting of 16 performance tests that assess form constancy, color constancy, sequencing, object completion, figure ground discrimination, body image, inattention, and spatial awareness. Clients are asked to perform a variety of tasks that assess these capacities. The majority of tasks are to be performed within 3 minutes. Scoring is based on accuracy of task completion and the time taken to complete each task. The test can be completed in approximately 1 hour. However, if the client is fatigued, the RPAB can be administered over two sessions.

In order to interpret the results, the therapist must have an estimation of the client's premorbid intelligence. A study of 69 normal subjects indicated that although age was not found to be correlated with performance on the RPAB, intelligence was correlated with performance on 11 of the 16 RPAB tests. Normative data have been divided into the three broad categories of above average, average, and below average intelligence. Therapists need to establish the premorbid intelligence of their clients in order to compare client results with test norms. The authors suggest using the Mill Hill Vocabulary Scale Synonyms test to estimate the client's premorbid intelligence (Cockburn et al., 1983; Whiting et al., 1985). Clients who score below the expected level for their estimated premorbid intelligence on three or more of the subtests are considered to be experiencing perceptual problems.

Test-retest reliability was established using a sample of 19 clients with stroke who were assessed 1 year after discharge. The clients were assessed on two occasions 4 weeks apart. Eleven of the 16 items were found to have a test-retest reliability of $\rho = 0.67$ or over using the Spearman rank-order correlation coefficient. Lack of variation in the scores for two subtests prohibited reliability calculations for these items. The three other items were revised and retested and are reported to be reliable. Inter-rater reliability was established with three therapists each rating video recordings of RPAB administration with six clients. Kendall coefficients of concordance for agreement between the raters ranged from 0.83 to 1.00 (Whiting et al., 1985; Bhavnani et al., 1983). Concurrent validity was established by comparing the scores of 57 clients on the RPAB with 11 other assessments of perception. Most of the RPAB tests correlated well with the 11 assessments known to be good measures of visual perception. Scores on the RPAB from persons with and without brain damage were compared and it was found the assessment did discriminate between these two groups. After these studies, the authors reported the RPAB to be both reliable and valid (Whiting et al., 1985).

A comprehensive manual is provided with the kit detailing instructions on administration, scoring and score interpretation, information on the reliability and validity studies conducted, and the normative data collected from a population of 69 subjects aged 16 to 69 years. The manual also provides a series of case studies that assist therapists in interpreting test results and develop treatment suggestions. For further information on the RPAB, the reader is also referred to Jesshope, Clarke, and Smith (1991); Matthey, Donnelly, and Hextell (1993); and Sloan et al. (1991). A shortened version of the RPAB is available and takes approximately 35 minutes to administer (Lincoln & Edmans, 1989).

How to obtain this assessment. Published by NFER-Nelson Publishing Company Ltd., Darville House, 2 Oxford Road East, Windsor, Berkshire SL4 1DF, UK. Phone: 01753-858961. Or obtain through: Western Psychological Services, 12031 Wilshire Boulevard, Los Angeles, CA 90025. Phone: 1-800-648-8857.

7. The Behavioural Inattention Test (BIT) (Wilson, Cockburn, & Halligan, 1987a)

The authors state that the BIT was developed to assess clients for the presence of unilateral visual neglect and to provide the therapist with information concerning how the neglect impacts upon the client's ability to perform everyday occupations (Wilson, Cockburn, & Halligan, 1987b). In this book, unilateral visual neglect is referred to as *unilateral neglect* (visual modality) and is discussed in more detail in Chapter 9. However, in summary, unilateral neglect may be defined as the failure to attend to a hemi-space or the body on the side contralateral to the lesion, despite intact sensory abilities. This standardized assessment incorporates many test items that have been used in the past in a nonstandardized way to examine for the presence of neglect (Wilson, Cockburn, & Halligan, 1987b).

The BIT consists of nine activity-based subtests (picture scanning, menu reading, map navigation, address and sentence copying, card sorting, article reading, telephone dialing, coin sorting, and telling and setting the time) and six pen and paper subtests (line crossing, star cancellation, letter cancellation, figure and shape copying, and line bisection) (Wilson, Cockburn, & Halligan, 1987). The authors report that the assessment is both reliable and valid. According to the BIT manual, the validity of the assessment was established in two ways. Initially the BIT scores of 80 clients were compared with their scores on other assessments of neglect (not reported in the manual) yielding a correlation of $r = 0.92$. A comparison was then drawn between client scores and therapist responses to a short questionnaire, again drawing a high correlation of $r = 0.67$ (again, methodology was not thoroughly reported in the manual). The BIT manual reported that inter-rater reliability was established by having two raters score 13 subjects (Wilson, Cockburn, & Halligan, 1987a). The correlation between assessors was reported to be $r = 0.99$. Test re-test reliability was established by assessing 10 subjects on two occasions, 15 days apart. The two administrations of the test yielded a correlation of $r = 0.99$. Cermak and Hausser (1989) offer a critical review of this assessment and suggest that more research is required to establish its reliability and validity. Clear instructions are provided in the manual for both assessment administration and interpretation of results. Normative data (based on a sample of 50 subjects) are also provided in the manual (Wilson, Cockburn, & Halligan, 1987a).

How to obtain this assessment. Thames Valley Test Company, 7–9 The Green, Flempton, Bury St. Edmunds, Suffolk IP28 6EL, England. Phone: +44 128 472 8608. Fax: +44 128 472 8166.

8. Loewenstein Occupational Therapy Cognitive Assessment (LOTCA) (Itzkovich et al., 1990)

The LOTCA was developed at the Loewenstein Rehabilitation Center in Israel in 1974 for use with people who have experienced a stroke, traumatic brain injury, or tumor. The purpose of the tool is to measure the basic cognitive functions that are prerequisites for managing everyday living tasks (Itzkovich et al., 1990). The test was developed for use by occupational therapists and does not require specialized training. The assessment consists of 20 subtests in four areas: orientation, visual and spatial perception, visuomotor organization, and thinking operations. The majority of items are scored from 1 (low ability) to 4 (high ability). A scoring sheet is used to document client performance on each subtest. Detailed instructions are provided for administration, including administration to clients with expressive language deficits.

The reliability and validity data for this assessment was published by Katz et al. in 1989. Construct validity was demonstrated through the use of exploratory factor analysis, which showed that a three-factor solution explained 60% of the variance associated with performance. Internal consistency reliability was demonstrated through alpha coefficients of 0.87 for perception, 0.95 for visuomotor organization, and 0.85 for thinking operations. Inter-rater reliability was reported to range between $r = 0.82$ and 0.97 for the 20 subtests. Concurrent validity was demonstrated when all subtests differentiated at the 0.0001 level of significance between the control group and a client sample (Katz et al., 1989). Therefore, the tool is able to distinguish between persons with and without brain damage. Criterion validity was established by comparing LOTCA scores with those obtained on the Weschler Adult Intelligence Scale with a correlation of $r = 0.68$. Normative data are also available. In summary, this tool is used throughout the world, and several studies have been published to support the use of this assessment battery with clients who have had a head injury and stroke (Cermak et al., 1995; Katz, Hefner, & Reuben, 1990).

How to obtain this assessment. Further information: Professor Noomi Katz, School of Occupational Therapy, Hebrew University, Mount Scopus, PO Box 24026, Jerusalem 91240, Israel. The assessment can be purchased through Sammons or Smith & Rolyan Catalogues.

9. Rivermead Behavioural Memory Test (RBMT) (Wilson, Cockburn, & Baddeley 1991)

The RBMT was developed in 1985 and revised in 1991 at the Rivermead Rehabilitation Center in Oxford, England. The battery was designed to assess a person's everyday memory abilities. This assessment offers the therapist an initial evaluation of the client's memory function, an indication of appropriate areas for treatment, and enables the therapist to monitor memory skills throughout the treatment program. The assessment has four versions so that the test can be re-administered to the same client without practice effects' biasing results. The assessment contains 11 categories with nine subtests. Each subtest presents a series of items that the client is required to memorize and recall later in the assessment. Test results can be interpreted in one of two ways. The first interpretation is used as a screening method. Clients' raw scores are totaled, and the client can be considered to pass or fail the assessment. The second interpretation requires the results for each subtest to be standardized, and a standardized profile score is recorded. Standardized scores of 0 to 9 may be interpreted to mean that the client has severely impaired memory; scores of 10 to 16 indicate moderately impaired memory; scores of 17 to 21 indicate poor memory; and scores of 22 to 24 are considered normal. The RBMT can be administered in approximately 30 minutes without specialized training by occupational therapists, speech-language pathologists and psychologists.

Face validity was measured by asking therapists to complete a 19-item memory checklist for a sample of clients. Results were correlated with subtests in the RBMT, with significant positive correlations. Construct validity was demonstrated when control subjects received considerably higher scores on the RBMT than the client group did. Concurrent validity was established by comparing client RBMT scores with scores on other memory assessments such as Corsi Blocks (Milner, 1971) and the Recognition Memory Test (Warrington, 1984). Correlations ranged from 0.2 to 0.63, revealing an acceptable overall correlation (Wilson, Cockburn, & Baddely, 1991).

Studies have demonstrated both parallel-form, test re-test, and inter-rater reliability. Although only small numbers of clinicians have participated in these reliability studies, excellent results have been achieved. For example two raters simultaneously scored 40 clients with 100% agreement. To establish parallel-form reliability, two randomly chosen versions of the assessment were administered to 118 subjects. The average correlation between the assessments was $r = 0.77$ for the screening score and $r = 0.86$ for the standardized score. Test re-test reliability was established at $r = 0.78$ for the screening score and $r = 0.85$ for the standardized profile score (Wilson, Cockburn, & Baddely, 1991; Wilson et al., 1989).

Limitations associated with this assessment include lack of differentiation between short- and long-term memory and the artificial nature of having to recall a lengthy list of items without contextual cues (as occurs in normal situations). It is also suggested that subtests such as orientation, route, date, and faces should not be administered to clients with perceptual problems. In summary, the RBMT is a quick and reliable assessment of a client's everyday memory abilities, including recall of directions, appointments, names, and faces. For further reading on the RBMT, the reader is referred to Cockburn, Wilson, and Baddeley (1991) and Malec, Zweber, and DePompolo (1990).

How to obtain this assessment. Thames Valley Test Company, 7–9 The Green, Flempton, Bury St. Edmunds, Suffolk IP28 6EL, England. Phone: +44 128 472 8608. Fax: +44 128 472 8166.

NONSTANDARDIZED ASSESSMENTS, BEHAVIORAL OBSERVATIONS, AND HYPOTHESIS TESTING USING FUNCTIONAL ACTIVITIES

Nonstandardized assessments do not have a uniform procedure for administration and scoring, operational definitions, a formal approach to interpret data, or known reliability or validity. Nonstandardized assessments cannot be relied on to accurately measure change in client performance over time or determine the effectiveness of a therapy program. However, they may still provide clinicians with useful information and supplement the information gained through standardized assessment (Box 3–3). Occupational therapists often want to gather information about both the partic-

---

BOX 3–3. THERAPIST REASONING—NONSTANDARDIZED ASSESSMENTS

Sometimes I find I can't gather all the information I need about how the client is managing using standardized assessments alone. Although I know I need to administer some standardized assessments so I can monitor change in my clients' performance, I still use some nonstandardized assessments, which provide supplementary information about the client's performance. These assessments are usually quicker to administer than the standardized ones. With these assessments, I find I am relying much more on my professional judgment to evaluate findings. For more inexperienced therapists, I usually recommend sticking with administering a complete standardized assessment or using the structured approach to hypothesis testing (outlined in text).

ular problems the client is experiencing and how these problems impact on the client's occupational performance. Because there are few assessments that specifically address how problems impact on the clients' occupational performance, the therapist may choose to use a nonstandardized assessment or checklist, observe the client's behavior during an activity, or use a hypothesis-testing approach to gather more information about the nature of the client's problems. Findings from these nonstandardized approaches to assessment must be interpreted with caution.

Tabletop Assessments and Checklists

When using a bottom-up approach to assessment, a variety of nonstandardized tabletop assessments can be used to examine for the presence of particular cognitive or perceptual problems. For example, in the assessment of **unilateral neglect,** occupational therapists have been using nonstandardized assessments such as the Draw-A-Clock test, Crossing-out Letters test, Human Figure or Face test, and the Alternating Simultaneous Stimuli test for a number of years. Several of these tests have now been standardized for use as part of BIT (Wilson, Cockburn, & Halligan, 1987a). Other nonstandardized assessments that clinicians may use include the Solet Test of Apraxia (Solet, 1974); item-recognition tests to assess for visual object agnosia; stereognosis tests, in which a client's vision is occluded and he is asked to identify objects; or the Self-Awareness Questionnaire (Gasquoine & Gibbons, 1994), which assists a therapist to determine a client's level of understanding of their problems. Although there are very little empirical data to support the use of any of these assessments, they are often clinically useful and are quick and easy to administer. Chapters 4 to 11 will alert the reader to the use of any nonstandardized assessments and discuss their use.

Hypothesis-testing Approach to Evaluation

Another nonstandardized approach to evaluation involves the use of **hypothesis testing.** The hypothesis-testing approach has been taught to students for several years at The School of Occupational Therapy, La Trobe University, Australia. A number of staff members in the school, including this author, have contributed to its development. Although this approach has many similarities to the four-stage model of problem solving outlined by Elstein, Shulman, and Sprafka (1978) and described in Fleming (1994b), the hypothesis-testing approach outlined here tests each hypothesis by manipulating variables and observing change in client performance. The hypothesis-testing approach described here has similarities to the dynamic interaction approach to assessment developed by Toglia (1989). In both of these assessment procedures, the therapist selects a functional activity to undertake with the client and proposes a hypothesis, which is then tested. Although the hypothesis-testing approach cannot replace standardized assessments, it remains useful for therapists who are not trained to use assessments such as the A-ONE or AMPS and for students and less-experienced therapists to use in conjunction with other standardized assessments. The aim of the hypothesis-testing approach is to obtain:

1. A detailed knowledge of the impact of the problem on the client's performance in daily living activities
2. An understanding of the variables (client, task, and environment) that impact on client performance
3. A knowledge of the type of therapeutic input and structure (i.e., therapist variables) that facilitate client performance
4. Information for the therapist to use to determine which cognitive or perceptual problems are impeding performance in daily living activities

A summary of the stages in the hypothesis-testing approach are provided in Figure 3–1. Each of the stages is described below.

1. Client Observations and Identification of Problem Areas
In the first stage in the procedure, the therapist develops a functional description of the client's problem. For example, in the first few days after the client's admission, the therapist observes that the client seems unable to adopt the dressing technique used each morning. The therapist documents this problem.

2. Analysis of Client Strengths and Weaknesses
The therapist considers all the information gathered to date. In addition to the problem areas that are being revealed, the therapist considers the client's strengths. Client strengths are important because they can be used in the treatment program to **motivate** the client, as a building block to regain lost abilities, or to compensate for lost abilities.

3. Hypothesis Formation
At this point, a single hypothesis (or multiple hypotheses) is generated. Hypotheses are plausible explanations for the client's problem. For example, the therapist might hypothesize that the client was unable to use the new dressing technique because:

1. He was unable to *remember* and therefore unable to *learn* the steps in this dressing technique, or
2. He was *impulsive* in his actions and disregarded the steps in the procedure.

HYPOTHESIS TESTING SUMMARY

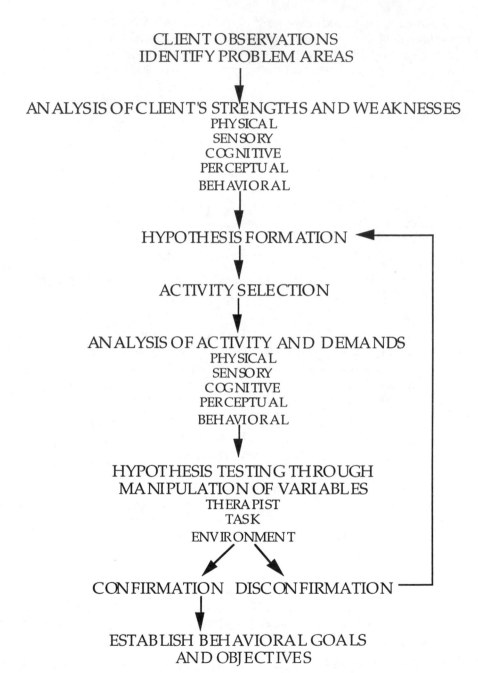

Figure 3–1. The hypothesis testing approach for evaluating cognitive and perceptual dysfunction.

These hypotheses are not rigid expectations of what the therapist thinks is wrong with the client; rather, they are proposals that he seeks to refute or confirm by further exploration. There are two main advantages in doing this. First, it helps the therapist to narrow down the possibilities and direct assessment toward more specific functions, therefore providing direction for the selection of standardized assessments. Second, considering the range of possible reasons for the client's difficulty prevents a therapist from jumping to a premature conclusion concerning the nature of the problem.

4. Activity Selection and Analysis

A suitable ADL is selected to test the hypothesis or hypotheses. This **activity** could be the same one in which problems were observed (as in step 1), or it could be a different activity such as bathing, grooming, or a kitchen task. The therapists should be familiar with the activity and have thoroughly analyzed it. This becomes very important once the therapist begins to manipulate task demands. **Activity analysis** (related to treatment) is discussed later in this chapter.

5. Hypothesis Testing

At this stage, the therapist structures the selected activity in order to control some of the variables present in the activity and manipulate or alter the relative presence or absence of others. In this way, changes can be introduced that allow the therapist to exclude alternative or competing explanations or hypotheses for the client's difficulties. The aim in the hypothesis-testing phase is to manipulate certain variables related to the activity to produce information in relation to the hypotheses formed. This will lead to confirmation or rejection of the hypotheses. The variables that can be manipulated in any activity include:

- Client variables—factors operating within the client that may influence performance (e.g., level of anxiety or degree of fatigue)
- Environmental variables—factors present in the environment that may influence performance (e.g., background noise or distractions)
- Task variables—factors present in the task that may influence performance (e.g., length of time the task takes to complete or the familiarity of the task)
- Therapist variables—factors operating as a result of therapist presence or input (e.g., the nature of the input [pictorial or verbal] or the therapist's relationship with the client)

Using the earlier example of the client who has difficulties using a new dressing technique, the therapist needs to manipulate the specific task demands in order to test his hypotheses. In relation to the first hypothesis, the occupational therapist could provide the client with a memory aid to see if it leads to an improved performance. For example, the therapist could write out the steps involved in dressing and place these next to the client's bed. Written instructions could be supplemented by photographs taken at each stage of the procedure. These instructions downgrade the memory demands of the task; therefore, if the client's difficulty is remembering the procedure, improved performance should be facilitated. If the client's performance was significantly improved by using this written guide, then the therapist will have some support for the first hypothesis, which was that the client had difficulty with the memory demands of the activity. However, if this type of prompt did not lead to an improvement in performance, it may be that memory demands are not the cause of the difficulty.

In regard to the second hypothesis, the therapist could question the client regarding his recall of the dressing procedure. It may be that the client is able to tell the therapist the steps involved but is unable to put this knowledge into action. This would suggest that memory functions were sufficiently intact to be able to complete the procedure. The therapist could then try various techniques to slow down the client's movements when dressing, that is, prevent his impulsive actions. For example, the therapist could do this by getting the client to verbalize each step in dressing out aloud before carrying it out. The therapist could physically slow him down by preventing incorrect actions and by guiding correct ones. If these types of techniques lead to an improved performance, and if in the process the therapist has done nothing to aid or prompt the client's memory, then the therapist has evidence to support the second hypothesis and refute the first.

6. Hypothesis Confirmation or Disconfirmation

At this stage, the therapist should evaluate the data and accept or reject each hypothesis. The therapist may, of course, decide that the information he has does not fit any of the hypotheses, and he may return to stage 1 to redefine the problem and generate new hypotheses. On the other hand, the therapist may think that the hypotheses were sound but that the action taken did not adequately test them; therefore, the therapist should go back to stage 3 and make further structured observations. Of course, as well as assisting the therapist to decide which hypothesis to accept, the activity will also provide information on how to facilitate the client's performance in everyday occupations. For instance, in carrying out the dressing task, the therapist may settle on the second hypothesis because he finds that the client's performance in dressing is greatly enhanced if he asks the client to state actions before performing them. The method of having the client verbalize his actions can therefore be seen as an important one in influencing performance. The therapist can use this knowledge in other settings or tasks, thereby facilitating the client's performance in a wide range of occupations. The therapist should confirm and supplement the information gained through the hypothesis-testing approach by using standardized assessments.

7. Behavioral Goal and Objective Writing

After the client's problem areas have been defined, the therapist can proceed to write **behavioral goals** and **behavioral objectives** (often referred to as *long-term* and *short-term* goals). Writing behavioral goals and objectives is not unique to the hypothesis-testing approach and should follow all assessment procedures. Some brief notes on goal and objective writing are made after the final section on assessment, which examines evaluating the clients in the home or workplace.

SITE VISITS AT THE CLIENT'S HOME OR WORKPLACE

The therapist may conduct one or more visits to the client's place of residence or workplace, with or without the client, during therapy (Box 3–4). The purpose of a home evaluation is to determine if the client will be able to live safely and comfortably in his chosen environment (e.g., see Allen, Earhart, & Blue, 1992, pp. 263–266). This includes an assessment of environmental barriers and supports. The therapist often conducts a nonstandardized assessment or uses a checklist when evaluating the client's home. Examples of these can be found in Christiansen and Baum (1997); Cooper, Rigby, and Letts (1993); and Unsworth (1998).

If a client previously had a job, the therapist may conduct several on-site work visits to meet with the client's employer, explore return-to-work opportunities, establish the nature of the client's work, and evaluate any environmental or task modifications that may be required to assist the client's return to work. Several standardized workplace assessments are available for therapists, including the Americans with Disabilities Act Work Site Assessment (Aja, Jacobs, & Hermenau, 1992) and the Job Analysis During Employer Site Visit (Demore-Taber, 1995). Findings from home and work assessments may lead to structural adjustments to the environment, modifications in the way activities are performed, or a recommendation that the client moves to another form of housing or place of employment. The role of home and work assessments in relation to discharge planning are discussed in the treatment section of this chapter. For further information on home and work assessment, the reader is referred to Cooper, Rigby, and Letts (1995); Christiansen and Baum (1997); and Jacobs (1995).

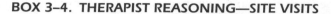

BOX 3–4. THERAPIST REASONING—SITE VISITS

When plans for the client's discharge are being formulated, I usually consider if a home or work visit is necessary. Such visits are usually needed when modifications to the physical environments will be required or when changes in the ways activities are conducted will need to be worked out. It's ideal if the client can come along on these visits. Sometimes it's not physically possible for the client to join me, and sometimes the client and I will agree that I should meet his or her employer alone. I usually take a home or worksite checklist with me when I go on a visit. These checklists are useful for making sure I don't miss any details. Because my clients have cognitive and perceptual deficits, my primary concerns when evaluating the home or workplace relate to safety. During a home evaluation I usually seek to answer the following questions:

- Can the client safely use appliances to heat the house?
- Is the client safe to use cooking appliances in the kitchen?
- Can the client keep the house locked and secure?
- Will the client be safe in the bathroom (e.g., using hot water, using electric appliances in wet areas)?

These issues must all be addressed before the client can return home.

If a client is returning to work, then he is generally managing quite well; therefore, I focus on how his residual cognitive and perceptual problems might affect his work. During a worksite visit I might examine:

- What are the physical work hazards?
- How will the client manage to get along with colleagues?
- Will the client manage the full work routine?
- How well do the client's capacities and abilities match the demands of the job?

Again, each of these issues must be raised and dealt with before the client resumes his duties.

≡ ESTABLISHING PROBLEM AREAS AND WRITING GOALS

FORMULATING THE PROBLEM LIST

Having evaluated the data gained from standardized and nonstandardized assessments, the therapist and client generate a list of strengths and problems. The problem list is prioritized to reflect the client's goals, immediacy of the problem, and time and attention that must be paid to the problem during intervention. Understanding why intervention for some problems takes precedence over others can best be viewed in the context of the client and his unique combination of problems, strengths, goals, values, and family support. Clinician and client reasoning behind the priority assigned to some of the problems experienced by a variety of clients is explored in the case study chapters.

All three kinds of clinical reasoning may be used by the therapist when forming the problem list. For example, whereas procedural reasoning is used to define a client's problems interactive reasoning is used when negotiating the problem list and the priority to be assigned to each problem with the client. Conditional reasoning is used throughout the process as the therapist considers the client's medical status, how he was living and what he was able to do prior to attending occupational therapy, as well as the client's and therapist's shared vision of what the future may hold.

WRITING GOALS AND OBJECTIVES

Some brief notes on goal and objective writing are made here to provide background information for the case study chapters. Okkema (1993) suggests that writing realistic goals is one of the biggest challenges faced by therapists because it takes great skill to integrate all the information required. Goals and objectives should reflect the client's strengths, problems, prognosis, and expected level of recovery. The best goals and objectives reflect the shared aims and values of the client, his family, and the therapist. Incongruency between client, therapist, and family goals requires careful negotiation and creativity so that a therapy plan that is motivating and satisfactory to all parties may be implemented. Using an assessment such as the Canadian Occupational Performance Measure (COPM) (Law et al., 1994) can ensure that the goals are client- rather than therapist-driven.

For the purpose of this book, a *goal* is a statement about a long-term aim that the client will achieve through participation in the therapy program. Goals are generally concerned with reducing the impact of disability and handicap on the client's life and optimizing quality of life. Therefore, goals are concerned with occupational performance areas. Goals may take a month, several months, or even a year to be achieved. In many texts, goals are referred to as *long-term goals*. An *objective* is a short-term aim that the client can achieve in one or several therapy sessions. An objective is more precise than a goal because it includes the desired outcome and the ways

Table 3–4. Goal and objective writing

BEHAVIORAL GOAL AND OBJECTIVE TOPIC	WHAT TO WRITE	THERAPIST REASONING
Who will do the task	The client's name	—
Given what	The therapeutic activities and approaches used by the therapist	I need to generate the therapeutic activities and approaches (e.g., verbal feedback, discussion with the client or instruction) I can use to facilitate my client's skill development. The activities and approaches I write here will guide my treatment. These activities will facilitate skill development or the particular ability documented in the "does what" section below.
Does what	What the client will be able to do	This is the performance that the client has difficulty with and needs to be able to do. I might write the activity that will be achieved (e.g., making a sandwich) or the skill that will be developed (e.g., problem solve a solution). This component of the goal or objective encapsulates what my client and I want to achieve.
How well	The level of performance to be achieved	This is the first part of measuring the standard that the client will achieve. I need to write how well the client will perform the "does what" component of the objective. This may reflect the "quality" or "amount" of the client's performance.

(continues)

(continued)

Table 3-4. Goal and objective writing		
BEHAVIORAL GOAL AND OBJECTIVE TOPIC	**WHAT TO WRITE**	**THERAPIST REASONING**
By when	The time frame in which the performance is to be achieved	This is the second part of measuring the standard that the client will achieve. I need to determine the time frame in which the client will complete the "does what" part of the objective.

it will be measured. In many texts, objectives are referred to as *short-term goals*.

There are several approaches to writing goals and objectives, and therapists often have quite different styles in formulating and writing them. This is evident in the case study chapters, in which a number of examples of goal-writing styles can be seen. Often the approach taken reflects the aim of the writer. For example, if the goal or objective is to be used for reimbursement, then it will be client-driven and will state what the client is to achieve and how this will be measured (Trombly, 1995b). However, if the aim is to write a goal or objective that assists the therapist to plan treatment as well, then the behavioral goal and behavioral objective writing approach may be useful. Behavioral goals and objectives are written using the who, given what, does what, how well, by when method. This method was discussed by Whalley Hammell (1994). The main difference between these goal-writing styles is that behavioral goal writing includes a section outlining the activities and therapeutic techniques to be used. This method helps students and novice clinicians consider the total therapy program at all times. Another advantage of using this approach is that outcomes of the therapy intervention are clearly documented in the "how well" and "by when" sections; therefore, the success of the therapeutic intervention can be readily measured. An explanation for each of the components of the behavioral method of goal and objective writing and some of the reasoning behind them is provided in Table 3-4. The following is an example of a behavioral objective written with a client who has planning difficulties, so that she can get to the local shops in a future therapy session.

Who	Jane Doe
Given what	Explanation of the task, a road map, bus timetable, therapist assistance to organize the task, a day planner devised by the therapist, and verbal prompts
Does what	Will use a road map and bus timetables to plan how and when to get to the local stores from the hospital, by walking and taking the bus, for lunch
How well	So that she has the route she will take to get to the stores and determine the time she will need to leave the hospital to get to the bus stop in time for late morning bus
By when	On completion of two 30-minute occupational therapy sessions

≡ AN OVERVIEW OF INTERVENTIONS

Having identified problem areas, goals, and objectives provides the parameters and guidelines for intervention. *Intervention* is the process of working with the client to assist him in achieving enjoyable, competent, and effective engagement in his everyday living occupations. Although the term *treatment* is commonly used when working with clients who have cognitive and perceptual problems, many occupational therapists are now adopting the broader term of intervention. Both terms are used in this text. The purpose of intervention with clients who have cognitive and perceptual problems is generally to assist the client to return to living in the community and achieve the highest quality of life possible. When planning intervention, clinicians often ask a series of questions such as those listed in Table 3–5. The answers to these questions help shape the interventions used.

INTERVENTION PRINCIPLES IN COGNITIVE AND PERCEPTUAL DYSFUNCTION

Intervention principles are guidelines that support practice. The principles used by therapists may differ depending on the theoretical approaches they adopt. However, in general, intervention principles for clients with cognitive or perceptual problems include the following:

- Intervention is conducted within a theoretical framework.
- The therapist is able to articulate if he or she is using a remediation, adaptation, or combination approach in therapy.

Table 3–5. Therapist considerations when planning intervention

INTERVENTION PLANNING-RELATED QUESTIONS	THERAPIST REASONING
What are our mutually agreed goals and objectives?	The objectives that have been developed by my client and me will guide therapy. In planning treatment activities, I need to keep these objectives uppermost in my mind.
What activities has the client expressed as being important or of interest or enjoyable?	I want to make sure that the therapeutic activities selected are motivating and enjoyable for the client as well as offering opportunities for skill development. This will provide opportunities for success for the client and will keep the client motivated in therapy.
What resources do I have available (time and materials)?	When planning a therapy program I need to consider how much time my certified occupational therapy assistants (COTAs) and I have available each day for individual and group therapy. I also need to consider what equipment and tools I have and the suitability of the environment for therapy activities.
Can I include the family in treatment?	Is the family willing and able to be involved in the therapy program? In addition, have I adequately educated the family about the nature of the client's problems, their management, and the role of occupational therapy?
How much research support is there for a particular therapy approach?	Have I adequately researched the therapeutic approaches/tasks I want to use with the client? I need to be able to justify my treatments and indicate whether there is sufficient evidence to warrant their use. Although I am aware that there is only a limited literature to support the treatment of cognitive and perceptual dysfunction, I need to ensure that my treatments are based on documented research.
Will the skills acquired by the client in one therapy activity generalize to others?	In order to maximize therapy, it's important to ensure that gains made with the client in one task or environment generalize to others. I need to reinforce skills in a variety of tasks and settings to ensure they generalize. Answering this question is particularly important if I am using a bottom-up approach to therapy.

- A range of occupations or activities should be used as intervention.
- If a remediation approach is used, opportunities are provided for the client to generalize skills learned in one activity or environment to others.
- Opportunities are provided for both individual and group therapy.
- Whenever possible, the client's family and friends should be included in the intervention process.
- Mechanisms for the evaluation of intervention must be in place before intervention begins.

Some of the issues relating to these principles are described below.

APPROACHES TO INTERVENTION

In Chapter 1, the two main approaches to intervention were described as *adaptive* and *remedial*. Neistadt (1990) described the adaptive approach as relying on teaching the client to modify the environment and the ways in which tasks are completed and to use intact skills to complete activities they are having difficulty with. Client strengths are acknowledged and built upon and it is assumed that the client will learn to do tasks in a different way. The remedial approach is based on the belief that the human brain is capable of recovery through neural plasticity and reorganization of function where new brain areas take over from areas that have been damaged. Intervention aims to stimulate recovery by retraining specific components of lost abilities using tabletop or computer-based activities. Clinicians can adopt either or both of these approaches in their intervention. Some clinicians often commence the therapy program by using a remediation approach. After the client's skill recovery has plateaued and discharge is planned, compensation strategies may be adopted to facilitate the client's successful return to community living.

One of the main issues that has plagued researchers and clinicians alike who use a remedial approach to intervention is whether or not skills learned in one activity and environment generalize to others. When using adaptive and compensatory strategies, this issue is not so important. Compensatory and adaptive strategies are often activity dependent, and Neistadt (1990) suggests that these approaches actually reduce the need for the client to generalize skills. In the past, therapists using remedial approaches assumed that **generalization** of skill occurred. However, research suggests that this may not be the case (e.g., Jongbloed et al., 1989). Therefore, it is important for clinicians to reinforce skills gained in one task or environment to others. This may include the clinician's discussing ways to generalize the skill with the client and practicing the same skill in a variety of activities during the same intervention session to encourage skill generalization. More recently,

Neistadt (1994a, 1995a) has taken another approach to this problem and has been examining clients' capacity to learn after brain damage. Neistadt argues that both adaptive and remedial strategies may work well with clients depending on their ability to learn. Although remedial approaches require "far transfer" of learned material, adaptive approaches require only "near transfer." Neistadt (1995a) suggests that assessing a client's learning capacity is very important when choosing an approach to therapy.

THE USE OF GROUPS

Although the focus of this book is on providing individual occupational therapy programs to clients who have cognitive and perceptual problems, most therapists include their clients in some group activities. Chapter 11 deals specifically with conducting groups with clients who have cognitive and perceptual problems and outlines several different kinds of groups. Groups may meet to work on specific skill areas (e.g., communication, concentration, or social skills) or to provide an opportunity for members to share experiences and support each other. One of the main advantages of groups is that they reduce the need for the therapist to always provide feedback to the client. Instead, group members offer both support and critical feedback to each other. Feedback from peers is very powerful and can be extremely useful to clients, particularly when behavior change is required. The reader is referred to Chapter 11 and Sohlberg and Mateer (1989), Okkema (1993), and Prichard and Bernard (1995) for further ideas and information on conducting groups with clients who have cognitive and perceptual problems.

THE ROLE OF EDUCATION

Many occupational therapists who work with clients who have cognitive and perceptual problems state that they use a "three-pronged" approach to intervention: remediation, adaptation, and education. Each of these approaches can be incorporated into the intervention plan in different ways and with different emphasis. Remediation and adaptation approaches have been previously discussed. Education is an important component of all therapy programs. The client and his family are educated concerning the client's problems and the implications of these on his daily occupations (Box 3–5). Clients with cognitive and perceptual problems often lack insight and therefore may not be able to make use of this education immediately. Family members are also open to education at different times. For example, when the client is first in the hospital after trauma, stroke, or neu-

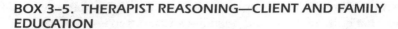

BOX 3–5. THERAPIST REASONING—CLIENT AND FAMILY EDUCATION

Throughout a client's rehabilitation, I like to spend time talking with him or her about what has happened, providing as much factual information as possible. My clients are often slow to absorb this information, so it often helps to write it in a day book or diary. I need to provide my clients with a lot of support during this time because the information is difficult to deal with and emotionally draining. I also spend time with the significant people in the client's life so they feel they know what is going on both in terms of the client's medical condition and what we are doing in therapy and why. Sometimes it's hard for partners or family to hear what therapists have to say; sometimes they are just relieved to be told anything. Most of the time it's really helpful to keep family and others up to date regarding therapy progression because these people are important to the client and can really reinforce what you are doing in therapy.

rosurgery, the family is usually more focused on survival, speech, and the ability of their family member to walk. After the client is in rehabilitation, it may take some time for the family to understand what the cognitive and perceptual problems are and the impact of such problems on day-to-day function. Often, it is only after an outing or spending some time in therapy that family members begin to understand the implications of the client's problems. At this point, family members are particularly receptive to information about the client's problems and strategies they can use to facilitate recovery.

ACTIVITY SELECTION, ANALYSIS, AND GRADING

Many occupational therapy texts contain excellent descriptions of how to select therapeutic intervention activities or occupations. The reader is referred to Christiansen and Baum (1997), Hopkins and Smith (1993), and Trombly (1995) for further information in this area. Either the client or therapist may be primarily responsible for activity selection. The three main approaches to activity selection are:

1. For the therapist to choose activities based on the challenges they present and the opportunity they provide to stimulate the client
2. For the client to choose motivating and interesting activities
3. For the therapist and client to choose activities together based on therapeutic value and client interest

The method of activity selection often depends on the model of practice used by the therapist and his commitment to the concept of client-centered practice. After an activity has been selected, an activity analysis must be conducted to determine the components of the task, whether the task will stimulate the client appropriately, and how different aspects of the activity can be manipulated to provide maximum therapeutic value for the client. Activity analysis helps confirm if the activity selected is in fact the best one to use with the client. Experienced clinicians conduct activity analyses almost simultaneously as they generate ideas for intervention. In the case study chapters, expert clinicians present their activity analyses aloud so their reasoning can be examined. There are several excellent books on activity analysis, and the reader is referred to Allen et al. (1992a); Breines (1995); Lamport, Coffey, and Hersch (1993); and Levine and Brayley (1991).

An essential component of activity analysis is the ability to grade the activity. **Grading** refers to any modifications made to the activity to ensure it is at the "just right" level so that the client is optimally challenged (Berlyne, 1969; Csikszentmihayli, 1975). Activity grading is usually done before the client commences the task. However, as the therapist proceeds with the activity, constant adjustments may be required to ensure the client remains optimally challenged throughout the task. The therapist can grade three main aspects (referred to as *variables*) of an activity: therapeutic input (i.e., the way the therapist interacts with the client), the activity itself, and the environment in which the activity takes place. The types of grading related to these variables are summarized in Table 3–6. The case study chapters reveal clinician reasoning associated with activity grading. As a general

Table 3–6. Different ways of grading an activity

VARIABLE	TYPE OF GRADING
Therapist	Verbal cueing
	Visual cueing
	Feedback
	Physical assistance or guidance
Task	Time taken/duration
	Number of steps or items
	Degree of complexity
	Rate
	Familiarity
Environment	Number of distractions
	Appropriateness of context

guide, activities require upgrading when the client is not optimally challenged by the activity and downgrading when the activity is too difficult, overstimulating, or frustrating for the client.

DISCHARGE PLANNING

Throughout the therapy process, but particularly toward the end of a client's in-patient rehabilitation, the therapist, client, and his family needs to consider the client's lifestyle on discharge. Toward the end of the program, the therapist places greater emphasis on ensuring the client's successful transition to home (or other long-term housing), work, and driving (if appropriate). Although evaluations of home and work may be conducted earlier in the client's rehabilitation, thorough evaluations are required before discharge. Moreover, the therapist needs to determine if the client requires outpatient services or referral to other day-therapy programs.

Housing

Although a client's discharge has usually been under consideration since his admission to in-patient care (McKeehan, 1981), discharge housing plans are typically formulated after the client's progress has plateaued and gains are no longer being made in therapy (Box 3–6). At this point, the therapy team (including the client and his family) considers the best match between the client's skills and the demands and support provided by different forms of housing (Unsworth, 1995, 1996). The importance of housing in our lives cannot be underestimated. Housing provides status, security, comfort, and is the focus of family and social life. Whereas appropriate housing can promote independence and well-being, a mismatch between accommodation type and the person's habits, skills, and personality can lead to isolation, hardship, and unsatisfactory reliance on others (Wilson & Calder, 1990).

There are two major types of housing available to persons with disabilities: supported accommodation and community-based accommodation. *Supported accommodation* may be defined as any accommodation that provides personal care and medical services to persons on a consistent or continual basis; it includes nursing homes, skilled nursing facilities, and sheltered or group housing. Community-based accommodation includes private homes, retirement villages, caravans, hotels, and rooming houses. Although all these community housing options provide a relatively independent community lifestyle, support is still available. If an individual

> ## BOX 3-6. THERAPIST REASONING—HOUSING PLANS
>
> Before a client's discharge, I usually present the team (which includes the client and his or her family) with information relevant to housing, such as the client's accommodation choice, current abilities, problems, and family supports. Other team members, such as the nurse and social worker, also contribute a lot to the discussion that follows. The team considers all the issues, and we negotiate suitable housing and formal support services to the client and his family or partner. I find I am using all three forms of reasoning when trying to work out with the client where the best place to live is. Determining the best match between the client's skills and the demands of different types of housing is basically procedural. I draw on a lot of skills when I interact with the client and family. Sometimes the family doesn't want the client to return to live with them after an injury but doesn't want to admit it to the client. This can make communications really difficult. Throughout the discharge process I use conditional reasoning as I consider what the client's future will be like given the context of their past and what has happened to them more recently. I think that housing is very important to quality of life, so I find I spend a lot of time working out the best option with the client and his or her family.

requires assistance with personal and instrumental ADLs to retain his community living status, formal support networks are available, including home help services, personal care attendants, home maintenance services, transport, paramedical services, food services, respite care, and home nursing (Unsworth, 1993, 1995). Interventions that facilitate a client with cognitive and perceptual problems to return to community-based housing usually center around enabling the client to carry out ADLs in an acceptable and safe manner.

Return to Work

Conducting work-site evaluations was discussed previously in this chapter. Intervention focuses on ensuring that the client makes a smooth transition to his full- or part-time job and is capable of resuming his old duties or taking responsibility for modified or new ones. Several of the case study chapters explore return-to-work issues. In addition, there are several excellent texts on assisting clients return to work (including clients with cognitive and perceptual problems), and the reader is referred to Jacobs (1991, 1995), Jacobs and Bettencourt (1994), and Berg Rice (1998).

Driving

Finally, a very important area for evaluation and possible intervention before a client's discharge is the client's ability to drive safely. Although most assessments are conducted at the beginning of a therapy program, driving evaluation is usually undertaken closer to discharge when the client's status is stable and any long-term cognitive and perceptual problems have been identified. Driving is central to our independence in the community and is an ADL that most of us take for granted; therefore, returning to driving is often very important to clients after they are discharged from the hospital. Internationally, the laws concerning a client's ability to drive after acquired brain damage vary greatly. However, in general a client's vehicle insurance policy may not be valid unless he has informed the insurance company of any long-term disability or license conditions and followed up with any medical evaluations requested by the company. In many countries, it is often the role of the occupational therapist to assess a client's ability to drive and provide any retraining required after accident or injury. Driving assessment and retraining require therapists to use all their skills because the client's physical, visual, cognitive, perceptual, and psychosocial status must be taken into consideration.

Occupational therapists have an important role to play in assisting clients with the physical aspects of driving, including vehicle modification and transfer techniques. However, the largest role for therapists is in evaluating and in many cases retraining skills in the areas of vision, visual perception, cognition, perception, and communication. The majority of literature in the area of driver assessment and retraining is concerned with clients who experience cognitive and perceptual problems after head injury or stroke (e.g., Brooke et al., 1992; Galaski, Bruno, & Ehle, 1993; and Kortleing & Kaptein, 1996). Because of the specialized nature of conducting driver evaluations and retraining and the fact that few texts provide this material, brief notes are made here concerning driving assessment in the United States. Information is also provided regarding driving evaluation in Australia. Australia is one of the few countries where occupational therapists have been included in legislation as experts in this area. Occupational therapists who are not trained in driver evaluation need to refer their clients with cognitive and perceptual problems to occupational therapists who are qualified in this area.

The Association of Driver Educators for the Disabled (ADED) was formed in the United States in 1977. Today, approximately 60% of its members are occupational therapists (Pierce, 1996). This organization runs examinations to test occupational therapists, certified occupational therapy assistants, and driver educators who wish to become Certified Driver Rehabilitation Specialists (CDRS). The examination costs approximately $175. According to Pierce

(1996), before scheduling a client who has been referred for a driver evaluation, the therapist must ensure:

- The client has a valid license or learners permit
- The client has obtained physician approval for the evaluation
- The client meets Department of Motor Vehicles (DMV) standards for driving (including visual acuity, field of vision, and freedom from seizures)
- Funding is available for the driver evaluation and follow up (confirm in writing if a third-party payer is involved)

A driver evaluation process includes:

- A clinical evaluation and off-road assessment with the client (this may utilize specialized equipment such as the Elemental Driving Simulator or the Cognitive Behavioral Driving Inventory [Gianutsos, 1994])
- Vehicle evaluation, modification, and inspection
- Driver training and education in the evaluation vehicle and the client's own vehicle
- Licensing and/or formal notification to vehicle insurers

In Australia, occupational therapists have also been involved in driver evaluation and retraining for the past 15 years. Each of the states in Australia has slightly different legislation concerning driving with a disability and involves occupational therapists in different ways. As an example, an outline is provided concerning the role of occupational therapists and legislation in the state of Victoria (population, approximately 5.5 million). In Victoria, the state licensing authority (equivalent to the DMV) is VicRoads. Occupational therapists trained as disabled driver assessors are included in Victorian road and traffic legislation along with medical practitioners and ophthalmologists as having the necessary qualifications to perform disabled-driver assessments and supply this information to VicRoads.

Occupational therapists who wish to be trained as disabled-driver assessors undertake an 80-hour postgraduate course through the University's school of occupational therapy. The course comprises both on- and off-road intensive education. At the end of the course, participants complete several examinations and are then registered by VicRoads. Participating in the course and becoming a registered disabled-driver assessor costs approximately $1500. These occupational therapists are not trained to become driving instructors; rather, they are trained to work alongside driving instructors. There are several clinics in Victoria staffed by occupational therapists who are qualified disabled-driver assessors. These clinics are generally attached to head injury and stroke rehabilitation centers, and the majority of clients with cognitive and perceptual problems in Victoria are evaluated by these units before returning to driving.

MEASURING THE OUTCOME OF OCCUPATIONAL THERAPY INTERVENTION

Being able to measure the outcome of an occupational therapy intervention is important for several reasons (Box 3–7). First, the therapist wants to know if each intervention session is leading to an improvement in the client's performance. The therapist continually makes modifications during a therapy session to maximize the therapeutic value of activities used. This may include upgrading, downgrading, or changing the task. Second, knowledge of the outcome of different therapy approaches or programs can guide therapists to select the interventions that work best and are most cost-effective. A cost-effective program is one in which the outcome is greater than or worth the resources invested. Finally, data concerning the outcomes and effectiveness of an occupational therapy program can be used by clinical facilities to demonstrate to insurance companies the value of providing an occupational therapy service. A large enough sample of

---

BOX 3–7. THERAPIST REASONING—OUTCOME MEASUREMENT

Outcome measurement is very important in our clinic. In fact, it seems to be really important everywhere. My manager wants objective evidence that our interventions really make a difference in the client's ability to live independently. Although management and the insurers are interested to see degrees of recovery at a capacity/impairment level, evidence of reduced disability is seen as more important. I guess ultimately we are trying to ensure that the client will return home independent in activities of daily living (ADLs) and with a good quality of life, therefore placing as little financial burden on the community as possible. The need to demonstrate that my therapy is worthwhile has forced me to examine the standardized assessments available to measure change in my clients at a disability and handicap level. Although this chapter has reviewed a number of impairment-oriented assessments and there are a range of good assessments to gather information about a client's personal and instrumental ADLs (e.g., see AMPS [Fisher, 1997], Adult FIM [Guide for the Uniform Data Set for Medical Rehabilitation, 1993], Barthel Index [Mahoney & Barthel, 1965], and ALSAR [Williams et al., 1991]), there are not so many assessments of handicap. There is certainly a need for further research in the areas of assessment development and outcome measurement.

data that shows cost-effective outcomes for clients can be used to ensure that third-party payers or health insurance organizations continue to fund occupational therapy services.

The outcome of an occupational therapy program can be measured in several ways, including:

1. Reassess the client using standardized assessments to determine if improvements have been made.
2. Reexamine behavioral goals and objectives to determine whether these have been met.
3. Ask the client if he feels he has improved.
4. Ask the client's family or friends if they see improvements.
5. Evaluate if specific intervention strategies have generalized to other activities.

The most objective approach to measuring outcomes is through the re-administration of a standardized assessment, if the test manual indicates that this is appropriate. However, when reevaluating the client using a standardized assessment, the therapist must be aware that improvements may be caused by real change in the client or practice effects associated with test familiarity. Okkema (1993) suggests overcoming this problem by using assessments that have different forms for pre- and postintervention assessment. Another difficulty when documenting outcomes is demonstrating that change is due to the therapy and not to spontaneous recovery or the efforts of family and friends; this is best done through the use of control group studies. In this kind of research, clients are randomly assigned to groups in which one group receives therapy and the other does not. This kind of research is rare because of the ethical problems associated with withholding therapy from one group since therapy is believed to lead to improvements. Therapists have conducted alternative approaches to outcomes research using:

● Single case designs
● A waiting list of clients as a control group
● Assigning clients randomly to receive different kinds of therapy (overcoming the problem of a control group that receive no therapy)

Outcome measurement is an important and topical issue in therapy today, and several of the case study chapters in this book examine the outcome of interventions used. For further discussions on outcomes measurement in occupational therapy, the reader is referred to Ellenberg (1996), de Clive-Lowe (1996), and Rogers and Holm (1994).

☰ THE OCCUPATIONAL THERAPIST AS A TEAM MEMBER

To this point, only the role of occupational therapists in evaluation and intervention with clients who have cognitive and perceptual problems has been considered. However, the majority of occupational therapists working in this area are members of a multidisciplinary team. Team approaches rather than individual clinician care are recognized as the best practice for all clients, including those with cognitive and perceptual problems. Team members include the client and his family, a nurse, occupational therapist, speech-language pathologist, psychologist and/or neuropsychologist, physician/physiatrist, social worker, and possibly a physical therapist. Each team member has a unique contribution to make to the client's recovery (Unsworth, 1997). As part of a multidisciplinary team, the occupational therapist has the opportunity to discuss assessment and treatment ideas with other therapists and ensure a coordinated approach to client care. In particular, the speech-language pathologist, neuropsychologist, and occupational therapist can share important information about the client's language and communication abilities, the nature of the client's impairments, and the ways these impact on the individual's occupational performance. Team members provide support to each other when working with challenging clients, and team meetings provide a forum for information and idea exchange. Experienced therapists reflect on the variety of services offered to the client to ensure that service duplication is minimal and that all involved clinicians are working together with the client toward mutual goals. Although the emphasis of this book is placed on the work of occupational therapists, it is useful to consider the role and contribution of other team members to clients' habilitation and rehabilitation.

☰ SUMMARY

This chapter examined some of the procedures clinicians use when working with clients who have cognitive and perceptual problems and some of the accompanying reasoning. Starting with assessment, this chapter documented a variety of standardized and nonstandardized approaches to evaluating clients. Owing to the limited information in most texts about assessments that can be used with clients who have cognitive and perceptual problems, nine evaluations were reviewed. Next, the chapter summarized the reasoning that supports problem list formation and methods of goal and objective writing. Principles and approaches to intervention were documented to provide the reader with an overview of the rationale behind treatment programs. Many of the case study chapters refer to activity analysis and grading; therefore, an explanation of what activity analysis is and how activities can be graded was provided in this chapter. One of the final sections of the chapter explored discharge planning, which is the concluding component of any therapeutic intervention. Issues related to clients' housing, return to work, and driving were summarized. To conclude, brief comments were made concerning teamwork. Although this book is primarily concerned with the work of occupational therapists, we usually work as members of multidisciplinary teams. It is important to consider that the occupational therapy program is only part of the total habilitation or rehabilitation process experienced by the client. In summary, the purpose of the first three chapters has been to provide the reader with the background information required to work through the case study chapters that follow. Chapters 4 to 11 are now presented and provide the reader with insights into how therapists reason in their practice with clients who have specific cognitive and perceptual problems.

≡ REVIEW QUESTIONS

1. Describe five characteristics of a standardized assessment. Why is it important to have a formal base for interpreting data? What are two commonly used approaches to interpreting data obtained?
2. Several standardized assessments are described in this chapter. If the therapist suspects the client has memory problems, what assessment would be most appropriate to use? What other assessment techniques could also be used?
3. Describe how a therapist uses the hypothesis-testing approach to evaluate a client. List three advantages and three disadvantages associated with the use of a hypothesis-testing approach to evaluation.
4. What kinds of clinical reasoning does a therapist use when forming goals and objectives with a client?
5. Write a behavioral objective for a client who has a left unilateral neglect and wants to purchase a snack (e.g., sodas and cookies) for her family at the hospital cafeteria.
6. Review Table 3–6 and describe how the activity of making a beef, lettuce, and tomato sandwich could be both up- and downgraded.
7. When planning a client's discharge, what factors need to be considered?
8. Discuss what arrangements are in place or legal requirements exist in your state or county for clients with acquired cognitive and perceptual problems to be evaluated before resuming driving.

9. Describe five different ways the effectiveness of an intervention program can be documented. Why aren't nonstandardized assessments useful when conducting outcomes research?

☰ ACKNOWLEDGMENTS

I would like to thank Guðrún Árnadóttir, Leslie Duran, Anne Fisher, Ellie Fossey, and Alison Laver for reviewing and contributing to sections of the Review of Standardized Assessments component of the chapter.

4

Evaluation and Intervention with Concentration Impairment

CAROLYN UNSWORTH, PhD, OTR

- Alertness
- Alternating Concentration
- Attention
- Concentration
- Distraction/Distractibility
- Divided Concentration
- Focused (Selective) Concentration
- Generalization
- Hypoxia (Cerebral)
- Information Processing
- Instrumental Activities of Daily Living
- Prompt
- Sustained Concentration
- Topographical Orientation

On completion of this chapter, the reader will be able to:

- Define concentration and describe the three kinds of concentration discussed in this chapter
- Describe two theories of concentration and the anatomical basis for concentration
- List two standardized assessments an occupational therapist may use to screen for problems with concentration and two standardized assessments a neuropsychologist may use to assess these problems
- Outline five intervention strategies that clients with concentration problems can use to help them complete activities
- Describe five ways to upgrade or downgrade an activity when working with a client who has problems with concentration
- Successfully work through the Review Questions

≡ INTRODUCTION

The purpose of this chapter is to present the reasoning behind evaluating and then implementing an intervention program with a client who is experiencing problems with concentration. As the first case study chapter in the book, this chapter examines concentration because this skill supports and is a prerequisite for many other cognitive skills. Concentration is one of the most important prerequisites for memory (as discussed in Chapter

5), and together concentration (attention) and memory are the primary pre-requisites for learning (Wood, 1987). All clients need to be able to learn if they are to gain maximum benefit from rehabilitation; therefore, occupational therapists need to establish that a client has adequate concentration and memory skills to be able to proceed with therapy. The importance of the capacity to concentrate is often underrated by therapists, and many textbooks fail to adequately cover the topic. This chapter opens with a brief review of the features of concentration and the brain regions responsible for this function. The case of Jen-Lin is then presented. Jen-Lin experiences difficulties with concentration as a result of brain **hypoxia** after a drug overdose. The therapist's reasoning behind the overall intervention program for Jen-Lin is presented. In particular, an intervention session with Jen-Lin is detailed. The chapter concludes with a summary and some questions for the reader to answer.

WHAT IS CONCENTRATION?

Terminology

Although the terms *concentration* and *attention* are often used interchangeably, the majority of occupational therapy and neuropsychology texts dealing with cognitive problems after brain damage seem to adopt the term *attention*. However, because of the arguments presented by Stringer (1996), the terms *attention* and *concentration* are kept separate in this text for both conceptual and practical reasons. As Stringer explains, *concentration* is narrower in meaning than *attention*. Whereas *concentration* relates to directing thoughts and actions toward a stimulus or stimuli, *attention* is a broader term that also encompasses the capacity to detect and orient to stimuli (1996). Accordingly, the term *attention* is used in this text in relation to unilateral neglect, in which a client fails to attend to stimuli presented in a hemispace (described in detail in Chapter 9). Additionally, the term *concentration* is used in this chapter to avoid confusion with *attention deficit disorder*, which is generally used to describe a developmental disorder. Please note that although many of the texts cited in this chapter use the term *attention*, it has been changed to *concentration* to maintain consistency across the chapter. It is also important to note that concentration is related to, but separate from, arousal and **alertness** (Stringer, 1996). Being aroused and alert involves the capacity to maintain a state of wakefulness in which the individual is ready and able to respond to events in the environment (van Zomeren & Brouwer, 1994). Therefore, a capacity to concentrate is dependent on an adequate level of alertness (Stringer, 1996).

Definition of Concentration and Problems with Concentration After Brain Damage

Concentration is a difficult construct to define (Gray, 1990; Ponsford, Sloan, & Snow, 1995; van Zomeren & Brouwer, 1994). To effectively concentrate, an individual must be able to inhibit focusing on distracting stimuli and to shift focus to relevant features according to the task, past experiences, or needs. Concentration involves purposefully and voluntarily directing one's thoughts and actions toward a stimulus or stimuli (Stringer, 1996).

After brain damage, a problem with concentration is one of the most frequently reported deficits (Cicerone, 1996; Ponsford & Kinsella, 1991; van Zomeren & Brouwer, 1994). Even clients with mild brain damage often complain of slowed thinking, being more easily distracted, and having trouble doing more than one thing at a time (Cicerone, 1996). Researchers classify concentration problems in different ways. For the purposes of this chapter, **concentration** (called **attention** in many of the cited texts) is classified according to the writing of Stringer (1996), van Zomeren and Brouwer (1994), Sohlberg and Mateer (1989), Wood (1987), and Okkema (1993). In a broad sense, concentration has two dimensions: capacity and control. *Capacity* refers to the amount of information processing a person can do in a given time, and *control* refers to an individual's ability to direct concentration capacities (Weber, 1990). Furthermore, concentration is generally referred to as existing in three forms: sustained, focused (selective), and divided (alternating). Although not a hierarchy, it often seems that concentration is a continuum in which "alternating concentration" requires the greatest degree of skill (Okkema, 1993). Relevant features of each of these forms of concentration, as well as some of the problems that may arise after brain damage, are listed next. A feature common to all these forms of concentration is the possibility of **distraction.** In addition to environmental distractions from other people, noises, or activities, an individual can self-distract. For example, an individual may be putting cookies on a baking sheet, notice that his shirt is untucked, and then respond to this environmental distraction immediately rather than finishing putting the cookies in the oven, washing his hands, and then tucking in the shirt.

Sustained Concentration

Sustained concentration is the capacity to concentrate on relevant information during occupations. Sustained concentration implies that a person can maintain a consistent response during a continuous activity. A client who has problems with this kind of concentration may report that he starts to watch a television program and then "just drifts off." Sustained concentration capacities are more likely to be impaired in people with severe, rather than mild, head injuries. Sustained concentration is also referred to as a *concentration span*.

Focused (Selective) Concentration

The capacity to concentrate on an occupation despite environmental visual or auditory stimuli is referred to as **focused (selective) concentration.** To effectively engage in most occupations, an individual needs to be able to filter out what is important and to ignore what is not. A client who has to stop his dressing activity to talk to the therapist may be demonstrating difficulties with selective concentration. Clients who are easily disturbed by music or other forms of background noise may also be experiencing problems with selective concentration. Therefore, a problem with focused concentration is often referred to as **distractibility.**

Divided and Alternating Concentration

Divided and alternating concentration are sometimes considered together; however, **alternating concentration** is the capacity to move flexibly between tasks and respond appropriately to the demands of each task, and **divided concentration** is the capacity to respond simultaneously to two or more tasks. Divided concentration is required when more than one response is required or more than one stimuli needs to be monitored (Mateer, Kerns, & Eso, 1996). The main difference between selective and divided/alternating concentration is that a selection of stimuli is required to be ignored in selective concentration. However, in divided/alternating concentration tasks, all stimuli are relevant but the individual is required to provide different responses and levels of response to each stimulus (van Zomeren & Brouwer, 1994). Clients who experience problems with divided/alternating concentration usually show a decrease in performance in one task when a second is added. For example, a decrease in performance may be noted if a client is required to write down a phone message as it is relayed by a caller. Clients who have difficulty with these forms of concentration may have great difficulties with more complex activities of daily living (ADLs), such as cooking a meal or driving.

Although concentration can be divided into the categories of sustained, focused (selective), and divided/alternating, there is limited empirical evidence to support problems with these specific forms of concentration in individuals after brain damage. van Zomeren and Brouwer (1994) reviewed more than two decades' research investigating concentration deficits and concluded that in experimental testing situations, clients' performance on concentration tasks seemed most markedly affected by a slowed information-processing speed. Although these specific forms of concentration deficits described here may not be present in testing situations, they do seem to appear in more complex settings, such as those presented in ADLs in the community (Ponsford & Kinsella, 1992).

Summary

Given their often subtle presentation, clients' problems with concentration are not always recognized by therapists. Left untreated, such problems can cause significant difficulties for clients, both in their rehabilitation programs and as they try to reintegrate into their communities after hospitalization (Sohlberg & Mateer, 1989). No single intervention strategy to overcome concentration deficits will work for all clients. Many researchers agree that **generalization** of training does not occur from specific therapy tasks to other ADLs (Stringer, 1996). Ponsford, Sloan, and Snow (1995) conclude that strategies to overcome a variety of cognitive problems including concentration are more likely to be of lasting benefit if they are directly related to and applied in real-world settings.

THEORIES OF CONCENTRATION

Problems with concentration can accompany brain damage resulting from many causes, including cerebrovascular disease producing stroke, traumatic brain injury, demyelinating disease (such as multiple sclerosis), central nervous system infections, compromised brain metabolism, hypoxia (e.g., after near-drowning), and exposure to toxic substances (Stringer, 1996). Despite the fact that so many people experience problems with concentration after brain damage, the underlying basis for this problem is far from clear (van Zomeren & Brouwer, 1994).

Although there is little agreement concerning the underlying mechanisms of normal concentration, several of the more prominent theories are briefly reviewed in this chapter. For more details on these theories, the reader is referred to van Zomeren and Brouwer (1994). One feature that many theories have in common is that concentration is equated with **information processing.** Information-processing capacity is defined as ". . . the amount of information that can be attended and responded to in a finite period of time" (Sohlberg & Mateer, 1989, p. 113). Broadbent (1958) introduced the idea of "selectivity" in information processing. This theory postulated that when concentrating or attending, an individual selectively responds to one event while inhibiting responses to others. Therefore, the brain was believed to process information one piece at a time, or serially (Sohlberg & Mateer, 1989). However, a flaw in this model was that processing may occur in different modalities simultaneously.

Whereas Broadbent continued to refine his theory, Shriffin and Schneider (1977) partly solved the problem by describing a two-process model of information processing: controlled (conscious) and automatic processing (van Zomeren & Brouwer, 1994). Whereas some tasks, particularly when they are overlearned, seem to be executed automatically, others (particularly tasks that an individual is learning) require conscious or controlled processing (van Zomeren & Brouwer, 1994). When learning a task, an individual relies on feedback and therefore constantly concentrates on the task. This controlled concentration continues until the individual masters the task (Sohlberg & Mateer, 1989). When performance becomes automatic, the individual's actions are managed by prearranged instruction sequences and he or she is free to concentrate on other aspects of the task or on a different task. Therefore, automatic processing is said to occur in parallel (van Zomeren & Brouwer, 1994). Whereas automatic processing occurs in parallel and places very limited demands on the individual, controlled processing is thought to occur serially (Sohlberg & Mateer, 1989; van Zomeren & Brouwer, 1994).

Shriffin and Schneider (1977) also suggested that there are two forms of concentration problems: divided attention (concentration) deficits (DADs) and focused attention (concentration) deficits (FADs). DADs are believed to result from speed limitations when trying to consciously process material. For example, if too much information is presented too quickly when we are trying to learn a new skill, we miss important components and may not learn the skill properly (van Zomeren & Brouwer, 1994). FADs occur when automatic processing tendencies conflict with the responses demanded in a task (Sohlberg & Mateer, 1989). For example, when driving an American car, the headlight switch is usually located on the right side of the controls; however, if a person previously drove a European-made car, in which the controls are on the left, he will need to consciously attend to this difference. If the driver turns on the windshield wipers in error (located on the right side), then a DAD is present (van Zomeren & Brouwer, 1994).

Whereas Shriffin and Schneider's (1977) theory of concentration relies on an information-processing approach, Shallice (1982) proposed a cognitive schema theory to explain concentration. Shallice presented a model of human behavior in which all activity is viewed as the unfolding of mental schema (van Zomeren & Brouwer, 1994). "Triggers" (i.e., perceptual stimuli) are required for schema to become active, but it is possible that many triggers could be activated simultaneously, resulting in chaotic behavior. Shallice (1982) proposed that two adaptive mechanisms control relations between schemas: contention scheduling and supervisory attention control.

The supervisory attention (concentration) system supervises the running of specialized, or non-routine, programs. This system also contains mechanisms that operate when new action sequences are required. Therefore, the supervisory attention system is responsible for selecting alternate strategies. Selection of which programs or schemas to run is determined by the supervisory attention system together with "contention scheduling" (Sohl-berg & Mateer, 1989). Contention scheduling selects action strategies based on the strongest perceptual triggers, controlling which stimuli will be se-lectively concentrated on and is ideally suited for routine behavior. At this stage, more research is required to determine exactly how schema selection occurs and why (van Zomeren & Brouwer, 1994).

In summary, the work of several key researchers, such as Broadbent (1958), Shriffin and Schneider (1977), and Shallice (1982), has increased our knowledge of concentration processes in normal individuals (and in those after brain damage). These theories form the basis for most work in this area today (e.g., see Cicerone, 1996; Weber, 1990). However, a great deal more research and theorizing is required before we can begin to fully understand the mechanisms that underlie concentration.

BRAIN REGIONS RESPONSIBLE FOR CONCENTRATION

Multiple brain regions are thought to be responsible for producing con-centration, but it is beyond the scope of this text to fully review these or the supporting research evidence. The reader is again referred to van Zomeren and Brouwer's excellent text (1994) for a more comprehensive review of this area. However, in summary it appears that concentration is brought about by the reticular formation, which regulates arousal; the various sen-sory systems, which bring and code relevant sensory information; and the limbic and frontal regions, which underlie the drive and affective com-ponents of concentration. In reviewing a variety of empirical studies con-cerning brain regions responsible for concentration deficits, Stinger (1996) concluded that problems with sustained concentration are usually related to lesions in the caudate nucleus; lesions in the frontal, temporal, and pari-etal lobes; and combined basal ganglia and brainstem lesions. Poor per-formance with focused (selective) concentration or distractibility is often linked to lesions in the frontal and temporal lobes and medial cortical and limbic pathways. Finally, Stinger (1996) suggested that difficulties with al-ternating or divided concentration are generally linked with diffuse brain lesions and lesions in the frontal and parietal lobes. Cutting-edge research using positron emission tomography (PET) is also adding to our under-standing of the mechanisms that control and direct concentration. One brain structure currently under scrutiny for its possible role in guiding con-centration is the pulvinar nucleus of the thalamus. However, further re-search is required to examine how the pulvinar is involved in mediating concentration and its relationship with other brain regions also thought to be responsible for concentration (Bear, Connors, & Paradiso, 1996).

CASE STUDY: JEN-LIN

BACKGROUND

This section of the chapter provides background information on the case study presented to illustrate one therapist's reasoning concerning evaluating and conducting intervention programs with clients who have disordered concentration. Although the "problem" that has been identified as the topic for this chapter is concentration, this approach of identifying an impairment is somewhat at odds with the way the therapist described in this chapter identifies the "problem" as being at the disability level. Rather than defining the problem as being reduced concentration, the therapist views it as being the difficulties the client has in performing her ADLs. Therefore, the reader is alerted to the conflict of focusing the chapter around the impairment of concentration versus the functional difficulties the client has that result from the impairment.

INTRODUCTION TO JEN-LIN

Although Jen-Lin was born in Vietnam, she immigrated to the United States at 5 years of age with her uncle, aunt, two cousins, and grandmother. Her parents died when she was 4 years old, and her aunt and uncle raised her. She is currently 35 years old and lives with her boyfriend, Peter, in an inner-city area. She sees her aunt, uncle, and cousins frequently. Jen-Lin works as a sales assistant in a store selling women's clothes. Both Jen-Lin and her boyfriend occasionally use the illegal narcotic cocaine. Jen-Lin was admitted to the emergency department at a large city hospital after an accidental overdose of this drug. Jen-Lin was with her boyfriend at the time of the overdose, and he called the ambulance some time later when he became aware that she was not breathing properly. Respiratory failure, thought to result from the inhibition of the medullary centers in the brain, can result from cocaine overdose (Dackis & Gold, 1990). The ambulance officers were able to revive Jen-Lin, but she experienced a brief period of hypoxia resulting in diffuse, mild brain damage. A computed tomography (CT) scan did not reveal any specific lesion sites. Often neurological clients who seem to recover quickly are discharged back into the community, where they may experience major problems in managing their ADLs. However, one of the doctors noted that Jen-Lin seemed to be having problems, and she was discharged to the rehabilitation facility the next day. On admission to the rehabilitation facility, Jen-Lin was able to walk and had normal control of her upper limbs. However, she appeared a little confused and could not recall what had happened to her.

THE THERAPY SETTING

After acute care, Jen-Lin was admitted to a dedicated rehabilitation facility with 50 beds. This state-funded rehabilitation facility specializes in evaluating and treating clients after acquired brain damage and spinal cord injury. Although it is unusual, clients may reside at this facility for up to 6 months and transfer from ward-based accommodation to independent living apartments before discharge to the community.

INTRODUCTION TO THE OCCUPATIONAL THERAPIST AND TREATMENT MODEL

Michael is a senior occupational therapist who works on one of the three main units at the rehabilitation facility. He supervises two junior occupational therapists and has had this job for 8 years. Michael uses a top-down, or compensatory/adaptive, approach to therapy and rarely uses standardized assessments with his clients. However, the hospital administration is putting increasing pressure on all therapists to use outcome measures, so Michael is now investigating standardized assessments that may be able to assist him in objectively documenting change in his clients' status over the course of their rehabilitation.

In Box 4–1 Michael provides a description of his approach to therapy which is "top-down," or adaptive and compensatory. He contrasts this approach with one that is more "bottom-up," or remedial. Michael's description is quite useful because it provides the reader with a comprehensive review of information regarding the approaches to intervention taken by all therapists in this book. At the moment, many occupational therapists are electing to use "top-down," or adaptive, approaches in therapy, having rejected "bottom-up," or remedial, approaches. However, it remains to be seen if this is a 1990s trend or a lasting shift in occupational therapy focus. In any case, many therapists confidently and competently work from a bottom-up perspective and have great success with their clients. Other therapists believe that it is possible to combine the two approaches (and we see examples of this in several of the chapters; refer in particular to Chapter 8, on evaluating and treating simple perceptual problems). This book strives to produce a balanced view and therefore presents a variety of approaches to evaluation and intervention with clients who have cognitive and perceptual dysfunction. Although Michael states that he relies on a variety of models to guide his

BOX 4–1. THERAPIST REASONING—SELECTION OF A THERAPEUTIC APPROACH

When I first graduated from occupational therapy school, I worked in a large, busy acute care hospital. I used a variety of remedial and adaptive approaches with my clients, who mostly had strokes, head injuries after motor vehicle accidents, or gunshot wounds causing damage to the brain or the spinal cord. But nowadays I mostly use the top-down or compensation/adaptive approach with clients. I suppose I came to using this approach because I found that my rehabilitation clients didn't respond particularly well to remedial approaches. I think that remedial approaches work better with clients who are in acute stages of recovery, but I have clients in therapy here for up to 6 months. These clients are working very slowly toward getting back to some sort of decent life in the community. The issues these clients face are about reintegrating into the community and this means facilitating the client to manage self-care and some basic instrumental activities of daily living (ADLs) (i.e., domestic and community activities) and having the social supports and leisure activities to have as good a quality of life as possible. I don't really see the point of targeting the underlying skills that the clients have problems with to any great extent. Rather, I want to look at each client's performance in activities that are important to them and work on these activities. My approach here has been very influenced by the writings of Giles (1992) and Giles & Clark-Wilson (1992), who describe the Neurofunctional Approach.

But having said all this, I think there are two limitations to using an adaptive/compensatory approach alone. First, I need to be able to interact with other team members, particularly the physiatrists and the neuropsychologists, and be able to "label" the client's "problems" as impairments as well as disabilities. In other words, I need to be able to confirm with colleagues that the client has a disorder of concentration or unilateral neglect or whatever, as well as to describe how this produces difficulties in performing self-care, instrumental (domestic and community) ADLs, or leisure activities. To overcome this problem, I'll use a hypothesis-testing approach when undertaking an initial activity with a client so I can determine what underlying skill deficits may be impacting on performance.

Another problem with using an adaptive or "top-down" approach in my work is that I don't use any standardized assessments. This is a concern at the moment because I'm under increasing pressure from my boss and the center's administration to demonstrate the outcome of occupational therapy on my unit. Because I work functionally, I've been investigating assessments that I can use with my clients that support this philosophy. It seems that AMPS (Assessment of Motor and Process Skills) (Fisher, 1997a) would be suitable, and I'm booked to do the course next month. I've also written to get the COPM (Law et al., 1994), and I'm following up on dynamic interaction assessment (Toglia, 1992b) to see if I can use this to document change in my clients' status over time. Since the early 1990s I've been influenced by Kielhofner's Model of Human Occupation (MOHO) (1995a) when working with clients. However, apart from the Interest Checklist (Kielhofner & Neville, 1983), I don't really use any of the assessments from this model either.

intervention, he believes that the neurofunctional approach as described by Giles and Clark Wilson (1992) offers him the most guidance when working with clients who have cognitive and perceptual problems. The neurofunctional approach to therapy was reviewed in Chapter 1, and aspects of this approach are described in this chapter in relation to therapy conducted.

DATA GATHERING

Michael reviewed Jen-Lin's medical record and spoke briefly to the nurse in charge of the unit before conducting an initial interview. This provided Michael with basic information concerning her medical and social background and her current status and behavior. The diagnosis noted in her medical file was mild diffuse brain damage after hypoxia due to drug overdose.

INITIAL INTERVIEW

Michael describes the purpose of an initial interview in Box 4–2. Michael uses interactive reasoning to try to get to know the client as a person and to begin to develop rapport with this person.

REPORTING INITIAL FINDINGS

Michael made the following entry in Jen-Lin's medical file after the initial interview:

Initial Interview:
Jen-Lin appears oriented to person and city but is not oriented to month or day. Reports a sketchy version of events that led to her hospitalization. Appears to be easily distracted (by the other client in the next bed and noises outside the room) and had difficulty recalling events from the previous day. Jen-Lin reported that she had trouble concentrating. Further evaluation in the area of cognitive and perceptual function is required. Jen-Lin's interests include clothes and fashion, shopping, gardening, and cooking. She works as a sales assistant in a women's clothing store. Communication notebook introduced and explained. Introductory occupational therapy information placed in notebook for boyfriend and other visitors. Requested they consult with Jen-Lin and bring in clothes for her to wear other than a nightgown.

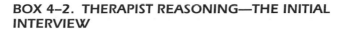

BOX 4–2. THERAPIST REASONING—THE INITIAL INTERVIEW

When I first meet the client, it's a good opportunity to begin to get to know him or her as a person and for them to get to know me. I start by introducing myself and providing a very basic description of my role at the center. I do a quick check of the client's orientation by asking him about who he is, where he is, the time and date, and so on. Then I start to gather information about the client's interests (based on the Interest Checklist [Kielhofner & Neville, 1983]) and his lifestyle. I might gather some background information on family, friends, work, and how the client feels about these. I also take note of the client's appearance (clothes and grooming, symmetry of posture, and so on]) because this tells me a lot about how they are doing at the moment. Depending on what I have observed, I may do a really quick physical and sensory assessment just to see if there are any problems in that area. Depending on how the interview has gone, I may also have detected some cognitive or perceptual problems, and I might deliberately focus some questions to gain more information in this area. At the initial interview, I also usually introduce a communication book. Relatives and friends often come to visit later in the evening, so I leave a communication notebook on the bedside table as a means of conveying information to the family about day-to-day events so they can discuss these with the client. I also leave my phone number in the book so they can call me whenever they wish. I try to establish a good relationship with the client in the initial interview—this is important because we will spend a lot of time together in therapy, and I want the client to feel comfortable.

THE SELECTION OF STANDARDIZED AND NONSTANDARDIZED ASSESSMENTS

As discussed previously, Michael does not use any standardized assessments to determine the presence or severity of cognitive and perceptual problems. However, he noted problems in the area of concentration and memory in the initial interview, and many therapists use assessments such as the Loewenstein Occupational Therapy Cognitive Assessment (LOTCA) (Itzkovich et al., 1990) or Chessington Occupational Therapy Neurological Assessment Battery (COTNAB) (Tyerman et al., 1986) to formally assess these problems. In addition, Table 4–1 provides a description of some of the standardized assessments that are specifically designed to determine if a client has a disorder of concentration (referred to as *attention*) and the type or types of disorder (e.g., sustained, focused, or

Table 4–1. Standardized Assessments of Concentration

NAME	SOURCE	DESCRIPTION
Stroop Test	Stroop (1935)	Clients are asked to identify the colors in which a list of words are printed. The color ink used does not correspond to the meaning of the word. For example, the word blue might appear in red ink, and the client must inhibit the natural tendency to read the word instead of reporting the color of the text. This assessment detects difficulties with selective concentration.
Test of Everyday Attention (TEA)	Robertson et al. (1994)	Composed of eight subtests: elevator counting, elevator counting with distractions, elevator counting with reversal, visual elevator, telephone search, telephone search while counting, map search, and lottery.
Random Letter Test from the Mental Status Examination	Strub & Black (1985)	A total of 60 letters are read at the rate of one per minute. Target letters are read at spaced intervals. The client is asked to indicate when the target letter is read.
Trail-making Test	US Army (1944)	The client is required to sequentially connect numbers (Part A) or letters and numbers (Part B) on a page of randomly placed numbers and letters. This assessment tests for divided concentration.
Symbol Digit Modalities Test	Smith (1982)	Using a code system, the client is asked to pair symbols with their corresponding number within 90 seconds. Normative data is available for individuals aged 18 to 78 years.
Paced Auditory Serial Attention Test (PASAT)	Gronwall (1977)	The subject is required to add pairs of digits presented at a predetermined rate. Sixty digits are presented in each trial. Based on the idea that concentrational problems will manifest when the amount of information to be processed per time available exceeds the individual's capacity. This assessment tests for sustained and divided concentration.

divided). All of these assessments have some data available to support their reliability and validity. Neuropsychologists generally administer the Stroop Test (Stroop, 1935), the Paced Auditory Serial Attention Test (PASAT) (Gronwall, 1977) and the Trail Making Test (US Army, 1944). In addition, neuropsychologists may administer various components of the Wechsler Adult Intelligence Scale-Revised (WAIS-R) Digit Span, or Spatial Span Subtest (Kaplan et al., 1991) to investigate problems of concentration (referred to as *attention*).

Rather than conduct a standardized assessment, Michael chose to undertake two nonstandardized functional evaluations with Jen-Lin: observations of ironing a shirt and making a sandwich. He chose these tasks in consultation with Jen-Lin given her need to take care of her clothes (to present well at work) and to take a sandwich to work each day. Michael reasoned that these evaluations would provide two types of information:

1. Jen-Lin's performance (abilities and problems) in both these ADLs, and
2. Details of the kinds of cognitive and perceptual impairments that might be limiting her performance. As stated earlier, Michael finds information on the impairments that limit a client's performance useful to present at the case conference team meeting.

The findings from the shirt ironing evaluation are documented below.

FUNCTIONAL EVALUATION: IRONING A SHIRT

Giles (1992) strongly emphasizes the importance of observation when evaluating clients. He points out that therapists often intervene too quickly before they have a chance to observe what the client can really do. To aid therapist observation, as well as begin to understand the kinds of impairments that might be limiting performance, a hypothesis-testing approach can be used (as described in Chapter 3). Michael used this approach with Jen-Lin during his evaluation of her ironing a shirt, and he wrote the results using three columns:

● Column 1 contains a description of the functional activity that is evaluated
● Column 2 contains observations and evaluation findings
● Column 3 contains competing hypotheses to explain evaluation findings. The best hypothesis is underlined or can be bolded

The findings of the shirt ironing evaluation are reported in Table 4–2.

(text continues on page 145)

Table 4–2. Observations of Jen-Lin Ironing a Shirt and Possible Hypotheses to Explain Performance

Context: This activity took place in the small client laundry room at the rehabilitation facility. The laundry room contains an iron and water jug on the shelf together with other laundry items such as washing liquid and fabric softener. The laundry also contains a separate dryer and washing machine, plus an ironing board. The laundry is a quiet room, and when the door is closed, it is free from distraction.

ACTIVITY PHASES	OBSERVATIONS	THERAPIST REASONING AND HYPOTHESES
Jen-Lin to set up the task of ironing a shirt in the laundry	Jen-Lin commenced by taking the shirt to the ironing board. She commented that she needed the iron and went over to the shelf. However, she began to pick up and look at several other items on the shelf. After a few minutes, Michael cued Jen-Lin verbally, by asking her what she was looking for. Jen-Lin looked blankly at Michael and then while looking around the room she saw the ironing board and shirt, which seemed to prompt her to say, "Oh . . . I'm looking for the iron," which she then located straight away.	Giles (1992) suggests that it is important to assess what the client would normally do, so I usually get the client to set up the task, rather than having everything ready. I think Jen-Lin is having problems concentrating on what she was doing. It looks like a problem of **selective concentration** because she was very distracted by the other items on the shelf when looking for the iron.
Attending to the iron (adding water and connecting to electricity)	Jen-Lin plugged in the iron and turned it on. She also checked the heat setting and commented that her shirt was cotton. She then stood back and commented that the iron would need to warm up. Jen-Lin did not put water in the iron, and Michael asked her about this.	Jen-Lin showed good problem-solving skills again by commenting that the iron needed to heat up. I was unsure whether she usually put water in the iron or not, and some irons don't require water, so I decided to check this with her.

(continues)

Table 4–2. Observations of Jen-Lin Ironing a Shirt and Possible Hypotheses to Explain Performance

ACTIVITY PHASES	OBSERVATIONS	THERAPIST REASONING AND HYPOTHESES
	Jen-Lin replied that she usually put water in the iron and asked Michael if there was a water jug. Again, Jen-Lin scanned the shelves for a long time until Michael cued her to find the small plastic jug.	Again, Jen-Lin seemed distracted by the items on the shelf and seemed to be having a problem with **selective concentration.**
Laying out the shirt	After several moments, the iron was ready to use, yet Jen-Lin did not start the task. She asked Michael questions about the hospital and how long he had been there. Eventually the iron hissed and steam rose from the top, which seemed to draw her back to the ironing task. She started by laying out a sleeve to iron.	Again, external cueing (this time from the iron) seemed to be required for Jen-Lin to continue with the task. I did not want to cue her this time because I really wanted to see how long it would take for her to return to the shirt. She seemed **distracted** by the conversation.
Ironing the first sleeve	Jen-Lin began ironing the sleeve. Michael asked Jen-Lin about how she usually ironed a shirt, the order and so on. She stopped what she was doing and told Michael that she usually ironed the sleeves, then front and back, and then the collar last.	I wanted to get an idea of how Jen-Lin usually ironed a shirt so I could get some idea of what her performance should be like, so I asked her about this. I also wanted to see if she could manage talking and ironing at the same time. I suspected she also had a problem with **divided concentration** and therefore would not be able to do this. She stopped the ironing and set it down to respond (I noted that the iron was set down safely but will need to watch for safety issues).

(continues)

(continued)

Table 4–2. Observations of Jen-Lin Ironing a Shirt and Possible Hypotheses to Explain Performance

ACTIVITY PHASES	OBSERVATIONS	THERAPIST REASONING AND HYPOTHESES
Ironing the second sleeve	Jen-Lin stopped ironing the second sleeve and looked up as Michael scratched his face. She oriented her gaze to his hand. She asked him how long he had been married. She did not stand the iron up this time when she stopped ironing. Michael suggested that Jen-Lin look at whether the iron was safe or not and then suggested that it was probably better that she finish the ironing and then they could talk some more.	Although Jen-Lin seemed to be doing a good job with the ironing, she was quite distracted by my scratching my face, and she stopped ironing. She probably noticed my wedding ring at this stage because she asked me how long I had been married. She seemed sidetracked by this irrelevant idea. This again signalled **selective concentration** problems. When she stopped ironing this time, she did not put the iron back in its correct position, which was a safety hazard.
Ironing the back of the shirt and the front panels	At this point, the back of the shirt front became a bit tangled with the sleeves. Jen-Lin swore loudly and slammed the iron down on the table. She immediately apologized.	At this point Jen-Lin needed to straighten the shirt with one hand and iron with the other. Again, a **divided concentration** problem became evident as she could not manage both of these. I think her swearing outburst showed more than a usual response to frustration, possibly signalling a problem with **adaptive behavior.** It was good to see that she apologized—it seems that she has some insight into this behavior.

(continues)

Table 4–2. Observations of Jen-Lin Ironing a Shirt and Possible Hypotheses to Explain Performance

ACTIVITY PHASES	OBSERVATIONS	THERAPIST REASONING AND HYPOTHESES
Ironing the collar and hanging up the shirt	Jen-Lin did not seem to have any particular difficulty with the final phases of ironing the shirt, although she appeared to be fatiguing. After hanging up the shirt, Jen-Lin stopped and asked Michael questions about the facility and other questions similar to those she had asked at the beginning of the session.	By this time Jen-Lin was looking a bit tired, and I expected her performance to deteriorate accordingly. However, she managed to iron the collar and hang up the shirt. I was not surprised that she asked me questions similar to those she had asked just half an hour earlier. Given that she seems to be having problems with **concentrating,** she is therefore probably not going to **remember** new information. She did seem to manage the whole task, and I don't think she is having problems with sustained concentration. This is consistent with her diagnosis of mild brain damage.
Packing up the iron	Jen-Lin held her shirt in her hand and declared she was ready to take it back to her room. Michael asked her if everything was packed up from the task. Jen-Lin looked around her and noticed the iron and that it was still on. She tried to unplug it with one hand while still holding the shirt but couldn't manage it.	At this point I think Jen-Lin was tired, and I cued her to put the shirt down so she could unplug the iron and empty the water. Again this showed signs of **divided concentration** deficit.

(continues)

Table 4–2. Observations of Jen-Lin Ironing a Shirt and Possible Hypotheses to Explain Performance

ACTIVITY PHASES	OBSERVATIONS	THERAPIST REASONING AND HYPOTHESES
Returning to her room after therapy	Jen-Lin seemed unable to find her way back to her room from the laundry room despite having walked the route on several occasions. She commented that she could not seem to find her way back. Michael cued her to identify a landmark near her room so that she could use the hospital signs to assist her to get to that point. She eventually used the hospital garden courtyard signs to find her way to her room (Jen-Lin's room is located right next to the courtyard).	Although Jen-Lin seems to be having trouble with **topographical orientation,** I think it's really because she doesn't **concentrate** on which way she is going so that she can't find her way around the hospital. Her performance improved significantly when I cued her to use the signs to find her way to the courtyard. Her room is just near the courtyard, and she located her room easily from there.

STRENGTHS AND PROBLEMS

From the shirt ironing and sandwich making evaluations and the interview with Jen-Lin, Michael concluded that Jen-Lin would have difficulties completing the majority of the more complex domestic and community ADLs. Jen-Lin and Michael identified that the most important functional problems she was experiencing were:

- Clothes maintenance (ironing and repairs)
- Managing retail tasks at the clothing store where she works (i.e., customer interactions and demands, managing the phone, and managing money)
- Cooking simple meals
- Finding her way around the rehabilitation facility (Michael noted the need to assess **topographical orientation** on their outings in the community as well as in the hospital and to determine whether this problem was compounded by or due to reduced concentration)

From the hypothesis-testing approach taken in the shirt ironing evaluation, Michael concluded that the impairments that underpinned Jen-Lin's functional difficulties related to:

- Being unable to ignore distractions (i.e., focused concentration)
- Being unable to do more than one thing at a time (i.e., divided concentration)
- Reduced short-term and long-term memory (see Chapter 5) and new learning (both probably stemming from concentration problems)
- Being unsafe while undertaking tasks and behaving appropriately, such as outbursts of swearing (i.e., adaptive behavior problems/executive abilities) (see Chapter 6)

These problems were confirmed by the neuropsychologist's report from standardized testing and seem consistent with a diagnosis of mild brain damage.

Jen-Lin's strengths included:

- Some insight into her problems; therefore, she was motivated and cooperative in therapy
- A supportive boyfriend who visited her regularly and seemed eager to assist in the therapy program
- Normal motor and sensory capacities (some slowness detected initially quickly resolved)
- Normal speech and language
- An employer holding her job for her

LONG-TERM GOALS AND SHORT-TERM OBJECTIVES

Together Michael and Jen-Lin negotiated the problems they would work on in therapy. Some compromises were necessary because Jen-Lin could not really understand the extent of the problems she would have when returning to work. Michael and Jen-Lin agreed that they would examine these problems further.

The following long-term goals were established:

- Jen-Lin will be independent in managing maintenance of her clothes
- Jen-Lin will be able to cook meals (using her recipe collection)
- Jen-Lin will be able to return to her job at the clothes store at least part-time
- Jen-Lin will be able to find her way around the facility and her community

A variety of short-term objectives were set for each therapy session relating to these long-term goals. In particular, the following objectives were set for three sessions specific to task described below (sorting recipes).

Jen-Lin, given a structured environment, verbal cueing from the therapist, a schedule for taking rest breaks. and written instructions to help her to concentrate, will be able to:

- Successfully devise a system for organizing her loose recipes
- Organize the recipes according to her system
- Assemble a card system in a box and arrange her recipes

INTERVENTION STRATEGIES AND ACTIVITIES

Although Jen-Lin is experiencing some memory problems, occasional outbursts of swearing, and difficulties finding her way around, the emphasis of this chapter is on problems with concentration. Therefore, the intervention section is more directed at this impairment and the resulting problems Jen-Lin has in managing at home and returning to work. Since Michael follows a neurofunctional approach to therapy, the intervention described below is mainly adaptive, or "top-down," in nature. For other treatment ideas that are remedial, the reader is referred to Wood (1987); Mateer, Sohlberg, and Youngman (1990); and Okkema (1993).

GENERAL INTERVENTION STRATEGIES

In general, the following ideas are helpful when using a top-down, or adaptive, approach to working with clients who have concentration problems:

- One therapist works with the client at a time (multiple therapists or assistants provide too many opportunities for distraction).
- The therapist needs to cue the client verbally when he is about to make an unexpected move or, when another distraction is imminent, the therapist needs to redirect the client's attention to the task.
- Activities that are interesting to the client will increase capacity to concentrate.
- Self-talk can be a useful strategy for the client to keep himself on track. For example, teach the client to cue himself to concentrate: "I must really concentrate and finish this [label] component of the activity." This may be enhanced by having the client verbalize the steps of the activity aloud. This can be downgraded to sub-vocal after the client is accustomed to this approach.
- Verbal feedback is important so the client can adjust his performance and maintain adequate concentration.
- Provide information in short blocks with pauses so that the client can absorb information. Teach the client to request that other people present information in this way.
- Make checklists with the client for tasks he undertakes regularly. Practice using these to ensure the client has success in completing tasks.
- Provide a diary or notebook so clients can write down important information (this strategy assists with concentration as well as memory).
- Grade activities. Table 4–3 contains a variety of ways to downgrade activities when working with clients who have concentration problems. (This table builds on Table 1–9.) To upgrade activities, simply remove some of the assisting mechanisms or prompts.

(Sohlberg & Mateer, 1989; Cohen & Mapou, 1988; Ponsford, Sloan, & Snow, 1995; van Zomeren & Brouwer, 1994; Zoltan, 1996).

SELECTION OF THERAPEUTIC ACTIVITIES WITH JEN-LIN

Michael and Jen-Lin discussed the kinds of activities that they would use in therapy. The highest-priority activities related to their goals of managing her clothes, returning to work, cooking meals, and finding her

Table 4–3. Grading Activities with Clients with Concentration Problems

If using a remedial approach, upgrade as client skill improves.
If using an adaptive approach, upgrade as the client puts strategies in place to
  compensate for difficulties.

VARIABLE	WAYS TO DOWNGRADE ACTIVITY DEMANDS AND THEN GRADUALLY INCREASE THESE
Therapist	• Provide visual or verbal prompts to assist or encourage the client to concentrate and gradually withdraw these.
	• Provide visual or verbal prompts to assist or encourage the client to shift focus from one aspect of the task to another in a logical way and gradually withdraw these.
	• Provide the client with feedback regarding performance.
	• Provide information to the client in short sentences with pauses in between sentences so the client has the time to process the information. Gradually increase the amount of information and the speed with which it is delivered.
Task	• Build regular rest breaks into the task and reduce these as performance improves.
	• Attempt the activity when the client's energy levels are the highest (e.g., at a time of day when the client is refreshed), then attempt when the client is more fatigued or when there are other competing demands.
	• Provide repetition of information or instructions for the task and gradually withdraw this.
	• Reduce the amount and complexity of information to be dealt with and then gradually increase the complexity of information.
	• Change activities regularly to maintain interest and then spend increasing amounts of time on activities.
	• Provide more than adequate time for the activity to reduce the stress of time pressure and gradually reduce the time available to a more reasonable period.
Environment	• Modify the environment to reduce the number of distractions or move to a quiet room. Gradually introduce normal distractions such as music or other people talking nearby.
	• Conduct activities in an appropriate environment. For example, cooking is done in the kitchen (generally there is no need to upgrade this by changing environments).

way around. In addition, Michael and Jen-Lin identified several other leisure activities that they could use in therapy. These activities related to gardening (one of her leisure activities) and managing her recipes. Jen-Lin seemed reluctant to do gardening at first but became more interested when Michael showed her the outdoor courtyard area with raised garden beds (for wheelchair access) and the small shed with all the necessary gardening equipment. Jen-Lin explained that she had thought they would only be able to pot small plants in the therapy department. Michael noted that this showed good problem-solving skills. Jen-Lin saw several other clients doing woodwork and ceramic activities and said she did not want to be involved in any of those. Michael explained that Jen-Lin would only be involved in activities that she was interested in or that she identified she had problems with.

Jen-Lin's boyfriend, Peter, brought in her recipe box, which was full of magazine and newspaper clippings of recipes and hand-written recipes from friends. He suggested that Jen-Lin had always complained that she could never find the recipe she wanted. Michael and Jen-Lin decided that they could organize the recipes as a therapy activity. Michael reasoned that Jen-Lin would need to follow recipes carefully in the future as a way to help her concentrate on cooking. It seemed to be important to have a well-organized recipe system that Jen-Lin could add to in the future.

Three days after Jen-Lin's admission, she and Michael tackled the task of creating an organized system for Jen-Lin's recipe's. Table 4–4 provides a description of Jen-Lin and Michael's development of the recipe box as well as some of Michael's reasoning connected with it. This activity was conducted over several therapy sessions. Although this activity requires the use of many cognitive and perceptual skills, it was also selected as an intrinsically interesting and meaningful task to Jen-Lin and an activity she would continue with in the future.

In addition, Michael and Jen-Lin set up a number of simulated work environments that demanded skills such as money handling and managing the phone. Michael eventually upgraded these tasks so that Jen-Lin had to deal with more than one task at a time, such as answering the phone while completing a customer sale. Toward the end of Jen-Lin's therapy, Michael arranged for Jen-Lin to spend some time in the therapy department office answering the phone and taking messages. Jen-Lin also spent several sessions working in the volunteers shop at the facility selling small craft items.

(text continues on page 156)

Table 4–4. The Activity of Making a Recipe Box: Strategies and Therapist Reasoning

This activity ran over five 1-hour therapy sessions over 3 days in an individual treatment room. In between steps 1 and 2, Jen-Lin and Michael shopped for necessary items at the local mall. Michael used this shopping session as a therapeutic activity and worked with Jen-Lin on money management, interacting with the store assistant, and finding her way to and from the mall. Over the course of the five sessions, improvements in Jen-Lin's performance were noted.

ACTIVITY STEPS AND PROBLEMS EXPERIENCED	STRATEGIES TO OVERCOME DIFFICULTIES	THERAPIST REASONING
1. Planning the task and gathering the equipment • unsure of where to start • difficulty finding the glue, scissors, and pen in the equipment cupboard	Devise a checklist of written instructions for the task with Jen-Lin; she can tick these off as the task progresses. Verbally cue Jen-Lin to find the items in the cupboard or have a written checklist of all the items that are to be collected. Provide regular feedback throughout the task.	Cooking is an activity that is meaningful to Jen-Lin and therefore motivating. She has expressed a wish to sort her recipes. I think that in the future she will need to follow her recipes carefully as a way to help her concentrate on her cooking. The task can also be structured so that it can easily be up- or downgraded in complexity. It is important to teach clients to break tasks down into steps so they can see what is to be done and manage the task more easily. As occupational therapists we are used to doing this all the time, so it's not too difficult to teach this to clients. Having a structured task means that there is less opportunity for the client to become "lost" with what he is doing and get distracted.

(continues)

(continued)

Table 4–4. The Activity of Making a Recipe Box: Strategies and Therapist Reasoning

ACTIVITY STEPS AND PROBLEMS EXPERIENCED	STRATEGIES TO OVERCOME DIFFICULTIES	THERAPIST REASONING
		try to provide immediate, noncritical feedback for all my clients on a regular basis. I try to let Jen-Lin know when she is doing well, as well as when she is having problems. I am also encouraging her boyfriend Peter and her family to provide feedback in this way as well. It is often the case that feedback from the family is more meaningful than from the therapist.
Shopping task: as a separate therapy activity, purchase a box with three sets of normal cards and one set of divider cards	The reader can devise therapeutic goals, strategies and reasoning behind this shopping activity.	
2. Devise a list (index) of all the categories of recipes required in the box	This written index will act as a guide for sorting out the recipes.	Since we had talked about the overall structure of the task, Jen-Lin had a pretty good idea how she wanted to structure the recipe box. She decided to divide the recipes into courses. Furthermore, she divided the main course recipes by the types of foods (e.g., fish, chicken, beef).
• seemed distracted by other activities going on in the therapy department	Work in a separate therapy room, which is isolated from the busy, noisy therapy department.	

(continues)

152

Table 4–4. The Activity of Making a Recipe Box: Strategies and Therapist Reasoning

ACTIVITY STEPS AND PROBLEMS EXPERIENCED	STRATEGIES TO OVERCOME DIFFICULTIES	THERAPIST REASONING
	Encourage Jen-Lin to use her strengths, such as problem-solving skills, to assist her in successfully completing the task.	She placed the index at the front of the box but quickly forgot the index categories she had created. I cued Jen-Lin to use her problem-solving skills to overcome this problem. She eventually decided that she needed the index on the table with her so she could follow it.
3. Sorting the recipes into categories (soups, starters, mains, desserts) • while trying to find the correct category for one recipe, Jen-Lin was continually distracted by the content of the recipes and their pictures • difficulty talking with therapist while doing the task	Teach the client to use self-instructional techniques and self-monitoring techniques to keep on track with tasks. This technique can be used with several activities, and when the client is used to this approach, he may eventually generalize this skill to a full range of activities. This component of the activity allows a lot of opportunity for repetition, which is important for clients who have concentration problems. Repetition provides more opportunity for material to be remembered. Cue client to concentrate on one task at a time and to chat with people only during breaks in the task.	Teaching clients to use self-instructional and self-monitoring techniques is quite demanding. Not all clients are going to get to the point where this will be possible. I am working with Jen-Lin to say aloud (verbalize) what she is doing as a way of keeping herself on track. Eventually we'll downgrade this to make it subvocal. Jen-Lin has been practicing to think about what she is doing every ten minutes or so. This way, when she does get off track she can bring herself back to what she was doing. I find that when clients have the opportunity to repeat components of activities, they are more likely to remember them. For example, having worked with the index system to sort recipes

(continues)

Table 4–4. The Activity of Making a Recipe Box: Strategies and Therapist Reasoning

ACTIVITY STEPS AND PROBLEMS EXPERIENCED	STRATEGIES TO OVERCOME DIFFICULTIES	THERAPIST REASONING
		(e.g., entrees or chicken dishes) for the past two sessions, Jen-Lin hardly needs to refer to this anymore. She has learned where each pile of recipes is placed. Although this is not a very functional example, I can see the same thing occurring in her other activities, such as money handling and clothes maintenance tasks.
4. Sorting recipes within categories (sorting dishes within the main course section such as fish, vegetarian, chicken, beef)	Verbal cueing to assist Jen-Lin to stay on track.	Jen-Lin is not usually distracted by herself so much as by other people. Although it is quite usual to ask others about themselves, it's the way Jen-Lin suddenly seems to notice something and stop what she is doing that really makes it seem like a distraction. It was the same when she noticed my wedding ring during the ironing assessment. The good thing is that when I point out this distraction to her, she is usually able to cue herself verbally to get back to what she was doing. Although she needs some help with this at the moment, she is certainly improving in using this technique.
• distracted by Michael's shirt		
• frustration outburst (on tearing one of the recipes) with swearing		

(continues)

154

Table 4–4. The Activity of Making a Recipe Box: Strategies and Therapist Reasoning

ACTIVITY STEPS AND PROBLEMS EXPERIENCED	STRATEGIES TO OVERCOME DIFFICULTIES	THERAPIST REASONING
		I find it best to ignore these outbursts. Jen-Lin seems to be aware they are inappropriate, and the number of outbursts is reducing.
5. **Writing recipe names onto tops of cards and gluing recipes onto them** • periodically stops gluing recipes onto cards and reads recipe or comments on a picture • distracted by noise outside the room, rises out of seat, and looks toward the door • appears to be fatiguing	Employ similar strategies to those outlined in Step 3 above. Try to alert Jen-Lin to possible distractions in advance so that she is aware of them but is able to keep working. A rest break system also needs to be introduced to maximize performance.	I think it's important for clients with concentration problems to take regular rest breaks. It's also really important to encourage clients to eventually monitor this themselves. I'll start the client off by suggesting a 5-minute break every 15 minutes, and by the time they are taking breaks only every 30 minutes or so, then I'll get the client to start to monitor it themselves.
6. **Write each recipe onto the main index card and then assemble the box with index at front and cards in their place**	Jen-Lin is experiencing very few difficulties and is taking regular rest breaks herself. This seems to be greatly increasing her capacity to concentrate on tasks.	I notice for the first time that Jen-Lin did not stop what she was doing (writing the names on the recipe cards) and look up when I asked her about Peter's work. Since she has been in rehabilitation for over a week now, I am deliberately trying to challenge Jen-Lin more to see if she can manage

(continued)

Table 4–4. The Activity of Making a Recipe Box: Strategies and Therapist Reasoning

ACTIVITY STEPS AND PROBLEMS EXPERIENCED	STRATEGIES TO OVERCOME DIFFICULTIES	THERAPIST REASONING
		doing more than one task at a time (e.g., converse and do a task). Jen-Lin really seems to be fatiguing by the end of her fifth session on this recipe box task. This final session took place in the afternoon when Jen-Lin has more trouble keeping on track with tasks. I'm impressed that she was able to monitor this and ask for rest breaks. Although tired, she wanted to finish the task so she could show visitors that evening. Jen-Lin commented that she was keen to show the completed box to her boyfriend Peter and to her aunt, who also loves to cook.

THE USE OF COMPUTERS IN RETRAINING CONCENTRATION

Although Michael does not use computers as part of his intervention, many occupational therapists do use them to assist clients in overcoming a variety of cognitive and perceptual deficits, including problems with concentration. Owing to the popularity and controversy surrounding the use of computers in the retraining of cognitive and perceptual skills, this area is briefly mentioned in this chapter. First, it must be noted that therapists who use computer programs to retrain clients in cognitive and perceptual skills are working from a "bottom-up," or remedial, perspective. That is, these therapists believe that recovery of concentration skills is possible through direct retraining activities. Although some researchers have demonstrated minor improvements in clients' performance on concentration tasks after computer retraining, many others have not found this to be the case (refer to reviews by Ponsford, 1990 and Gauggel & Niemann, 1996). Others suggest that even if there are improvements in performance, they may not generalize from computer tasks to other real-world activities such as dressing or shopping (Stringer, 1996). This reasoning explains why many therapists do not choose to use computer rehabilitation activities. However, programs that are commonly used in computer-based retraining of concentration are "React" and "Search" (Gianutsos & Klitzner, 1981). The reader is referred to Ponsford and Kinsella (1988) and Sohlberg and Mateer (1989) for information on using these programs. Advantages of including computer-based rehabilitation in a total intervention program include the objectivity, accuracy, and immediacy of feedback that a computer can provide. Moreover, the client gains feedback and information from a source other than the therapist. An overview of computer-enhanced cognitive rehabilitation is presented by Molloy (1994).

PROGRESS REPORT AND MEASURING THE OUTCOME OF THERAPY

Over a 3-week period, Jen-Lin made significant gains. Her performance on simulated work tasks increased significantly, as did her ability to maintain her clothes and cook meals using her recipe cards. Many of her concentration problems seemed to resolve. Spontaneous recovery of concentration problems after brain damage is frequently reported (Ponsford & Kinsella, 1988). In areas in which Jen-Lin was still having difficulties, further compensatory strategies were initiated. The rehabilitation team met to discuss her progress and unanimously agreed to recommend discharge. Before her discharge, she spent a weekend at home with her boy-friend, Peter. Before her weekend leave, Michael spent time with Jen-Lin and Peter talking about the kinds of strategies that had worked well in therapy (such as self-cueing) so they would both be aware of problems that might arise and ways they might solve various problems.

The weekend was very successful, and Jen-Lin and Peter reported only a few problems. For example, they had been to see a film in the evening and Jen-Lin said she was tired and found it hard to follow the plot. She and Peter decided they would try to see films in the afternoon when Jen-Lin was not so tired and that they would sit near the back of the movies so Peter could talk to her to help her with understanding the plot. Peter also reported that Jen-Lin seemed to have trouble sensing his moods. It has been proposed that these very subtle changes in clients after brain damage are due to an inability to concentrate on secondary cues. Clients are occupied with concentrating on the main cues and therefore miss more subtle information (van Zomeren & Brouwer, 1994). For example, Jen-Lin may be concentrating on Peter's sitting quietly and listening to music but may be unable to attend to the fact that he appears sad or unhappy.

Before writing Jen-Lin's discharge report, Michael reflected on how he documents the outcomes of therapy (Box 4–3). This approach was also described in Chapter 3.

DISCHARGE

The following discharge summary was placed in Jen-Lin's file:

Discharge Summary:
Jen-Lin has made many improvements over her 3-week stay on the rehabilitation unit. Four long-term goals were set relating to clothes maintenance, cooking meals, returning to her job, and finding her way around the facility. With written cues, Jen-Lin is now able to care for her clothes. Using a set of recipes created in therapy, Jen-Lin is able to cook meals with only distant supervision for safety. Plans have been made for Jen-Lin to be involved in a graded return-to-work program, which will be monitored. She is independently able to find her way around the facility. Jen-Lin and her friends and family also report improvements and are pleased that Jen-Lin is returning home. Jen-Lin will attend occupational therapy as an outpatient for 1 hour per week each second week for 2 months to ensure she maintains gains made in therapy at home.

Several days before Jen-Lin's discharge, Michael also suggested that the couple might like to spend some time with the facility's counselor to

BOX 4–3. THERAPIST REASONING—DOCUMENTING CLIENT OUTCOMES

When I'm trying to document the outcome of therapy with a client, I usually go back to the goals we set and determine whether or not these have been met. I also ask the client about his or her perceptions of progress, and finally I ask the family about the improvements they have noted. I am going to take the AMPS course and use the COPM (as described earlier). If I find these assessments useful, then I'll administer them at the client's admission and discharge and use this as another indicator of outcome. In summary then, the way I determine if change has occurred is to:

● evaluate if intervention goals and objectives have been met,

● ask the client and their family about their perceptions of improvements, and

● reassess using standardized assessments if appropriate.

However, the limitation with these approaches to measuring outcome is that I'm simply documenting that change has occurred. What I also need are some ways to determine whether these changes are due to therapy or to other factors such as spontaneous recovery or the influence of friends and family on the client.

discuss drug use. Although they refused this service on the grounds that they would not be using drugs in the future, Michael reinforced that this service was available should they decide to use it any time in the future. Jen-Lin was discharged after 3 weeks as an inpatient. She agreed to visit Michael as an outpatient once every 2 weeks for a 1-hour appointment to review her progress and deal with any problems.

FUTURE RECOMMENDATIONS

To try to maximize Jen-Lin's successful reintegration into home and work, Michael was involved in supervising a return-to-work program he had negotiated with Jen-Lin and her employer. To begin, Jen-Lin returned to work for only 2 hours per day for 3 days each week. This was in the mornings, when Jen-Lin felt her concentration was at its best.

One problem that Jen-Lin and Michael had worked on overcoming in therapy was ignoring distractions from background music. Jen-Lin knew that music was always played in the store. She and Michael devised a system in which she would carry a small clipboard in the store to write down customer requests and to keep track of the women in the store. She also wrote down phone messages and orders on this clipboard. At the end of each day she reviewed her notes and followed up on any orders to be placed. Each item was checked off on completion. She also carried small cards in her pockets detailing all her work tasks and the items connected with each as a **prompt.** Although she rarely used these, she felt safe because they were in her pocket. After 3 weeks, Jen-Lin felt confident enough to discard these. Gradually, over an 8-week period her work hours were increased until she was working 5 hours a day, 5 days per week. Jen-Lin felt this was enough for her at that time, and her employer was sufficiently happy with her work to agree to this plan indefinitely. This work routine was to be reviewed in 6 months' time.

Peter agreed to drive Jen-Lin to the clothes store and pick her up afterward on the days she was working. However, in the long term, Michael noted that Jen-Lin would need a driving assessment to determine her suitability to return to driving. Michael was relieved that Jen-Lin agreed that she was not yet ready to drive. Many clients lack the insight to know when they cannot drive, and this can cause considerable difficulties for the client and therapist at discharge.

SUMMARY

Many clients, particularly those with concentration problems, may not realize the full impact of their difficulties until they try to resume their lives on discharge from rehabilitation. Clients with concentration problems (and resulting difficulties with memory and learning) can appear so normal that family and work colleagues forget to make simple concessions such as structuring the environment or providing occasional cueing or feedback. Concentration problems are an important area for therapists to assess and treat. Simple solutions can make a world of difference to how clients manage their ADLs. This chapter presented background information on normal concentration and problems with concentration after brain damage. It presented the case study of Jen-Lin to illustrate one occupational therapist's approach to evaluation and intervention of a client who has problems with concentration.

REVIEW QUESTIONS

The seven questions that follow the case study "Harry" can be used to guide intervention with any client who has a cognitive and perceptual problem. However, use these questions to devise an occupational therapy intervention for Harry:

The client: "Harry," a 48-year-old man.

Medical details: Harry experienced a closed-head injury with loss of consciousness for 2 days and posttraumatic amnesia for 6 days after a motor car accident 10 weeks ago. The CT scan showed frontal hematoma, contusions, and subarachnoid blood; lesion in right parietal lobe; fractured base of skull; severe scalp lacerations (L); pneumothorax; and lung contusion. Currently, Harry is an inpatient at a rehabilitation hospital. He is receiving occupational therapy, physical therapy, and speech-language therapy.

Social situation: Harry's wife was killed in the car accident. He has a home in the suburbs and two children, a 13-year-old son and a 15-year-old daughter. (The children were not in the car at the time of the accident.)

Education: Completed an arts degree at community college.

Employment: Employed as a senior floor salesman for a liquor merchant. Duties include supervision of three staff, serving customers, and accounts and inventory management. Staff supportive of his return to work.

Physical status: Walks independently without aids; full control of upper limbs.

Cognitive status: Ten weeks after the accident, Harry is oriented and alert; however, he has difficulties remembering lengthy instructions. He needs external cues to follow the therapy program and is slow to learn new skills, requiring frequent repetition and practice. Harry requires either supervision or assistance with all ADLs. He demonstrates intact perceptual skills during activities such as cooking. Harry is slow to organize himself in all activities and unable to consider numerous elements in a task simultaneously. He is generally unable to recognize errors but is able to correct them. He often seeks assistance rather than solve problems on his own. He has occasional angry outbursts and has made inappropriate comments to staff. He also exhibits some difficulties in social situations. For example, he tends to talk over people and doesn't wait his turn in a conversation. Harry has superficial insight into his cognitive problems and can understand their implications if given concrete examples (e.g., slowness affecting work efficiency).

1. Provide a background summary that includes all relevant information.
2. What standardized and informal assessment methods might an occupational therapist use to assess this client's capacities and abilities?
3. As a result of conducting both functional and standardized assessments, you find that Harry has problems with several personal and **instrumental activities of daily living** (IADLs). In order to identify the specific problems that he has in an activity (and the cognitive deficits that produce these difficulties), use the hypothesis-testing approach. Use a three-column table to present this information.

- In column one, write a functional activity that the client has problems with
- In column two, write your observations and evaluation findings
- In column three, write your competing hypotheses; underline the best hypotheses for each problem

4. Write a list of functional problems the client has and possible impairments. (From your hypothesis testing above, column three of your table will provide you with this problem list—these will be the underlined hypotheses). In addition to this, provide a brief list of strengths (include information from the history as well as standardized assessments and hypothesis testing).
5. Based on your problem list, devise two long-term treatment goals. For each goal, write two behavioral objectives that can be achieved in one intervention session
6. Select one treatment activity for the client for a 45- to 60-minute intervention session. This activity will address one or more of your objectives. Provide a rationale for the selection of this activity (both therapeutic and other reasons). Provide information on the cognitive, motor, and sensory demands of the activity.
7. In a table, write out each step for the activity. Next, describe the problems that the client might have with this activity. In the third column, provide details of the intervention strategies you would use to address this client's cognitive difficulties at each step. Be specific in your strategies, providing a clear understanding as to how they could be integrated into your chosen activity. For example, do not say, "Provide client with external verbal cues"; instead, clarify *how* and *when* you would provide external verbal cues. Specify how you would upgrade and/or downgrade the step or strategy based on the client's performance *during* each activity step.

≡ ACKNOWLEDGMENTS

I would like to thank my colleague Ursula Winzeler for discussions that helped to refine the hypothesis-testing format used in this chapter.

5

Evaluation and Intervention with Memory and Learning Impairments

BEATRIZ C. ABREU, PhD, OTR, FAOTA

- Anterograde Amnesia
- Contextual Interference
- Contextual Congruence
- Learning
- Macro Perspective
- Memory
- Metacognition
- Metamemory

- Micro Perspective
- Quadraphonic Approach
- Retrograde Amnesia
- Taxonomies

On completion of this chapter, the reader will be able to:

- Define memory and learning
- Describe the anatomical basis for memory and learning
- Outline at least three taxonomies used to classify disorders of memory and three taxonomies used to classify disorders of learning
- Describe the features of the quadraphonic approach to therapy
- Successfully work through the Review Questions

≡ INTRODUCTION

The aim of this chapter is to present an approach to assessment and treatment of clients whose memory or learning capacity has been affected by brain injury. It begins by outlining some of the rudimentary knowledge from which a therapist draws: the basics of neuroanatomy and neurophysiology and a catalogue of memory and learning taxonomies. It then addresses current research trends in the areas of memory and learning. Finally, the case study of Evelyn is presented. The case study opens with a review of the theoretical basis for the quadraphonic approach for the evaluation and treatment of memory and learning impairments. The evaluation and intervention procedures used with Evelyn illustrate how to incorporate the quadraphonic approach in a clinical setting.

☰ THE THEORY OF MEMORY AND LEARNING

WHAT IS MEMORY AND LEARNING?

Broadly defined, **memory** is the capacity to store experiences and perceptions for recall and recognition. At the neurocellular level, it is a functional property of any nervous system component that aids in retaining information (Farber & Abreu, 1993; Fuster, 1995). Memory has been broken down into three activities: acquisition or learning, storage or retention, and retrieval or recall (Wickelgren, 1977). **Learning** has been described as a relatively permanent change in the capacity for responding that, resulting from practice and experience, persists with time, resists environmental changes, and can be generalized in response to new tasks and situations (Schmidt, 1988). Learning allows an individual to cope with the ever-changing demands of the environment (Farber & Abreu, 1993). Like memory, learning is an internal process: it can only be inferred based on observed behaviors (Schmidt, 1988). Researchers differ on the relationship between learning and memory. From one perspective, learning is only the initial stage of memory and, thus, is of a lower order (Lezak, 1995). However, although some have described learning as a higher process than memory, others have argued that they are of the same rank order (Fuster, 1995; Schmidt, 1988; Wickelgren, 1977).

Another issue among researchers is the relationship between learning, memory, and intelligence. One group traced the historical view of these relationships. In the 1920s, there was widespread agreement regarding a link. In the 1940s, the prevalent view was that learning was less a function of intelligence than of practice. In the 1960s, researchers came to understand learning as a non-unitary phenomenon. They believed that learning consists of different combinations of multiple processes that may or may not be linked to intelligence (Campione, Brown, & Bryant, 1985). Although theories and views have changed over time, neuroanatomical and neurophysiological processes are widely accepted. This chapter reviews some of them.

THE NEUROANATOMY AND NEUROPHYSIOLOGY OF MEMORY AND LEARNING

The nervous system is an organized constellation of nerve or neural cells and associated non-neural cells that function to receive, integrate, and transmit the impulses that comprise perception. Neurons act as this system's communicators, not by relaying impulses through direct contact but by bridging tiny gaps or synapses through chemical or electrical means. In the case of chemical synapses, neurons secrete substances that transverse the gap; in the case of electrical synapses, neural communication involves a flow of electrical current.

One traditional perspective of the nervous system, the hierarchical view, which is illustrated in Figure 5–1, identifies higher and lower centers as levels of control. A more recent and complex perspective, the dynamic systems theory view, better reflects reality by proposing a nervous system in which the levels of control are not fixed but change with time and can function in a nonlinear manner (Skarda & Freeman, 1987; Freeman, 1991; Kelso & Tuller, 1981). Although it does not deny the hierarchical view, it adds to it, incorporating new information about how environmental and other factors affect the order of nerve activation (Reed, 1989a, 1989b). Therefore, the therapist can benefit from using both perspectives (Gray, Kennedy, & Zemke, 1996).

Any part of the nervous system that receives, integrates, or transmits impulses contributes to learning and memory. This is accomplished through a dynamic and complex process that involves "feedforward" as well as feedback mechanisms and interaction between the different senses and the areas of the nervous system. It also shows both self-organizing and pattern-forming characteristics (Thelen, 1995). A comprehensive description of the nervous system is beyond the scope of this chapter; however, some of the brain structures and their relationships with learning and memory are discussed in this chapter.

Brain Structures

Following is an overview of four of the major structures of the cerebral cortex (i.e., the frontal, parietal, temporal, and occipital lobes) and the limbic system and the contributions of each to memory and learning. Figure 5–2 shows the basic structure of the brain, which includes the four lobes of the cerebral cortex. The frontal lobe, making up nearly one third of the cerebral cortex starting at the lateral fissure and extending to the central fissure, facilitates organization of memory (Fuster, 1993; Lezak, 1995; Moore, 1993). Frontal lobe impairment has been tied to general memory decline in individuals over the age of 70 years (Schacter, 1996; Strayer & Kramer, 1994; Young, 1996). The parietal lobes have been associated with tactile memory. This is based on the fact that clients who are unable to recognize features such as roughness, shape, and size, or who have astereognosis (i.e., the inability to recognize objects by touch) commonly have parietal lesions (Fuster, 1995). Visual-spatial memory and spatial attention have also been linked to the parietal lobe (Fuster, 1995; Moore, 1993). The temporal lobes process auditory input via the thalamus and play a part in auditory and

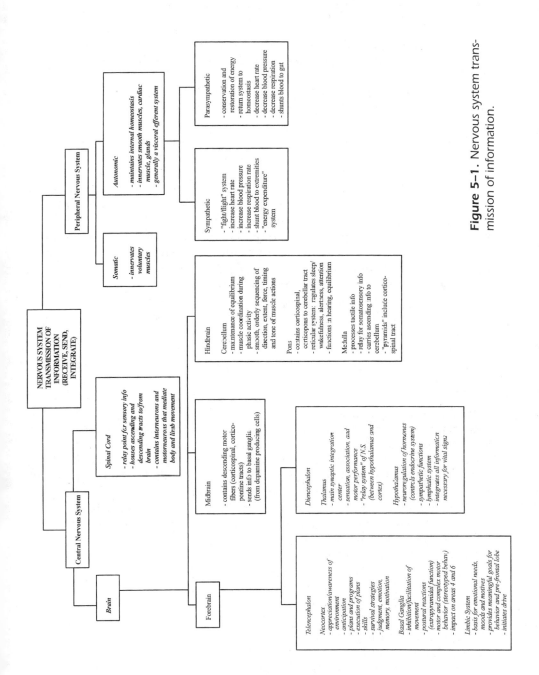

Figure 5–1. Nervous system transmission of information.

visual-object recognition (Fuster, 1995; Moore, 1993). Some evidence implicates the temporal lobe in visual memory as well as auditory memory (Fuster, 1993).

The limbic system is a functional arrangement of brain structures associated with memory and learning, motivation, olfaction, visceral functions, and a wide range of emotions (Cytowic, 1996; Moore, 1993). One of the functions of the limbic system is to modulate the emotional continuum of frustration, anger, rage, and violence (Moore, 1993). All structures within the limbic system coordinate function with the prefrontal lobe, anterior temporal lobe, hypothalamus, and other structures to assist in the process of learning and memory. In addition, the limbic system assists in the interpretation of an individual's external and internal world (Cytowic, 1996; Farber, 1982). This interpretation is modulated by the person's drive, automatic responses, and hormonal activity (Cytowic, 1996). Hormonal activity is a good example of the inseparable interplay between memory and the limbic system. Hormones are complex chemical substances produced by a variety of organs that possess a regulatory affect on other organs. The effect of hormonal activity on memory is not totally understood; however, the level of this activity in structures such as the hippocampus and the amygdala directly affects memory.

Two anatomical structures of the limbic system are the hippocampus and the amygdala. The hippocampus structures, located within the temporal lobes (see Fig. 5–2), are often described as an important memory system (Cohen & Eichenbaum, 1994). In particular, they are said to play an essential role in declarative memory (Squire, 1987; Squire & Alvarez, 1995; Squire & Zola-Morgan, 1991). (For an explanation of different types of memory, see the "Catalogue of Memory and Learning Taxonomies" section of this chapter.) The hippocampal memory function has been identified as temporary storage based on the fact that hippocampal synapses change quickly. The storage of information then gradually becomes fixed by a process called *memory consolidation*. This process may entail repeated transmission by these structures of identical messages, leading to permanent storage—independent of the hippocampus—in the neocortex (Squire & Alvarez, 1995). This serves to remind us that there is no single memory system but instead multiple and interactive systems.

The hippocampus is also hypothesized to assist associative learning and temporal and spatial navigation (Cohen & Eichenbaum, 1994). Evidence for hippocampal functions comes from studying the effects of animal and human lesions (Squire & Alvarez, 1995; Wilson, 1987). For instance, retrograde amnesia (i.e., the loss of memory acquired before injury) can result from damage limited to the hippocampus (Squire & Alvarez, 1995). The amygdala (located next to the hippocampus) is also believed to play a role in emotional memory. Referred to as the brain's emotional computer, it

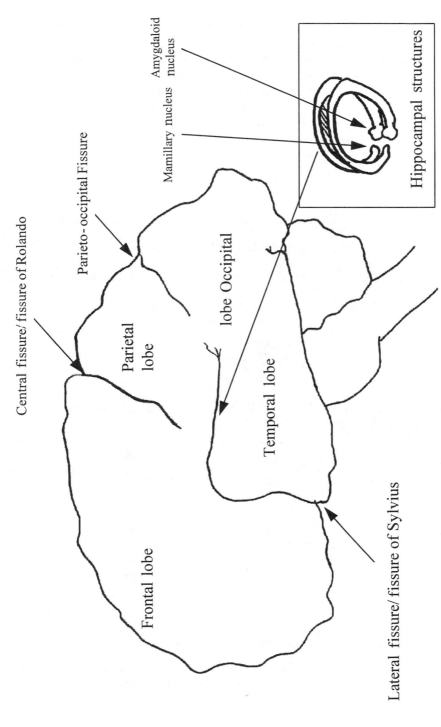

Central fissure/ fissure of Rolando

Parieto- occipital Fissure

Amygdaloid nucleus

Mamillary nucleus

Hippocampal structures

Parietal lobe

lobe Occipital

Temporal lobe

Frontal lobe

Lateral fissure/ fissure of Sylvius

Figure 5–2. Lateral view of the brain, including the four lobes of the cerebral cortex.

has been linked to determinations of "flight or fight" responses (Damasio & Damasio, 1989; Schacter, 1996). The release of stress-related hormones signaled by the amygdala can account for the power and lasting memory of emotional or traumatic experiences because these hormones appear to influence neuroregulation and memory development. Finally, the occipital lobe receives visual input through the lateral geniculate nucleus of the thalamus and interacts with the other lobes to bring about comprehension of visual environments. Clients with occipital lobe lesions may encounter cortical blindness, visual field cuts, and problems with visual-spatial memory and visual object identification.

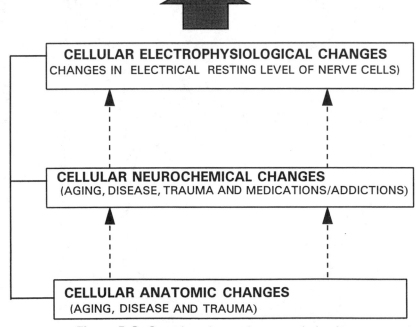

Figure 5–3. Overt learning and memory behaviors.

Practical Applications

Even from such a brief overview, it can be seen how a therapist may draw upon his or her understanding of the nervous system when working with clients who have memory and learning problems (Farber & Abreu, 1993). For instance, Figure 5–3 illustrates the relationship of overt behavior to chemical and anatomical changes in the synapses, which seem to be the structural elements in which change underlies behavioral changes. By analyzing the behavior of brain-injured clients, the therapist can infer what is happening at the neural level. The opposite is also true: from knowledge of the neuroanatomical and neurophysiological changes suffered by a client, the therapist can infer some of the obstacles that need to be addressed during an intervention program. Some therapists interpret a client's occupations and daily routines as a reflection of the nervous system's ability to self-organize and form patterns (Gray, Kennedy, & Zemke, 1996). This knowledge is thus a building block. By itself it is limited in its application, but it forms a critical part of the therapist's total outlook.

MEMORY AND LEARNING DEFINITIONS AND TAXONOMIES

One way of clarifying the complex concepts of memory and learning is by breaking them down into taxonomies. **Taxonomies** are orderly classifications based on commonalties or relationships. There is no universally accepted taxonomical system of memory and learning. Systems differ according to many factors, including the discipline from which one approaches the concepts of memory and learning, the methodology used, and the researcher's individual perspective. Taxonomies also evolve over time because of increased scientific understanding. Thus, numerous taxonomies have been developed (e.g., refer to Atkinson & Shiffrin, 1968; Baddeley, 1992; Cohen, 1991; Cohen & Eichenbaum, 1994; Fuster, 1995; Hertel, 1996; Llinás & Churchland, 1996; Monnier, 1975; Schacter, 1996; Schacter & Tulving, 1994; Squire, 1987). Descriptive outlines of memory and learning taxonomies are depicted in Figure 5–4 and are described below.

Memory Taxonomies

Several useful ways to classify memory include classifications according to sensory modalities, temporal characteristics, activities of daily living (ADLs), negative symptoms or amnesia, and mixed factors such as emotions and metacognition. Each of these is discussed briefly.

LEARNING TAXONOMIES

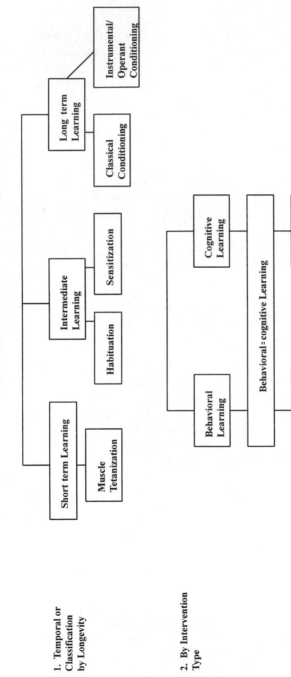

Figure 5–4. Learning taxonomies.

Sensory Modality Taxonomy

Sensory modalities are transmission channels for sense-generated impulses. These impulses are processed in the brain and can often develop into memory. These are divided into four categories: olfactory and gustatory, auditory, visual, and tactile and kinesthetic.

Olfactory and Gustatory Olfactory and gustatory sensations, which are each carried to the brain by different cranial nerves, are interrelated. For example, some odorous substances are able to stimulate the sense of taste (Monnier, 1975). Chemical analysis of food, which affects feeding behavior, is performed by olfactory as well as taste receptors. However, whereas the olfactory sensations are transmitted by the olfactory nerve I, the gustatory sensations are transmitted by three different cranial nerves: the 7th facial nerve, the 9th glossopharyngeal nerve, and to a lesser extent, the 10th vagus nerve (Monnier, 1975).

Unlike memories generated by other senses, those based on olfaction do not proceed through the thalamocortical pathway; rather, they project directly into the hippocampal system. The olfactory receptors, located near and connected to the emotional memory site called the *limbic system*, process input and adapt at a rapid rate. This close association with the limbic system enhances these receptors' capacity to create emotional memories. Thus, whereas malodorous substances can elicit nausea and vomiting, fragrant substances can cause feelings of sexual arousal (Monnier, 1975).

Olfactory memory has been studied by analyzing the effects of lesions on specific areas of the brain in both humans and animals. For example, humans who have undergone complete cerebral commissurotomy can smell and distinguish different foods but cannot name the odors (Heilman & Valenstein, 1993). This deficit is called *anosmia*, which is a loss of the olfactory sense that can be specific or general. Conversely, whereas hyperosmia is an extremely high sensitivity to smell and taste, hyposmia is decreased, but not lost, sensitivity. Likewise, studies of hippocampal lesions in rats revealed olfactory memory impairments (Eichenbaum, 1996). Other factors that affect olfactory sensitivity are older age, food deprivation, and drug use (Farber, 1982; Monnier, 1975).

The gustatory cortex projects to the orbitofrontal cortex at the base of the frontal lobe (Fuster, 1995). The gustatory receptors, or taste buds, are located on the tip and lateral margins of the tongue, on the palate, in the mucosa of the lips and cheeks, and on the floor of the mouth (Farber, 1982; Monnier, 1975). These receptors process a range of sensations derived from the four elemental tastes: bitter, sour, salty, and sweet. The tongue also feels temperature, pressure, and pain (Monnier, 1975). Humans with lesions in the orbitofrontal region have been found to have a condition called *ageusia*, an impairment of the gustatory system involving an inability to recognize familiar tastes (Fuster, 1995). Animal studies have shown that rats with lesions of the gustatory nerve lose interest in food and consequently die (Monnier, 1975). Therapists use gustatory memories in feeding clients and in coma treatment by employing the preferred tastes of individuals for stimulation and arousal (Farber, 1982).

Auditory Memory The auditory system converts the mechanical energy of sound waves on the eardrum into electrical impulses. These impulses are carried through the eighth cranial nerve to the thalamus and to the auditory cortex. Sound has several characteristics, including tone, intensity, and loudness. Speech requires particularly complex auditory detection and interpretation. Thus, auditory memory is often divided into two classes: verbal and nonverbal. Whereas verbal memory involves linguistic processing, nonverbal memory, such as the memory of music, does not (McAdams, 1996).

The auditory cortex is located in the temporal lobes. In the majority of humans, the left temporal lobe is dominant. Whereas lesions in this area cause verbal auditory memory deficits, lesions on the nondominant right temporal lobe have been linked to poor performance in nonverbal auditory memory, often resulting in the loss of musical memory (Gazzaniga & LeDoux, 1981; Springer & Deutsch, 1989). Conditions of auditory memory impairment include anomia, the loss of memory for names; acoustic agnosia, the loss of memory for nonverbal and nonmusical sounds; and amusia, the loss of music memory (Fuster, 1995).

The motor and receptive centers for speech and language are located in the parts of the brain called *Broca's area* and *Wernicke's area*. Broca's area, which is in the frontal lobe, focuses on expressive control of speech. Wernicke's area, which is on the border of the left temporal and the left parietal lobes, focuses on speech reception. Damage to parietotemporal areas has been associated with learning disabilities with regard to reading and writing.

Visual Memory The visual system converts the energy of light waves, which are projected from the retina, into electrical impulses. They are carried through the second cranial nerve to the thalamus and to the visual cortex (Abreu, 1981; Farber, 1982). The motor aspects of eye movements—which are controlled by six muscles, themselves supplied by the third, fourth, and sixth cranial nerves—are also critical to the visual memory bank. Light has several characteristics: luminosity or brightness, color or hues, magnitude, form, position, direction, distance, and symbolization (Monnier, 1975). Visual memory can be divided into memory for the appearance of objects and their location; memory for routes and maps, spatial layouts, and landmarks; and memory for complex events.

The visual cortex is located in the occipital lobe. Thus, prosopagnosia, or visual memory impairment for familiar faces, is sometimes associated with occipitotemporal lesions (Cytowic, 1996). Visual memory entails a great amount of neuroanatomical interaction: not only do the occipital and the temporal lobes play a role, but so do the parietal and the frontal lobes (Fuster, 1995). In humans, temporal lobe lesions have affected tasks involving form, distance, depth perception, and spatial relationships. They have also been tied to agnosia, or the loss of memory for objects and persons (Gazzaniga & LeDoux, 1981; Springer & Deutsch, 1989).

Tactile and Kinesthetic Memory There are three distinct processes that contribute to tactile and kinesthetic memory. First, mechanical indentations of the human skin (from which input is processed by a variety of receptor nerve cells called *exteroreceptors*) stimulate the sense of touch (Monnier, 1975). Second, kinesthetic sensations of position, movement, and tension in an individual's body parts are detected by a variety of receptor nerve cells located in the joints, muscles, and tendons (Monnier, 1975). Third, in practical terms, tactile and kinesthetic sense and memory processes are inseparable from motor memory (Fuster, 1995), which itself is anchored in a variety of sensory memories. For instance, stereognosis, or haptic sensation, is the capacity to discriminate an object by tactile and kinesthetic analysis, such as finding a key in a pocket full of different objects. However, this process must involve the movements of reacting and touching those various objects.

Whereas tactile memory has its representation in the parietal lobe, kinesthetic memory is represented in the parietal lobe and in the motor cortex. It has been suggested that the frontal lobe cortex is the supreme organizer for action and, therefore, is the seat of motor memory (Fuster, 1995), but this is not well established. Some of the impairments attributed to the tactile and kinesthetic memory system are astereognosis, autotopagnosia, and unilateral neglect (Fuster, 1995). Astereognosis is the inability to recognize objects by touch with vision occluded (discussed in detail in Chapter 8). Autotopagnosia is the inability to point to one's own body parts, although individuals with this impairment can name body parts if someone else points to them (Fuster, 1995). Unilateral neglect of body parts is considered a spatial attentional impairment that relates to the parietal cortex (see Chapter 9).

Temporal Taxonomy

The temporal component of memory, which relates to duration, is composed of three types of memory storage (Atkinson & Shiffrin, 1968). The first, sensory memory, is extremely brief in duration and may be subdivided relative to two associated sensory modalities: iconic or visual memory, and echoic or auditory memory. The second type of memory storage, short-term memory, involves a longer but limited duration of retention and functions in part as a transfer mechanism to the third type, long-term memory. A further subcategory of long-term memory is prospective memory, which enables individuals to carry out specified actions at future targeted times.

Long-Term Memory Taxonomy

Long-term memory can be broken down into two major categories, declarative and procedural (or nondeclarative) memory. Declarative memory stores facts and events that are experienced through verbal or other explicit means, such as spatial maps. It forms the basis for an individual's capacity to compare, contrast, and make inferences (Cohen & Eichenbaum, 1994; Llinás & Churchland, 1996) and is typically evaluated by means of expressive language. Declarative memory can be subdivided into episodic memory, which stores personally experienced events, and semantic memory, which deals with famous people, events, and facts. Procedural memory stores knowledge of procedures and rules and underlies the capacity to acquire particular skills. It may also be characterized as the nonconscious acquisition of bias and adaptation. It is primarily judged by performance. Independent from hippocampal influence, procedural memory is intact even in dense amnesiacs. Nondeclarative or procedural memory can be subdivided into skills, priming, simple classical conditioning, and operant conditioning (Tulving & Schacter, 1990). Procedural memory has implications for restoration of performance and function because it can be accessed separately from other forms of memory.

Short-Term Memory Taxonomy

One model subdivides short-term memory into a control system for limited processing capacity and two subordinate storage systems. The first system, the phonological, retains and manipulates speech-based information. The second system, the visuospatial, does the same for information based on sight and other senses that contribute to spatial perception (Baddeley, 1992).

Real-World Memory Taxonomy

The real-world taxonomy is based on Cohen's *Memory in the Real World* (1991), which describes memory in five categories important to daily living: (1) memory for plans and actions; (2) memory for places, objects, and events; (3) memory for people, faces, and names; (4) memory for personal experiences; and (5) memory for conversation.

Negative Symptom Taxonomy

The negative symptoms taxonomy could also be called a *taxonomy of amnesia*. Two types of amnesia have been distinguished, retrograde and anterograde.

Retrograde amnesia is the inability to use information acquired before an injury, illness, or onset of amnesia. **Anterograde amnesia** is the inability to acquire and retain new information (Cohen & Eichenbaum, 1994; Cytowic, 1996; Hodges & McCarthy, 1995). Recently, retrograde amnesia has itself been broken down into two types, loss of memory of personal events and loss of memory of personal facts. Based on clinical evidence, some brain-injured individuals exhibit loss of memory for events such as the previous year's holidays but retain memories about facts such as their educational background, marital status, and occupation (Mayes et al., 1994; Schnider et al., 1996; Squire & Alvarez, 1995).

Mixed Memory Taxonomies

Mixed taxonomies are arbitrary classifications created by the author and include two different, unrelated types of memory, emotional memory and metamemory.

Emotional Memory Emotional memory is the retention of an emotional event (Hertel, 1996). Three types have been distinguished: eyewitness memories, flashbulb memories, and repressed memories. Eyewitness memories, or memories of emotional situations witnessed firsthand, can range from accurate to poor depending on such wide-ranging factors as automatic system arousal, hormonal changes, and attentional focus (Hertel, 1996). Flashbulb memories are memories of personal experiences connected to events that are not witnessed firsthand but reflect the individual's own experience during the original event (Hertel, 1996), such as the memory of what one was doing when President John F. Kennedy was assassinated. Repressed memories are associated with abuse and trauma. There are many questions regarding this type of emotional memory and the process by which it is "recovered." For instance, some propose that repressed and then recovered memories can be falsely created through social encounters or therapeutic interventions.

Metamemory Metamemory is an individual's subjective knowledge about his capacity to acquire, retain, and recall information (Cavanaugh & Perlmutter, 1982; Koriat, 1994; Parkin, Bell, & Leng, 1988). It is grounded in judgments about familiar past information and is based on new information (Cornoldi & De Beni, 1996; Leonesio & Nelson, 1992; Metcalfe, 1993; Nelson & Narens, 1992; Reder, 1996). Three types of **metamemory** have been distinguished: metamemory regarding task, metamemory regarding one's self or one's own memories, and metamemory regarding memory strategy (Bjork, 1994). For example, students preparing to study for examinations may reflect on the task before them in terms of what they need to commit to memory; they may reflect on the state of their own memory in terms what they already know; or they may reflect on the best strategy for studying or acquiring new memory. The relationship of metamemory to memory itself is a source of controversy. Some researchers consider them separate and distinct processes, with the former monitored in the frontal lobe (Reder, 1996).

Learning Taxonomies

As seen in Figure 5–4, learning has been classified in at least three ways: in temporal terms, according to type of intervention, and by modality. Each of these is described briefly.

Temporal Taxonomy

One way to distinguish the types of learning is along temporal lines in the sense of the longevity of learning's effects (Schwartz, 1985, 1991).

- Short-term learning occurs when a repeated stimulus causes a simple increase or decrease in the number of responses at the cellular level, for example, when the repetition of a high-frequency sound leads to a change in the number of muscle contractions (Kandel, 1976).
- Intermediate-term learning occurs when a repeated stimulus leads to a progressive increase or reduction of the neural impulse discharge that controls response (Schwartz, 1985, 1991). This progressive reduction in response has been called *habituation* and can act to save energy by weakening response to less relevant stimuli in order to allow focus on more relevant tasks presented by the environment (Farber & Abreu, 1993). Many brain-injured individuals often exhibit an inability to habituate, responding to all stimuli with equal intensity.
- Long-term learning, or conditioning, occurs when a repeated stimulus leads to a behavioral stimulus-response pattern. Two types of conditioning have been distinguished, classical conditioning and instrumental conditioning. The first occurs when responses are brought on by indirect associations, such as when rehabilitation devices like wheelchairs (which are associated with injuries) generate negative feelings. Instrumental conditioning, on the other hand, occurs when a stimulus is directly associated with a response. An example is the behavioral effect of report cards.

Intervention Type Taxonomy

Three categories of learning have been distinguished based on different types of intervention or applied stimuli: behavioral learning, in which behavior is altered through the use of simple rewards and punishments; cognitive learning, in which behavior is altered through the use of ideas; and behavioral-cognitive learning, a combination of the first two types.

Modality Taxonomy

There are two types of learning in terms of modality or therapeutic agency. Whereas motor learning is the acquisition of skilled movements as a result of practice (Schmidt & Bjork, 1992), verbal learning is the acquisition of memory through spoken information.

Application of Taxonomic Understanding

The classification systems described for memory and learning might be more or less interesting or useful according to one's perspective. For instance, the sensory modality taxonomy may be a useful guide for an occupational therapist or for anyone dealing with brain-injured clients. Within many of the taxonomies outlined previously, memory and learning systems operate separately but interactively—that is, although systems such as long- and short-term memory perform different tasks, they work simultaneously and culminate in a perception of unified or cohesive memory (Schneider, 1993). Likewise, if everyone on a therapeutic team understands the breadth of memory and learning taxonomies (and thus the complexity of memory and learning processes), they are better able to work toward a total and cohesive intervention.

☰ CURRENT RESEARCH TRENDS

A survey of current memory and learning literature suggests two general research trends. The first is human oriented (covering differences between experts and novices) and the other is technologically oriented. Both are of interest to students as well as to practicing therapists. The importance of discussing research trends and methodologies is based on the assumptions that expert practitioners take into consideration how data is collected and from which population the data is derived (e.g., normal individuals, special individuals, animals, or machines) before considering the application of the findings. This section highlights research trends considered relevant to memory and learning.

EXPERT/NOVICE DIFFERENCES IN MEMORY AND LEARNING

In the main area of research, clinical psychologists are studying the differences in memory and learning in experts (i.e., those skilled in acquiring and retaining information) and novices (i.e., those less proficient in these tasks) with an emphasis on the role of experts' metacognitive processes. A parallel body of work is being undertaken by educators who are looking at memory and learning differences in teachers and students (Brown, 1987; Chi et al., 1994; Chi, Feltovich, & Glaser, 1979; Flavell, 1979; Glaser, 1990a; Gobbo & Chi, 1986; Hong, 1995; Loxterman, Beck, & McKeown, 1994; Perfetti, 1995; Wertsch, 1985; Winne, 1995). It should be understood that in this context, people may be simultaneously expert in some areas and novice in others and that each person's place on the expert–novice axis evolves over time.

Expert learners have been found to have various characteristics: they analyze information more deeply in constructing memories (Gobbo & Chi, 1986; Kintsch, 1994); they are industrious in adapting strategies and setting goals for extending their knowledge (Winne, 1995); and they demonstrate superior short-term, semantic, and general memory (Haenggi & Perfetti, 1994; Posner, 1988). One author (Glaser, 1990b) defines expertise-based knowledge as deriving from specialized knowledge, employing more inferences, using more abstract principles, and being self-regulating. **Metacognition** is an individual's subjective knowledge or beliefs about his or her own cognitive capacity, state, and processing strategies (Narens, Graf, & Nelson, 1996; Reder, 1996). Expert learners demonstrate a high use of metacognitive processing using more introspection strategies. They have a sharper sense of awareness and feeling of knowing that they know or do not know the solution to a problem.

The metacognitive activity of self-regulation, a self-monitoring of organizational learning strategies in order to increase the speed and efficiency of the learning process, plays a critical role in the expert–novice literature. However, researchers disagree about the nature of this self-regulation, as they do about metacognition as a whole (Reder, 1996). Some view it as a personality trait and others view it as a cognitive process or as an instructional technique for complex problem solving (Benardi-Coletta et al., 1995; Slife, Weiss, & Bell, 1985; Swiderek, 1996; Wilson et al., 1993; Winne, 1995). Not all researchers even agree that metacognition necessarily aids in memory and learning. In some instances it has been suggested that metacognition is a hindrance (Wilson et al., 1993).

There are at least two ways in which this exploration of novice–expert differences may prove useful in the practice of occupational therapy. First, special-populations research has identified similarities between brain-injured clients and novice learners. Some studies suggest that self-regulation aids in the learning processes of the cognitively impaired (Blackmer & Mitton, 1991; Benardi-Colletta et al., 1995; Paris & Winograd, 1990; Winne, 1995). Therefore, subsequent theoretical developments may lead to developments in practical treatment routines that will reduce the complexity of learning and ease the client's acquisition and retention of information (Leinhardt, Weidman, & Hammond, 1987). Second, this research may prove useful by helping therapists understand their own learning processes. This is important given that teachers or therapists structure their lessons or treatments based, at least in part, on their understanding of their own learning processes (Abreu, 1990, 1994; Hattrup & Bickel, 1993; Leinhardt, 1990; Simmons & Resnick, 1993). Such practical applications of metacognitive insights, although advocated by several occupational therapists, need further studies for validation and evaluation (Abreu, 1998a, 1990, 1994; Abreu & Toglia, 1987; Neistadt, 1992; Parham, 1987; Peloquin, 1996; Toglia, 1991, 1993a).

TECHNOLOGY APPROACHES TO UNDERSTANDING MEMORY AND LEARNING

The second main area of current research related to memory and learning revolves around the development and use of medical technology and intelligent machine technology (Dreyfus & Dreyfus, 1986; Glaser & Chi, 1988; Hobson, 1996; Klopfer, 1986; Nyberg et al., 1996; Papanicolaou, 1987; Roland, 1982; Schneider, Casey, & Noll, 1994; Schneider, Noll, & Cohen, 1993; Shute & Glaser, 1990). A brief description of both these types follows.

Neurological Technology

Brain imaging technologies, which have made it possible to identify neural structures involved in memory and learning, enable us to describe the interactions between these structures' pathways and even to detect neural dysfunction (Schneider et al., 1994; Weinberger, 1988). These technologies include positron emission tomography (PET), functional magnetic resonance imagery (FMRI), and magnetoencephalography (MEG). Portraying the brain in three dimensions, PET has revealed that learning and memory operate on multiple neural structures simultaneously (Damasio & Damasio, 1989). For example, the use of PET has linked the retrieval of episodic memory to activity in the right prefrontal lobe, anterior cingulate, bilateral medial temporal lobes, parietal lobes, and cerebellum (Nyberg et al., 1996; Squire et al., 1992). However, PET's use is limited by its use of radioactive agents (Schneider et al., 1994). FMRI involves sequential acquisition of images, resulting in sufficient resolution to track small areas of activation across neural systems (Schneider et al., 1994). MEG technology has allowed us to record brain activity in real time (Llinás & Churchland, 1996).

Research with another neurological technology, auditory event-related potential (ERP), is being used as a potential biological marker of cerebral and memory function (Omahony et al., 1996). The results of various investigations using this technology with clients with Alzheimer's disease, those with schizophrenia, and healthy individuals suggest that ERP may be useful in identifying frontal lobe dysfunction (Omahony et al., 1996), in predicting the severity of specific physiological and psychological abnormalities in schizophrenia (Levitt et al., 1996), and in determining the potential intactness of recognition memory in cases of suspected malingering (Ellwanger et al., 1996).

Another area of memory and learning research opened up by advances in neurological technology concerns the operation of the brain during sleep and dreaming (Hobson, 1996). A fascinating, counterintuitive, and potentially very useful hypothesis has arisen: neural activity during dreaming resembles the neural activity of an injured brain (Hobson, 1996). For example, both include an amnesia-like inability to recall, a temporal disorientation, scenarios with disparate elements, and visual imagery akin to hallucination (Hobson, 1996).

Neurological technology has allowed clinicians and researchers to better understand the complexities of the interactions between memory and learning at the neural level. Another form of investigation uses machine technology, sometimes called *intelligent machines*; it is discussed in the next section.

Intelligent Machines

Robots, expert systems, and other computerized programs are intelligent machines employed in the research of memory and learning (Churchland, 1995; Dreyfus & Dreyfus, 1986; Llinás & Churchland, 1996; Schneider & Graham, 1992). Some of these are so technical that they seem inaccessible to occupational therapists and other nonexperts. However, according to some neuroscientists, computational models form a potential bridge between disciplines interested in learning and memory (Llinás & Churchland, 1996).

Intelligent machine technology is controversial. Some deny the possibility of any human application of nonconscious machines. But, in fact, there is not an unbridgeable chasm between this area of research and the human-oriented research outlined previously. After all, intelligent machines are programmed and evaluated according to instructional strategies used by expert human beings. Likewise, researchers in education and cognition are developing guidelines for teachers based on computer systems that work like expert teachers (Klopfer, 1986). Conversely, however, these machines are constructed to emulate humans, so we should not be overly optimistic about expanding our understanding of memory and learning from their operation (Schneider & Graham, 1992).

The use of intelligent machines has allowed clinicians and researchers to better understand the use of instructional strategies and provide a potential bridge between the research laboratory and the rehabilitation practice. As can be seen from the previous discussion, human- and technology-oriented research provides stimulating and thought-provoking ideas for clinical practice.

CASE STUDY: EVELYN

The following is a case study that uses the quadraphonic approach to evaluate and treat a brain-injured client. The therapist's overall objective is to increase clients' opportunities and capacities for action, help them achieve their goals, and increase their level of satisfaction.

INTRODUCTION TO EVELYN AND THE THERAPY CENTER

Evelyn is a 20-year-old university student who lived at home with her parents and two younger brothers. She was struck by a car while driving her motorcycle to school. Although she was wearing a helmet, she suffered a severe closed-head injury and was admitted to the emergency room of a nearby hospital in a coma. Evelyn proceeded through the medical system, including a coma program and acute rehabilitation. She was discharged to a transitional living center, which is where this case study begins. The Transitional Learning Community (TLC) at Galveston (Galveston, Texas) is a nonprofit, 27-bed facility that specializes in post–acute brain injury rehabilitation. TLC's threefold mission includes direct care, education, and research in the field of brain injury. Therapists at this center use the quadraphonic approach to working with clients who have cognitive and perceptual problems. Although this approach was briefly described in Chapter 1, it is now presented here in detail.

THEORETICAL BASIS FOR THE QUADRAPHONIC APPROACH TO THERAPY

The **quadraphonic approach** to therapy, which will govern the case study outlined in the next section, integrates two orientations in the area of cognitive retraining. One of these is reductionistic in character, employing a micro perspective; the other is holistic or humanistic and proceeds through a macro perspective (Abreu, 1990, 1992, 1994, 1998a, 1998b; Abreu & Hinojosa, 1992; Duchek & Abreu, 1998). The descriptor "quadraphonic" stems from the fact that the micro orientation is guided by four theories and the macro orientation is guided by four characteristics unique to each client.

MICRO EVALUATION PERSPECTIVE

The **micro perspective** was originally designed as a cognitive frame of reference while the author was fulfilling a doctoral requirement (Abreu, 1981). This frame of reference focused on a client's foundational subskills or performance components using two theoretical foundations, information processing and teaching-learning. The micro perspective was later expanded (Abreu & Toglia, 1987). In 1990, the author integrated two additional theoretical foundations, neurodevelopmental and biomechanical, to form the micro perspective of the quadraphonic approach (Abreu, 1990). Micro perspectives have also been called *restorative* and *bottom-up* (as described in Chapter 1) (Abreu, 1994; Trombly, 1993; Wood et al., 1994).

Figure 5–5 depicts the micro perspective of the quadraphonic approach. The outer square is composed of the four complimentary theories, which are drawn upon to facilitate the design of therapeutic strategies. These four theories are:

1. The information-processing theory explains how the mind functions and how people perceive and react to the environment. For example, it assumes that there are three stages of processing within the nervous system: stimulus detection, discrimination and analysis, and response selection (Abreu, 1992; Klatzy, 1980; Light, 1990). It can be used to explain some post–brain injury behaviors in terms of dysfunction at one or more of these stages.

2. The teaching-and-learning theory explains how individuals use cues gathered from the environment to alter their capacity and methods of response, thereby increasing cognitive awareness and enhancing control. Two of the subcategories of this theory involve self-generated or natural learning (e.g., learning to sit or walk) and externally gener-

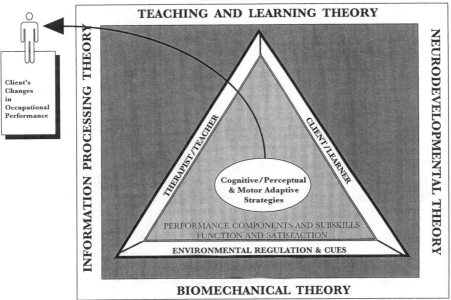

Figure 5–5. The quadraphonic approach—micro perspective. (Used with permission of Abreu, B. C. [1990]. *The quadraphonic approach: Course handouts.* Galveston, TX: Therapeutic Service Systems.)

ated or mediated learning (e.g., learning to read or write). Information-processing theory and teaching-and-learning theory serve to explain cognition insofar as it resides only in the brain. However, the brain cannot be artificially separated from the body, which is closely related to the cognitive-perceptual system. The second two theories, then, aim to give proper credit to this relationship between mind and body.

3. The dynamic neurodevelopmental theory views movement as a coordinated effort of multiple subsystems of the body combined with environmental variables resulting in action for a purpose or task (Bernstein, 1967; Thelen, 1995; von Bertalanffy, 1968). This action or motor coordination is produced by self-regulating and flexible reorganizing mechanisms at the neuronal and behavioral levels that are mutually dependent (Barton, 1994; Thelen, 1995). In other words, this theory now recognizes that different circumstances activate different nervous system structures and communication strategies (Reed, 1989a; 1989b).

4. The biomechanical theory views the body as a work or motion machine composed of muscles, bones, tendons, and ligaments. It employs kinematics to analyze the mechanical components of the body and kinetics to analyze motion with consideration of its interacting causal forces. This theory recognizes that changes in muscle tone are related to motor recruitment patterns and joint alignment (Ryerson & Levit, 1997). It enables the therapist to understand the integration of the nervous system and musculoskeletal systems with perceptual motor skills.

Guided by this four-part theoretical framework, the therapist and client develop cognitive, perceptual, and motor-adaptive strategies to enhance the client's performance and improve satisfaction (see Fig. 5–5). In developing these strategies, they must also consider the effects of three interactive forces, as depicted on the legs of the triangle surrounding the oval: the client, the environment, and the therapist.

- The client can be understood as a combination of four factors: the story of adaptation and loss, the stage of awareness, the stage of motor learning, and the stage of recovery and acceptance.
- The environment can be broken down into three components: physical, social, and cultural. The physical environment includes the activities, conditions, circumstances, objects, and people surrounding the client (Gentile, 1987). The social environment includes the client's social networks; family structure; perception of personal roles, rights, and duties; and community resources (Mosey, 1986). The cultural environment includes the traditions, values, norms, language, and symbolic meanings that are shared by the client and any group (Mosey, 1986).
- The therapist uses three types of reasoning to form an educated evaluation, plan an effective intervention, and reevaluate the plan as required. These are (1) procedural reasoning, or thinking on their own about a case; (2) interactive reasoning, or thinking along with the client; and (3) conditional reasoning, which occurs when the therapist considers brain injury in a broader social and temporal context that incorporates the client's view of the future (Fleming, 1991).

The **macro perspective** is used to develop adaptive strategies that are congruent with both sets of the three interactive forces outlined previously to enable the client to achieve goals and improve satisfaction.

MACRO EVALUATION PERSPECTIVE

Macro perspectives have also been described as *adaptive, functional,* and *top-down* (as described in Chapter 1) (Abreu, 1994; Zoltan, 1996; Trombly, 1993). This is a clinical orientation that relies on daily living, leisure, recreation, work, and other ordinary occupations as primary therapeutic modalities. The macro perspective used in this chapter was inspired by clinical practices at the University of Southern California Hospital, where the author attempted to integrate occupational science into occupational therapy practice (Wood et al., 1994). Figure 5–6 depicts the macro perspective. The outer square is composed of four characteristics of a client that can be subjected to narrative and functional analysis in order to explain and predict the client's behavior as follows:

1. The lifestyle status is a client's manner of communicating, working, and performing day-to-day operations. The factors that are considered are personal characteristics and the use of economic resources.
2. The life stage status is a client's physical, emotional, and spiritual standing or development. Relevant factors include age, marital status, accomplishments, and failures.

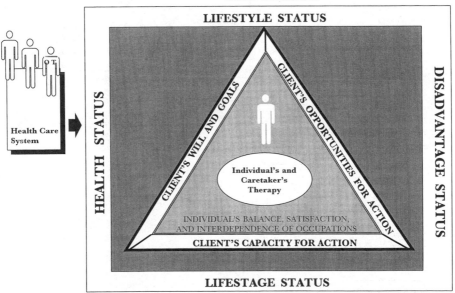

Figure 5–6. The quadraphonic approach—macro perspective. (Used with permission of Abreu, B. C. [1990]. *The quadraphonic approach: Course handouts.* Galveston, TX: Therapeutic Service Systems.)

3. The health status is the presence of premorbid conditions such as arthritis or back pain, as well as any changes in behavior or condition after the accident or illness.
4. The disadvantages status is the degree of functional restriction that results from impairment, including personal and social disadvantage. Examples are a client's inability to attend movies, shop, cook, or provide in any way for family members or others.

Based on analysis of these characteristics, an evaluation is made of the client's will and goals, opportunities for action, and capacity for action, as depicted on the three legs of the triangle in Figure 5–6. This information is then used to develop a therapy that is unique to the client's individual case, as represented in the oval at the center.

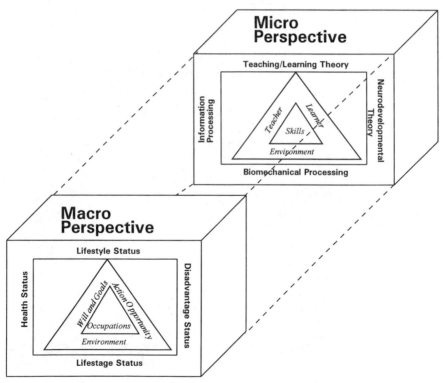

Figure 5–7. Quadraphonic approach evaluation model. (Used with permission of Abreu, B. C. [1997]. *The quadraphonic approach: Course handouts.* Galveston, TX: Therapeutic Service Systems.)

THE FLOW BETWEEN MICRO AND MACRO PERSPECTIVES

The quadraphonic approach to therapy is a holistic rehabilitation method that incorporates the reductionist orientation necessary for effective cognitive retraining with the holistic orientation necessary to produce an effective evaluation model. It rejects the rigid historical assumption that therapists must choose between holism and reductionism and assumes that both micro and macro perspectives are required because of the complexity of individual cases or clients (Fig. 5–7). The quadraphonic approach also treats these two perspectives as related; however, the relationship should not be understood as causal or directional in character (Wood et al., 1994). Perhaps the word that best describes the relationship is "confluence," the flowing together of two or more streams of thought (*Merriam-Webster's Collegiate Dictionary*, 1995). In the context of therapeutic practice, *confluence* denotes a fluid movement back and forth between the micro and macro perspectives, resulting in simultaneous attention to both performance components and whole-person functioning (Peloquin, 1996). Confluence is also an integral quality of the treatment model of the quadraphonic approach.

DATA GATHERING

MEDICAL RECORDS

The description in Box 5–1 presents the information the therapist gained from reviewing the client's medical chart.

INTERVIEW

In addition to medical data, the therapist needs to become familiar with the client's family, education, work history, leisure interests, narrative skills, and general communication capacity. Although the interview is a structured and focused process (Box 5–2), it should allow for improvisation in recognition of each client's uniqueness (Holstein & Gubrium, 1995; Josselson & Lieblich, 1995). Participants should be mutually attentive and take turns in the conversation. They should be open and should try to connect on the level of sentiment and emotion, as well as logic (Hartley, 1995). Box 5–3 discusses the actual interviews with Evelyn and her parents.

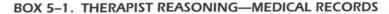

BOX 5–1. THERAPIST REASONING—MEDICAL RECORDS

I usually begin to gather data about a case by reviewing the client's current chart, complete medical history, and any additional documentation supplied on arrival at the treatment center. Evelyn's records indicated that on admission to the emergency room, she received a Glasgow coma score of 4. Initial computed tomography (CT) scans revealed multiple small hemorrhages, left parietal lobe contusions, and a small subdural hematoma (Horn & Zasler, 1996). Another CT scan performed 11 days later (after Evelyn emerged from her coma) showed contusions with right and left basal ganglia and left temporoparietal areas. A magnetic resonance imaging scan taken 3 months after the accident showed left subacute hemorrhages in the left temporoparietal regions and shear injuries in bilateral frontal and parietal areas. No operative procedures had been undertaken. Evelyn's history indicated no premorbid impairments. Since the accident, it was documented that her right side is weak.

EVALUATION AND ASSESSMENT

The evaluation of memory and learning proceeds through a series of eight tests. The first four are designed from the quadraphonic approach's "micro" perspective, corresponding to the four theories that define it: information processing, teaching and learning, neurodevelopmental, and biomechanical. The first two tests focus on memory and learning performance as functions of the brain; the second two focus on body performance factors that can affect cognition.

1. The Self-Reporting Awareness Test is an evaluative measure of a client's information-processing function or capacity to acquire memory. By testing a client's awareness of problems, it gauges his or her capacity to receive information from the outside world. This test is administered in conjunction with the other tests. Before taking each test, clients are asked if they think they have any problems in the area to be tested. After finishing each test, they are asked to evaluate how well they did and to predict how they will perform upon discharge based on their performance. Evelyn's answers to these three questions, administered in conjunction with her other seven tests, revealed that she had only a general sense that something was different since the accident. She required cueing (verbal prompts) to detect and correct memory and learning problems, and she had a very limited awareness of the ways her impairments would have an impact on her future.

BOX 5–2. THERAPIST REASONING—STRUCTURING AN INTERVIEW

I generally conduct a personal interview with the client and the family group to gather information about the client's family, education, work history, leisure interests, narrative skills, and general communication capabilities. I plan the interview questions in advance and often ask people who are to be interviewed to prepare and bring along certain information.

Some of the interview questions I ask have specific purposes in the "micro" sense. For example:

● I ask clients about their injury-related problems, which will indicate their self-awareness of disability.

● I ask about their independence as a test of self-reporting ability.

● I ask clients about any problems they might face in a future task, which will assist me to gauge their anticipatory awareness.

● Finally, I borrow the client's watch toward the beginning of the interview and ask what was borrowed at the end as a test of specific awareness.

The other questions I ask aim at understanding clients in a "macro" sense. For example, related to personality, I might ask:

● What are your personal strengths and weaknesses?

● What makes you happy or sad?

Related to the client's daily living needs, I might ask:

● How independent do you feel?

● What are your frustrations?

To get a feel for the client's state of mind I might ask:

● Are you satisfied with your personal roles as son or daughter, friend, and client?

● Are you satisfied with the therapeutic services available to you?

2. The Visual and Auditory Memory Test, actually a battery of tests, is based on teaching-and-learning theory. It evaluates short-term memory as a function of a client's capacity to organize information. An example of a visual memory test is to show a client a picture depicting two actions, one in the foreground and one in the background, for 30 seconds, after which the client is asked to describe what he or she saw. Most clients will miss one or the other action or details. After coaching the client on cognitive techniques or skills, the same test is repeated to gauge improvement with repetition and cued strategies. An auditory memory test proceeds similarly, with clients asked to re-

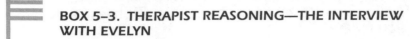

BOX 5–3. THERAPIST REASONING—THE INTERVIEW WITH EVELYN

At the interview with Evelyn and her parents, Evelyn told me that their goals were to return to school and regain the independence she was accustomed to displaying before the accident. Evelyn reported her personal strengths to be a high level of motivation and a willingness to fight against odds. She said that her greatest practical problem was an inability to move her right side, adding that people told her that she also cannot think as quickly as she could before the accident. She repeated these same problems when asked about her awareness of disability. I asked Evelyn if she could foresee any problems in returning to school, but she said she couldn't think of any. However, her parents said they thought she would have problems with being able to cope with lectures, organizing her schedule, and studying effectively. I also asked Evelyn whether she could manage her self-care activities, and she told me that she was independent in self-care. Again her parents contradicted this when they reported that they regularly needed to remind her of daily-living tasks. Evelyn said that her greatest frustration was having people tell her what to do. She took pleasure in listening to music, and felt sad at missing school. From these descriptions, it seemed to me that Evelyn and her parents were having some difficulties given their very different understanding of Evelyn's abilities, as well as the fact that Evelyn's parents were reminding her of what to do.

At interview's end, Evelyn recalled that the therapist borrowed something but not what it was. I gave her a cue in the form of a hint that she had been wearing it. Then Evelyn remembered her watch. After the interview, I asked Evelyn if I could meet with her parents privately. I usually find this helpful, particularly when the client (like Evelyn) has poor insight into his or her problems. Evelyn's parents were tired and worried. They told me that they had used up all of their financial resources and were about to go into debt. I documented all this information and spent some time talking about Evelyn's problems and how we would deal with them at the center. They seemed reassured by this. I also generated a referral for a case manager to administer Evelyn's case and a family psychologist to help Evelyn and her parents in their relationship.

call a story that has been read to them. The repeat test in both cases is more important than the original because it stands as a predictor for rehabilitation. When originally tested, Evelyn exhibited better auditory than visual short-term memory. She missed some details in recounting the story she had been read but recalled no details of it, and she recalled only one of the two actions depicted in the picture. The therapist offered input on strategies that could improve her performance and when she was retested, Evelyn improved in both areas.

3. The Postural Control Test, guided by neurodevelopmental theory, evaluates a client's muscular system by measuring the shift in the center of gravity as affected by a series of reaching activities.

4. The Body Alignment Test, guided by biomechanical theory, evaluates a client's skeletal system, using resting and dynamic postures, range-of-motion, muscle strength, and endurance tests. Problems in this area or in posture, as described in number 3, can interfere with perception, sapping energy that might otherwise be put toward cognition. When asked to reach objects placed at different angles and locations, Evelyn proved to be slow and demonstrated asymmetry, favoring her left side. The body alignment test confirmed that Evelyn's right side was weaker, but the range of motion in her upper extremity joints proved to be within normal limits.

The second group of four tests are designed from the quadraphonic approach's macro perspective, focusing on the four categories of a client's daily-living characteristics: lifestyle, life stage, health, and disadvantage.

5. The Storytelling Test is an in-depth extension of the interview. Clients are asked to share their beliefs, ethics, and values through the act of telling life stories. This test serves two distinct purposes. First, it is the most powerful test of episodic and semantic memory. (Referring back to the section on taxonomies, episodic memory concerns personally experienced events, e.g., how a student and her classmates dress at college; semantic memory concerns general world knowledge, such as the latest Paris fashions). Second, storytelling elicits valuable information about a client's personality, real-life setting, and possible "under life" behaviors (Josselson & Lieblich, 1995). "Under life" behaviors are behaviors that may not be typical of the individual but arise in the treatment or rehabilitation environment. In the process, it forms the basis of a therapist–client partnership.

Evelyn's storytelling revolved around the differences between how she organized her daily activities before and after the accident. Before the accident, she led a fast-paced life, conveyed in stories involving her motorcycle, activities with friends, and school. After the accident, she felt slower and told many stories reflecting problems with her parents over issues of dependency.

Evelyn also said that her family and friends tell her she has less empathy and motivation than she did before the accident. Both Evelyn's episodic and semantic memories seemed mildly impaired on the basis of a lack of details in many of her narratives. It became clear that she had developed a passive demeanor in her "under life" as a therapy client relative to her real-life assertiveness, which was evidenced by her stories from outside the treatment center.

6. The Simulated Occupations Test is used to evaluate clients' daily life disadvantages and their ability to cope with them. Simulated Occupations Tests are tests of clients' procedural memory and proceed by observing the clients performing ordinary tasks. When planning and preparing a lunch with the use of a written recipe, Evelyn was disorganized and displayed time-management problems. When planning and conducting a trip around the therapy center, she had the same problems, twice becoming disoriented. Finally, she was unable to balance a checkbook independently, requiring help in setting the materials up and coaching of various kinds throughout the activity.

7. The Satisfaction Test administered in the form of a survey, is used to evaluate clients' overall level of contentment with their lifestyle, life stage, health, and treatment. As had emerged in the original interview, Evelyn's greatest dissatisfaction related to her lack of independence and control and her absence from school. In addition, she was bothered by her new relationships with her family, in which she felt at a disadvantage, and with friends, from whom she felt distant.

8. The Picture and Object Test is used to gain deeper insight into clients' lives. They are asked to bring photographs and objects that symbolize who they think they are. This test is most critical with clients who have difficulty communicating but is also useful and revealing with other clients, who are then asked to describe the information imparted by the objects and pictures. Evelyn brought three photographs: one of a class outing to the beach, one of her on her motorcycle, and the third of her at a rock concert. She also brought a telephone and one of her student notebooks, which she had filled with notes she wrote before her accident. She could recall some, but not all, of the background stories of the photos; general notions, but few specifics, about the classes in which she had taken the notes; and many stories of telephoning friends before the accident, but none since.

CREATING A BASELINE

The results of these tests are used to create a baseline, or a quantitative assessment, of a client's current status. As an example of how this is done, consider the Visual and Auditory Short-term Memory Tests. The therapist divides each test into sections, assigning each a percentage of importance. For example, the memory test described previously could be divided into six segments: the capacity to recall the depicted foreground and background action after one 30-second viewing (10%); the capacity to recall the depicted foreground and background action after a second 30-second viewing (10%); the capacity to recall 20 related objects after one 30-second viewing (20%); the capacity to recall 20 related objects after a second 30-second viewing (20%); the capacity to recall 20 related words after a 30-second viewing (20%); and the capacity to recall 20 related words after a second 30-second viewing (20%). The client's performance on this test is assigned a numerical value based on these percentages, which is then combined with similarly obtained numerical values from other tests to obtain an overall picture of the client's status.

With other tests, such as the Simulated Occupations Test, the task of dividing it into parts, assigning percentage values, and assessing the client's performance is a more arbitrary process and is more beneficial when done by an experienced therapist. Using this overall picture, or baseline, the therapist assesses the potential and timetable for cognitive rehabilitation. Evelyn's baseline values were around 75 percent throughout the battery of tests, with some as low as 69 percent, but none exceeded 80 percent.

PROBLEM LIST

Based on analysis of all the information gained through the data gathering (interview and assessment procedures), eight problems were listed:

1. Impaired awareness of disability
2. Visual and auditory short-term memory deficits
3. Attention (concentration) deficits
4. Slight body misalignment and postural control dysfunction
5. Low endurance
6. Slight impaired communication
7. Frustration at a loss of control resulting in dependence on others
8. Confusing and unsettling feeling that she has lost part of herself

INTERVENTION GOALS AND OBJECTIVES

The therapist and other members of the rehabilitation team drew up a list of goals based on Evelyn's problems. A meeting was then held with the

BOX 5–4. THERAPIST REASONING—INTERVENTION GOALS

I met with Evelyn and her parents and outlined six long-term goals for improvement based on the problems I had identified. Evelyn and her parents agreed with these goals and that these long-term goals were to be met within 3 months, with corresponding short-term goals to be met within 6 weeks.

One long-term goal was for Evelyn to be able to program, operate, and converse on the telephone independently. Corresponding short-term goals were for her to access emergency and information services and use different area phone books. A second long-term goal was for Evelyn to be able to usefully attend a school lecture. Corresponding short-term goals were for her to take notes from a simulated lecture and complete a simulated lecture-based assignment.

These two goals were aimed at improving Evelyn's attentional and memory capabilities while at the same time increasing her sense of control and feeling of satisfaction. Some of the other goals addressed these same problems, and others were aimed at different problem areas, such as having a physical therapist oversee an exercise regimen to ameliorate Evelyn's misalignment and postural dysfunctions.

client and family group to discuss these goals and recommend guidelines for the frequency and duration of intervention (Box 5–4). The client and family were asked to express any concerns regarding the proposed program, after which a verbal contract was established specifying a given period of time in which the client would attempt to achieve the agreed-upon goals. Periodic reevaluation meetings were held throughout the intervention period, and a graduation ceremony was held when it was completed to recognize Evelyn's achievements.

THE QUADRAPHONIC APPROACH TREATMENT MODEL

The quadraphonic approach treatment model is based on creating a confluent environment designed to empower the client to increase the opportunity and the capacity for action, achieve goals, and increase satisfaction. There are four phases of the treatment model: planning, preparation, performance, and postperformance or review. Quantitative and qualitative standards of practice are used throughout the model, although they may differ based on many factors, including population and measurement techniques. This confluent treatment model requires constant reevaluation and revision. Following is a brief outline of the treatment model.

1. **Planning.** The treatment-planning phase is based on the goals identified in relation to the level of performance (the baseline) established during evaluation. This phase is used to determine the practice, feedback, and environment used for treatment.

- Practice is a scheduled, planned repetition of an action or a behavior. Practice is affected by the type of action, the amount of action planned, its duration, and its frequency.
- Feedback includes the response to practice provided from various sources, including the therapist, caretakers, the client, and technology. The amount and frequency of feedback is critical in treatment. The treatment guidelines used in this model are based on a 50 percent performance level. This means that if a client's baseline performance is established at less than 50 percent of the norm being used, the therapist uses constant feedback (100%). If and when the client reaches a baseline above the 50 percent level, the amount and frequency of feedback decreases.

The environment includes the client, therapist, and all of the relevant objects that surround them. If the baseline for the client is established below the 50 percent level, a congruent environment is used. If and when the client establishes a baseline above that level, a more complicated environment with more **contextual interference** is used for treatment. A congruent environment (providing **contextual congruence**) is a simple one that requires minimal processing demands with familiar objects in a nonrotated position. The duration of the engagement is brief and the speed of presentation is slow. A congruent environment is designed to match the task with the goal. An environment with a high degree of contextual interference is complex, requiring higher processing demands with unfamiliar objects presented in a rotated fashion. The duration of the engagement is lengthy and the speed of presentation is fast. This type of environment is designed to make the goal more difficult to achieve in order to strengthen the learning pattern. It has been found that an environment with a high degree of contextual interference decreases immediate performance during practice but benefits performance for generalization of learning.

2. **Preparation.** The object of preparation is to get the client emotionally and mentally ready to make the optimal use of treatment. The preparation phase includes the therapist's acting as a guide to

shape the learning effort of the client until the goal is achieved. It has three parts:

- The therapist and client must establish a trusting and relaxed rapport. This is accomplished through a collaborative relationship between the therapist and the client in which they use friendly conversation, relaxation, stress-reduction or meditation techniques, and self-help techniques.
- The client's attention must be focused on the target or goal to be accomplished. Attentional recruitment is used to help the client focus on the relevant features of the task. This can be aided by simple instruction, cueing, incorporating activities in the treatment to use multiple senses, or increasing the intensity of treatment (e.g., increasing the volume used in the performance phase).
- Strategies should be developed to maximize the client's capacity to organize or process information during treatment. Organization is the planning and design of strategies to process information and enhance learning; it is conscious or subconscious and internal (self-generated) or external. The therapist may help clients to organize information by breaking the information into parts, reducing details, or relating the information to what the client already knows. Using multisensory, metacognitive, and metamemory techniques, clients are trained to monitor and control their behavior by conscious verbal and mental awareness.

3. **Performance.** The major objective of the third phase is to improve the performance and satisfaction of the client. For example, the aim of Evelyn's performance phase is to improve her memory and learning capacity and increase her satisfaction with these skills. The quadraphonic approach uses contextual modifications for the client, the therapist, and the environment to improve performance. Figure 5–8 provides a list of contextual modifications. The performance phase is designed and carried out based on the client's baseline and goals and involves three actions: practice, feedback, and environmental modification:

- Practice consists of a planned repetition by the client of an action or behavior at a predetermined frequency for a predetermined duration.
- Feedback consists of a helpful response provided to the client during practice, whether by the therapist or some other source. The frequency of feedback varies. One feedback model is based on a 50 percent performance level: if a client's baseline performance is established at less than 50 percent of the assumed norm, the therapist employs constant

(text continues on page 202)

CONTEXTUAL MODIFIERS

Contextual modifications are cues that can originate from three primary sources - the therapist, the task / environment, and the client - and from an interplay among them that occurs during task performance. Although clinically these modifications interact closely, it is important to articulate and distinguish them for purposes of evaluation, treatment, and research.

Contextual Dimension	Standard Approach	Contextual Modification [Therapist/ Client / Task]	Outcome Successful	Unsuccessful
1. **Sensory modality:** The visual, verbal, tactile, or movement cues provided.	☐ Standard No modification of sensory input	☐ Give verbal repetition ☐ Give verbal cues [includes questions / probes] ☐ Give visual cue / non-verbal feedback ☐ Give tactile / kinesthetic cue ☐ Give pictorial represen-tation ☐ Give written cues ☐ Increase illumination, contrast, brightness ☐ Other [e.g. enlarge]	*Given:* Verbal repetition Verbal cues ☐ Visual cue / non-verbal feedback ☐ Tactile / kinesthetic cue ☐ Pictorial representation Written cues Increased illumination, contrast, brightness ☐ Other [e.g. enlarge]	☐ ☐ ☐ ☐ ☐
2. **Amount of Information:** The number of instruc-tion steps, choices, or pieces of information presented.	☐ Standard No modification to amount of information	☐ Cue to initiate ☐ Give one step at a time ☐ Reduce the number of steps ☐ Shorten the task ☐ Other	*Given:* Cueing to initiate ☐ One step at a time Reduced number of steps Shortening of the task Other	☐ ☐ ☐
3. **Complexity:** The level of difficulty of the pieces of information given.	☐ Standard No modification of level of difficulty	☐ Simplify by using concrete explanations ☐ Simplify by demonstra-ting ☐ Simplify by using familiar tasks ☐ Simplify by using self-related items ☐ Simplify by increasing the spacing between items or objects [non-scattered] ☐ Simplify by decreasing spatial traits or position of objects ☐ Other	*Given:* Concrete explanations ☐ Demonstrations ☐ Familiar tasks only ☐ Self-related items ☐ Increased spacing between items or objects [non-scattered] Decreased spatial traits or position of objects ☐ Other	☐ ☐ ☐
4. **Pace:** The speed and consistency with which information is presented.	☐ Standard No modification of pace	☐ Give slow presentation ☐ Give fast presentation ☐ Give predictable / stable presentation ☐ Give random / unpre-dictable presentation ☐ Other	*Given:* Slow presentation Fast presentation Predictable / stable presentation Random / unpre-dictable presentation Other	☐ ☐ ☐ ☐
5. **Duration:** The interval of time that the client is given in which to respond to an instruction.	☐ Standard No modification of duration of time	☐ Give 15 seconds ☐ Give 30 seconds ☐ Give 1 minute	*Given:* 15 seconds 30 seconds 1 minute	☐ ☐ ☐

Figure 5–8. Contextual modifiers.

Contextual Dimension	Standard Approach	Contextual Modification [Therapist/ Client / Task]	Outcome — Successful	Unsuccessful
6. **Safety:** The information that the client requires in order to perform safely.	☐ Standard No modification of set up, equipment, and safety demands	☐ Explain safety measures ☐ Explain preventive measures ☐ Explain dangerous consequences ☐ Explain emergency procedures ☐ Repeat preventive measure ☐ Other	*Given:* ☐ *Explanation of safety measures* ☐ *Explanation of preventative measures* ☐ *Explanation of dangerous consequences* *Explanation of emergency procedures* *Repetition of preventive measure* *Other*	☐ ☐ ☐ ☐
7. **Medications:** Substances used to affect client's cognitive function.	☐ Standard No medications	Names _____ _____ _____ _____	*Given:* ___ *medication* ___ *medication* ___ *medication* ___ *medication*	
8. **Personal History:** References to the client's needs, values, interests, or preferences.	☐ Standard request to perform	☐ Connect task with the client's interests / preferences ☐ Connect task with the client's hobbies ☐ Refer to client's needs / goals ☐ Refer to client's values ☐ Use personally relevant task ☐ Use personally concrete task ☐ Other	*Given:* ☐ *A connection made with the client's interests / preferences* ☐ *A connection made with the client's hobbies* ☐ *Reference to client's needs / goals* ☐ *Reference to client's values* ☐ *Use of a personally relevant task* ☐ *Use of a personally concrete task* ☐ *Other*	☐ ☐ ☐ ☐ ☐ ☐ ☐
9. **Posterial Readiness:** The bodily positions that facilitate the client's execution of a task.	☐ Standard position assumed by client	☐ Cue the client to position the Eyes Head / neck Limbs Hand Hips None Other	☐ *Given cueing to position* *Eyes* *Head / neck* *Limbs* *Hand* *Hips* *None* *Other*	
10. **Therapy Set:** Information given the client about the goal / performance of the task or therapy.	☐ Standard request to perform	☐ Explain goal / purpose of task ☐ Explain goal / purpose of therapy ☐ Explain role of the therapist ☐ Other	*Given:* ☐ *Explanation of the goal / purpose of task* ☐ *Explanation of the goal / purpose of therapy* ☐ *Explanation of the role of the therapist* ☐ *Other*	☐ ☐ ☐ ☐
11. **Awareness of a Problem:** Awareness of impairment, dysfunction, restriction, and/or personal or social disadvantage.	☐ Standard No modification of awareness capacities and limitations	☐ Give general cues that a problem exists ☐ Give specific cues when error happens or problem exists ☐ Give specific cues after error happens or problem occurs ☐ Give gentle confrontation about the undetected problem ☐ Give away the answer / solution ☐ Other	*Given:* ☐ *General cues that a problem exists* ☐ *Specific cues when error happened or problem existed* ☐ *Specific cues after error happened or problem occurred.* ☐ *Gentle confrontation about undetected problem* ☐ *An answer / solution* ☐ *Other*	☐ ☐ ☐ ☐ ☐ ☐

Figure 5–8. *Continued*

Contextual Dimension	Standard Approach	Contextual Modification [Therapist/ Client / Task]	Outcome Successful	Unsuccessful
12. **Error Detection / Correction:** Information provided the client relative to the presence of error.	☐ Standard Client initiates response to error in the absence of observable cueing.	☐ Cue for error detection ☐ Cue for error correction ☐ Client self cues for error detection ☐ Client self-cues for error correction ☐ Other	*Given:* ☐ *Therapist cueing for error detection* ☐ *Therapist cueing for error correction* ☐ *Client self-cueing for error detection* ☐ *Client self-cueing for error correction* ☐ *Other*	☐ ☐ ☐ ☐ ☐
13. **Feedback Type:** The structuring of corrective verbal information that the client is given in which to respond to an instruction.	☐ Standard No modification of feedback	☐ Give [KP] Knowledge of performance feedback: Corrective information about a component or part of task, test, or movement ☐ Give [KR] Knowledge of results feedback: Corrective information about the total or whole task, test, or movement goal ☐ Give positive feedback: Corrective information in form of approvals, assurances, reinforcers ☐ Give negative feedback: Corrective information in form of disapprovals or negative reinforcers ☐ Give private feedback: Corrective information in a confidential or private environment ☐ Give public feedback: Corrective information provided in a group view or community environment	*Given:* ☐ *Knowledge of performance feedback* ☐ *Knowledge of results feedback* ☐ *Positive feedback* ☐ *Negative feedback* ☐ *Private feedback* ☐ *Public feedback*	☐ ☐ ☐ ☐ ☐ ☐
14. **Organizational Strategy:** Organizational methods / guidelines provided.	☐ Standard organization offered	☐ Provide guidelines about where to start / end ☐ Provide guidelines about where to look ☐ Provide guidelines about what to say ☐ Provide rules and guidelines for behavior ☐ Reorganize information ☐ Client self initiates strategy: ☐ Other	*Given:* ☐ *Guidelines about where to start / end* ☐ *Guidelines about where to look* ☐ *Guidelines about what to say* ☐ *Rules and guidelines for behavior* ☐ *Reorganized information* ☐ *Self initiated strategy:* ☐ *Other*	☐ ☐ ☐ ☐ ☐ ☐
15. **Activity Phase Breakdown:** The phase during an activity when the client's functioning breaks down and the therapist offers feedback.	☐ Standard No modification through- out any phase of the test, task, or activity	Give feedback: ☐ Before preparatory stage ☐ At initiation stage ☐ At middle stage ☐ At end stage ☐ After completion	*Given feedback:* ☐ *At preparatory stage* ☐ *At initiation stage* ☐ *At middle stage* ☐ *At end stage* ☐ *After completion*	☐ ☐ ☐ ☐ ☐

Figure 5–8. *Continued*

Contextual Dimension	Standard Approach	Contextual Modification [Therapist/ Client / Task]	Outcome Successful	Unsuc- cessful
16. **Social Milieu:** Manipulation made to the client's social environment.	Standard No modification of social milieu. Client's family, friends, social, and institutional support system.	Seat the client near a friend Ask the client to help another Ask a client-helper to work with the client Ask a question to elicit interaction Other	*Given:* Seating near a friend A request to help another A client-helper A question to elicit interaction Other	[e.g. claims no fit]
17. **Therapist's use of self:** The conscious use of personal strength and interpersonal capacities.	Standard No deliberate use of personal interventions	Given expressive touch Use gentle humor Move closer to the client Actively listen to a client's concern Use encouraging words or gestures Give power of choice	*Given:* Expressive touch Gentle humor Proximity of the therapist Active listening Encouragement Choices	
18. **Voice Tone Changes:** The modification of verbal tone that the client is given.	Standard No modification in voice	Use a therapy voice: formal therapeutic language Use a directive voice: inter- personal control, command- ing Use a sympathetic voice: calm, confident, yet gentle Use a modulated voice: modified to increase understanding [i.e., slower, louder, shorter statements]	*Given:* Formal tone Commanding tone Calm and gentle tone Modulated tone to increase understanding Other	
19. **Expectations for Accuracy / Correctness:** The therapist's anticipation / expectation relative to the client's success or failure.	Standard expectations	Therapist anticipates task failure Therapist anticipates task success No anticipation Other	But therapist's expectation was a failure And therapist's expectation was a success In the absence of any particular expectation Other	

Note : A Formula

Client's performance was successful in _____ when given _____.
               (Indicate the task / module)   *(Indicate the contextual modifiers that helped*

Use of _____ did not help. Client's level of awareness of his or her
     (Indicate other modifiers used that were not successful)

problems / _____.
     (State client level of awareness)

Figure 5–8. *Continued*

feedback; if the baseline is established above the 50 percent level, the frequency of feedback will be less than constant and will decline fur- ther as the baseline increases (Fig. 5–9).

● The environment to be modified includes the client, therapist, and all of the objects that surround them during treatment. A congruent envi- ronment is a simple one; for example, an environment with familiar objects placed in a nonrotated position. Two other facets of congruency are brief duration and slow presentation. The congruent environment makes minimal cognitive-processing demands on the client. A complex

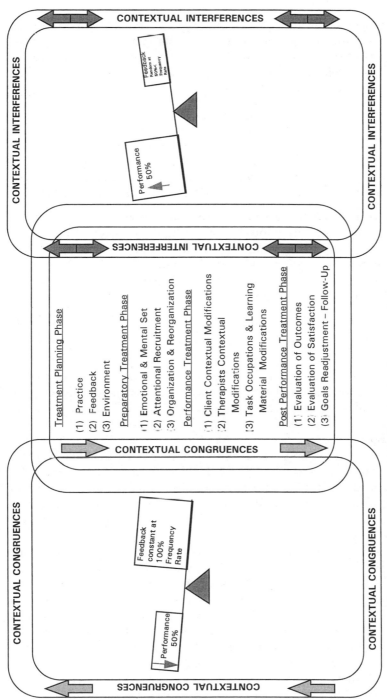

Figure 5-9. Quadraphonic approach treatment model.

environment, on the other hand, is marked by contextual interference, such as unfamiliar objects presented in a rotated fashion, longer duration, and fast presentation. This places higher demands on the client. Contextual interference makes the immediate treatment goal more difficult to achieve, but if used properly, it can strengthen the learning pattern (Abreu, 1995).

As with feedback, one model for environmental modification is based on a 50 percent performance level: if the client's baseline is established below the 50 percent level, a congruent environment is provided; as the baseline exceeds 50 percent, a contextual interference is introduced and it is increased as the baseline improves (see Fig. 5–9).

4. **Postperformance Phase and Review.** The postperformance phase is devoted to reviewing and documenting the progress the client has made toward increasing opportunities and capacities for action, achieving goals, and increasing the level of satisfaction. During this phase, the therapist, client, and family agree on a series of readjusted goals and objectives.

Using these four phases, treatment related to two of Evelyn's goals proceeded as follows:

1. **Goal of Telephone Proficiency.** *Planning and Preparation.* The therapist sought to help Evelyn focus her attention on the tasks at hand, screening out interruptions and distractions through coaching and cueing with regard to the endpoint or purpose of each practice session.

Performance and Practice. Beginning the first week, Evelyn spent a set period of time simulating calls to emergency services and soliciting help for telephone numbers and other information from the operator. She also practiced looking up and copying designated telephone numbers of friends from her personal directory. In the second week, she advanced to working with the city directory white pages, and in the third week, to dealing with yellow pages in different regional directories. In the fourth week, Evelyn began simulating ordering a pizza (sometimes she would really order a pizza to be eaten at the session's end) and calling repairmen and others who are commonly needed in everyday life. During week six, she was placed in an office setting and practiced taking phone messages for an imaginary boss. In week seven, she began programming the numbers of family members and friends into her phone. By week ten, she was locating the numbers of and calling other brain-injured people and sharing information and experiences.

Since Evelyn's baseline was around 75 percent, the frequency of feedback, delivered in the form of coaching and encouragement, was relatively low at 30 percent and grew even lower as Evelyn became adept at the various tasks (Bjork, 1994; Schmidt & Bjork, 1992). Contextual interference, on the other hand, was increased as the treatment period progressed and she improved her performance. This interference consisted of longer sessions on the phone, interruptions, the introduction of noise in her work area, and replacement of the simple phone in her message-taking environment with a multiple-line phone.

Postperformance and Review. Evelyn successfully completed her goals, and she, the therapist, and her parents decided that she was ready to proceed to more difficult ADLs, such as financial management.

2. **Goal of Usefully Attending Lectures.** *Planning and Preparation.* The therapist used anti-stress exercises to relax Evelyn before each session. Also, a strategy was devised to help Evelyn organize the lecture information. In the first 6 weeks of the intervention period, lectures were developed on topics she was familiar with and interested in, such as the history of rock and roll music. In the second 6 weeks, lectures were developed on topics that Evelyn could relate to through her previous experience as a nursing student and that could aid her metacognitive processes in the strategies of expert learners.

Performance and Practice. Each week, Evelyn attended a lecture, delivered by the therapist, in a real classroom. For 2 weeks, she simply listened and then discussed the lecture with the therapist. Beginning with week three, Evelyn took notes at the lecture, went over the notes afterward with the therapist, and then completed an assignment based on her notes. In the sixth week, she began writing summaries of the lectures from her notes. Beginning in the eighth week, she was given a quiz based on the weekly lectures.

More feedback was required in this area of the intervention program than in the telephone proficiency area, especially in carrying out assignments, writing summaries, and taking quizzes. Contextual interference (Bjork, 1994; Schmidt & Bjork, 1992) took the form of longer lectures, faster delivery, moving the client around the classroom from week to week, and using a blackboard to diagram selected lecture points.

Postperformance Phase and Review. Evelyn made progress over the 3-month intervention program and met her short-term goals but fell a bit short on her long-term goals, especially as judged from her performance on quizzes. Evelyn, the therapist, and her parents agreed to continue this area of treatment for an additional three months, with an end goal of Evelyn's being able to attend lectures for 2 hours a day.

MEASURING THE OUTCOME OF THERAPY

Outcome measurement is any attempt to quantify the quality of therapeutic services in terms of effectiveness or achievement of goals, efficiency or optimal rate of progress, and value or cost containment (Ellenberg, 1996; Foto, 1996). There are various standardized measures for different stages of recovery. Many service providers design their own. The outcome measurements used to evaluate Evelyn's treatment are discussed in Box 5–5.

COLLABORATION IN THERAPY

Intervention with brain-injured clients is a collaborative effort involving the entire rehabilitation team. This team incorporates the client and family group, as well as other professionals, who may include a case manager, family therapist or psychologist, physical therapist, recreational therapist, neuropsychologist, and vocational therapist. This collaboration not only allows constant monitoring of a client, if needed, but also provides a multiplicity of perspectives that is critical to treating the total client. In this light, the quadraphonic approach to occupational therapy,

---

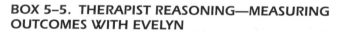

BOX 5–5. THERAPIST REASONING—MEASURING OUTCOMES WITH EVELYN

I chose two means of outcome measurement in the course of Evelyn's treatment: case management and a critical pathways timetable. The former involved a health care professional who coordinated and monitored all therapeutic services to ensure an efficient allocation of time and resources. The latter, as its name indicates, consisted of a timetable, designed by the rehabilitation team, that connected services and treatments with specific goals and target dates (Abreu et al., 1996).

Evelyn's intervention program met its critical pathways timetable and was satisfactory under the standards developed by the case manager. Although Evelyn retained minimal attention, memory, and learning problems, which appeared to increase in stressful situations, she had become fully aware of them and of the need to compensate. After four 3-month intervention periods, Evelyn returned to school and achieved general independence with the use of external memory aids such as checklists; outlines; and a personalized memory notebook, including a weekly calendar planner, a daily schedule, a "To Do" list, emergency numbers and addresses, and a diary section for her daily personal reflections.

which guided the case study in this chapter, is meant to broaden the perspective of the occupational therapy student, emphasizing the value of collaboration and showing the way to becoming a valuable collaborator rather than confining or limiting the student to one way of thinking or one view of therapy.

SUMMARY

This chapter has presented an overview of the theory of memory and learning and the use of the quadraphonic approach to assessing and treating clients who have problems with memory and learning. The case of Evelyn was used to illustrate some of the reasoning behind how an occupational therapist might use the quadraphonic approach when treating a client with a head injury.

REVIEW QUESTIONS

1. Identify primary areas of assessment addressed within the quadraphonic approach.
2. Describe an intervention plan from a "micro" and a "macro" perspective.
3. Discuss the possible practical applications for occupational therapy derived from an understanding of the human nervous system.
4. Using what you know of memory and learning taxonomies, discuss the relationship of memory and learning.
5. Discuss how current research into expert learning may help in the rehabilitation of brain-injured clients.
6. Discuss the differences between "micro" and "macro" perspectives of the quadraphonic approach. Also discuss how they are related.
7. Discuss the use of feedback and contextual interference in the treatment of a brain-injured client.

ACKNOWLEDGMENTS

I would like to express my gratitude to the research and editorial team of Diane Valdez, Jane Keel, Jeff Douglas, and Neil Huddleston for their help with the preparation of this chapter. I would also like to thank Dr. Brent Masel, the Moody Manor Foundation, Fort Lauderdale, Florida, and the Moody Manor Endowment for their support of this work. This chapter is based on the quadraphonic approach workshops formatted here in condensed form.

6

Evaluation and Intervention with Executive Functions Impairment

LESLIE DURAN, MS, OTR, and
ANNE G. FISHER, ScD, OTR, FAOTA

- Adaptation
- Collaborative Consultation
- Effective Performance
- Executive Abilities
- Executive Functions

- Markers
- Planning
- Purposive Action
- Temporal Organization
- Volition

On completion of this chapter, the reader will be able to:

- Define disorders of executive abilities, contrast executive abilities with executive functions, and describe the anatomical basis for disorders of executive function
- Describe behaviors typically seen in the performance of activities of daily living of clients with disorders of executive abilities
- Describe methodologies best suited to assess the performance of clients with disorders of executive abilities
- Understand the procedural, interactive, and conditional reasoning behind assessment of and intervention planning for clients with disorders of executive abilities
- Describe the AMPS
- Describe the use of the rehabilitative/compensatory model in guiding the evaluation process and intervention planning
- Successfully work through the Review Questions

≡ INTRODUCTION

The purpose of this chapter is to present the professional reasoning behind the assessment and treatment of a client who is experiencing disorders of **executive abilities.** The chapter opens with a detailed description of the expanded rehabilitative/compensatory model of practice. A summary of current literature describing the behavioral features and assessment methods of disorders of **executive functions** follows. The case of Curtis is then presented, including the therapist's top-down professional reasoning process when assessing the client, interpreting the test results, setting goals, and planning intervention based on the compensatory/rehabilitative model. In particular, the procedural reasoning process of interpreting the results of the Assessment of Motor and Process Skills (AMPS) is described in detail.

At the conclusion of the chapter, a second case study is presented and study questions are provided for the reader to answer.

WHAT ARE DISORDERS OF EXECUTIVE FUNCTIONS AND ABILITIES?

Executive functions are a subgroup of capacities and mental processes that occur within the brain. Disorders of executive functions can be considered impairments within the World Health Organization (WHO) classification of impairment, disability, and handicap (WHO, 1980). In contrast, executive abilities pertain to the behavioral manifestations of executive functions in the context of daily life task performances, including personal or instrumental activities of daily living (ADLs)—that is, disorders of executive functions, when they are manifested as disability, become disorders of occupational performance. The disruption of occupational performance concerns the occupational therapist.

Despite a growing interest in executive functions and their effects on daily life task performance, a precise and consistent definition of executive functions is not available in the literature. Although there is controversy regarding their classification, executive functions are sometimes described as higher-order cognitive functions (Glosser & Goodglass, 1990) or meta-cognitive functions (Katz & Hartman-Maeir, 1997; Winegardner, 1993). Others point out that executive functions cannot be equated with cognition (Lezak, 1995; Luria, 1966; Shallice & Burgess, 1991; Tranel, Anderson, & Benton, 1994). This view often also stresses the importance of considering the behavioral manifestations of executive functions as they pertain to the ability to perform daily life tasks (i.e., executive abilities; occupational performance). Compare, for example, the differences in the following definitions:

1. "The expression 'executive control functions' has increasingly been applied to a set of higher order cognitive processes. . . . These processes are critically involved in the selection, programming, and regulation of sensory inputs and motor output especially in nonroutine situations" (Glosser & Goodglass, 1990, p. 485).
2. Executive functions can be differentiated from behaviorally passive cognitive functions in that they "involve acting upon the environment" (Tranel et al., 1994, p. 134).
3. "Executive functions consist of those capacities that enable a person to engage successfully in independent, purposive, self-serving behavior" (Lezak, 1995, p. 42).

4. "Executive functions are the self-regulating and control functions that direct and organize behavior. Specific component areas include planning, decision making, directed goal selection, self-inhibiting, self-monitoring, self-evaluating, [self-correcting,] flexible problem solving, initiation and self-awareness" (Zoltan, 1996, p. 149).

Researchers who support the view that executive function cannot be equated with cognitive functions point out that many persons who demonstrate severe executive function disorders and associated problems with the performance of daily life tasks often perform within normal limits on neuropsychological tests of cognition, perception, language, and intelligence, including neuropsychological tests that are purported to assess executive functions (Lezak, 1995; Luria, 1966; Shallice & Burgess, 1991; Tranel et al., 1994). It appears that these persons are experiencing difficulties that often only manifest when they are engaged in the complex demands of daily life (Mateer, 1997).

Although the definitions we have presented are typical of those available in the literature, they fail to clarify what is actually meant by executive functions. One of the most comprehensive definitions has been presented by Lezak (1993, 1995), who has proposed that executive functions consist of the following four overlapping components:

1. *Volition:* the capacity to determine what one needs and wants to do and conceptualize a future realization of one's needs and wants. **Volition** requires the capacity to formulate a goal or an intention and then to initiate task performance. Self-awareness (i.e., body image as well as knowledge of one's capacity), awareness of the environment or context (e.g., use of environmental cues, time and place awareness), and social awareness (e.g., cleanliness and grooming, appreciation of social roles) also are critical.
2. *Planning:* "The identification and organization of the steps and elements (e.g., skills, materials, other persons) needed to carry out an intention or achieve a goal" (Lezak, 1995, pp. 653–654). **Planning** involves the capacity to look ahead and conceptualize change, conceive of alternatives, weigh and make choices, and develop a plan. Although some persons with executive function disorders are unable to either formulate realistic goals or intentions (i.e., volition) or plan, others may be able to formulate goals and initiate goal-directed task performance but are unable to realize their goals because of defective planning.
3. *Purposive action:* Capacities for productivity and self-regulation, including the ability to structure an effective and fluent course of action by initiating, maintaining, switching, and stopping complex action sequences in an orderly manner to realize a goal are called **purposive action.** Poor self-regulation can occur when there is a dissociation between intention

and action. Productivity may be reduced or erratic. The "problem becomes readily apparent in patients who 'talk a good game,' may even give the details of what needs to be done, but do not carry out what they verbally acknowledge or propose. Patients who do one thing while saying or intending another also display this kind of dissociation" (Lezak, 1995, p. 665).

4. *Effective performance:* The capacity for quality control, including the ability to monitor and correct one's behavior. Because ineffective self-monitoring and difficulty with self-correction are the primary features of the performance of persons with problems with **effective performance**, clients may not even perceive their mistakes, and others may identify them but take no action to correct them.

Hypothesized Neuroanatomical Substrates for Executive Functions

Executive functions have traditionally been associated with the frontal and prefrontal cortex (Glosser & Goodglass, 1990; Luria, 1966), but there is increasing evidence that they are not limited to these areas (Cummins, 1995; Schwartz, 1995; Tranel et al., 1994). The traditional tendency to equate executive function disorders with a "frontal lobe syndrome" is clearly depicted in the following description of the behavioral disturbances that can be associated with disorders of executive functions:

> Deficits in prioritization and temporal integration may lead to a "classic" frontal deficit, that is, the inability to plan and execute a sequence of behaviors needed to meet a goal. In the extreme, a client's behavior may be "driven" by irrelevant objects in the immediate environment because he or she cannot select only those stimuli and responses that are contextually relevant to the task at hand. In less extreme forms the deficit may be manifested by poor planning and sequencing, lack of foresight and anticipation, or grossly (and maddeningly) inconsistent behaviors relative to the client's past behaviors and stated goals. Clients with significant frontal injury may appear unable to visualize themselves in the future, grasp the relationship between long-term plans and the steps required to meet them, or to decide which actions fit most appropriately with a given goal (Hart & Jacobs, 1993, p. 3).

The current view is that these executive functions are mediated by reciprocal connections with other cortical and subcortical regions through the dorsolateral prefrontal-subcortical circuit (Cummins, 1995). Moreover, the evidence that certain executive disorders are seen only in clients with widespread and diffuse brain damage, as may be associated with traumatic brain injury and late-stage Alzheimer's disease, suggests that executive functions may involve both anterior and posterior brain regions (Schwartz, 1995; Schwartz, Mayer et al., 1993).

Current Research Trends

In contrast to the occupational therapist, whose primary focus of concern is occupational performance, the neuropsychologist has been the professional whose primary focus is understanding brain–behavior relations (Johnstone & Frank, 1995). Consistent with this focus, recent research among neuropsychologists has emphasized the development of theoretical models of the brain processes that underlie executive functions as well as the relation between executive functions and executive abilities (Levinson, 1995; Norman & Shallice, 1986; Schwartz, 1995; Schwartz et al., 1993; Shallice & Burgess, 1991). Understanding the relationship between executive functions and executive abilities is especially important to occupational therapists because of the widespread evidence that executive functions are difficult to identify using standard neuropsychological assessments but that decreased executive abilities can be seen in ADL task performance (Lezak, 1995; Luria, 1966; Mateer, 1997; Shallice & Burgess, 1991). These models may be helpful to the occupational therapist who seeks to answer the questions: What *are* executive functions and executive abilities? How do I recognize these problems in the persons with whom I work?

For example, Norman and Shallice and their colleagues (Norman & Shallice, 1986; Shallice & Burgess, 1991) have proposed a supervisory attentional system within the frontal lobe that controls one's ability to set goals, develop provisional plans, attempt solutions, and evaluate the effectiveness of the attempted solution. This is a process that leads to the formulation of goals that had not been anticipated (i.e., *unanticipated subgoal formation*) and subsequent modification of initial, provisional plans when something *unexpected, nonroutine,* or *unforseen* occurs. Provisional plans have **markers** associated with them. Markers are temporal, social, or task-related cues that inform a person that a performance error has occurred. More specifically,

> . . . a marker is basically a message that some future behaviour or event should not be treated as routine and instead, some particular aspect of the situation should be viewed as especially relevant for action. If the behaviour or event does occur later, then the marker would be triggered and this would lead to inhibition of the activity being carried out, the reassessment of the situation and so potentially the switching in or out of a particular course of action linked to a marker. Thus a task rule. . . would be realized through a marker becoming activated when the instructions are understood (Shallice & Burgess, 1991, p. 737).

Norman and Shallice (1986) and Shallice and Burgess (1991) propose that the supervisory system is activated in open-ended multiple subgoal situations when the person cannot rely on well-learned action routines to carry out an intended task. When a person experiences frontal lobe damage, the supervisory attentional system no longer functions normally. As long as the context and the contingencies of action are familiar, the person will function effectively, but

> . . . when the context or the contingencies are less familiar, loss of the [supervisory attentional system] influence on schema selection leads to rigidity of thought and action along well-trodden paths. Thus, faced with a novel task or task requirement, the patient may display a tendency to perseverate on familiar, but inappropriate, solutions (Schwartz et al., 1993, p. 63).

Loss of supervisory control can also result in environmental dependency (i.e., behavior driven or guided by the cues available in the social and physical environments), especially utilization behavior (i.e., the tendency to pick up and use objects visible in the environment) (Lhermitte, 1986; Tranel et al., 1994).

More recently, Schwartz and colleagues (Schwartz, 1995; Schwartz et al., 1993) described an action-based executive disorder characterized by "errors of action." In contrast to many authors' view (Norman & Shallice, 1986; Shallice & Burgess, 1991; Stuss, 1991), Schwartz and her colleagues assert that executive function disorders can be observed in routine, overlearned activities of daily living; task novelty is not required.

Schwartz et al. (1993) proposed that the components of action plans are schemas. Schemas are activated by either intentions (top-down activation) or an environmental event or affordance for action (bottom-up activation). Errors of action, or "action slips," may occur when (1) multiple intentions (or schemas) are active and the competition between them leads to confusion or blending of component actions sequences, (2) low level schemas are triggered by environmental events or affordances for action in the absence of an intention to perform the action (i.e., environmental dependency), or (3) premature loss of activation of a higher level schema results in inappropriate activation of lower-level component schemas (e.g., object substitution, utilization behavior, omissions, perseverations). Persons with disorders of executive functions have ineffective top-down activation and instead demonstrate an overreliance on bottom-up activation of schemas.

Assessment and Treatment Resources

Because of the previously mentioned problems associated with using neuropsychological tests to evaluate executive function, there has been a move toward naturalistic assessment of executive abilities (Schwartz et al., 1993; Shallice & Burgess, 1991). For example, Schwartz et al. (1993) stressed the advantages of implementing systematic analyses of a person's ADL task performances. In addition to noting the limitations of neuropsychological testing, they noted that "because the focus is on ADLs, such an analysis has more immediate relevance for treatment goals and procedures" (p. 65).

For the occupational therapist, there is another important consideration. Occupational therapists have tended to assess cognitive capacities to identify problems related to initiation, planning, problem solving, or other executive functions, but the occupational therapist's primary concern should relate to the ways executive function disorders impact on occupational performance. Therefore, it is more useful and efficient to assess the executive abilities through the direct observation of occupational performance.

The AMPS (Fisher, 1997a) is a standardized test that provides the occupational therapist with a method for detailed analysis of a person's executive abilities. There is strong support in the literature for the use of a tool like the AMPS for evaluating executive abilities. For example, Shallice and Burgess (1991) recommended that direct observation of ADL task performance involves observing a person perform complex daily life tasks (open-ended multiple subgoal situations). They also advocated for the need "to develop quantifiable analogues of the open-ended multiple subgoal situations" (p. 728) when the problems of persons with executive function deficits become manifest as decreased executive abilities. Many of the ADL tasks included in the AMPS provide open-ended multiple subgoal situations of sufficient challenge to detect, objectively measure, and quantify disorders of executive abilities. Although it is difficult to identify precisely the exact steps any given person might enact for any given ADL task in the AMPS, an example of the potential for evaluating a person's ability to efficiently and effectively implement and carry out a task that offers open-ended multiple subgoal situations is provided here using the AMPS task "tossed salad with dressing served in individual bowls—two or three people,"' which may involve the following steps:

1. *Planning*, during the AMPS interview, to prepare a salad with four ingredients (lettuce, tomatoes, cucumber, and radishes); add oil and vinegar salad dressing to the salad; serve the salad into three individual serving dishes; and clean up the workspace and put everything away.
2. *Choosing* the appropriate preselected ingredients from among alternative choices.
3. *Initiating* the gathering of the preselected ingredients.
4. *Initiating* and then *continuing* through to an appropriate and timely *termination* of the tearing of the lettuce and the cutting up of the tomatoes, cucumber, and radishes.
5. *Initiating* and then *continuing* through to an appropriate and timely *termination* of the addition of the salad dressing and the tossing of the salad.
6. *Initiating* and then *continuing* through to an appropriate and timely *termination* of the serving of the salad into the preselected number of serving dishes.

7. *Initiating* cleaning up the workspace, including putting unused tools and materials away, wiping the counter clean, and throwing waste in the trash container.
8. *Sequencing* of the steps of the task performance logically.
9. *Heeding* the essential goal of the task, including avoidance of behavior driven by environmental cues (environmental dependency).

Schwartz et al. (1993) described a system for coding action errors that provides additional support for the use of the AMPS to evaluate a person's executive abilities. In their coding system, "A-1s" are analogous to "actions" in the AMPS: *opening* the bottle of salad dressing, *pouring* the salad dressing onto the salad, and *tossing* the salad. An "A-2" is a grouping of A-1s into a task subroutine analogous to a "step" in the AMPS: *put salad dressing on the salad*. A-2s also have associated with them certain A-1s that define the A-2 subroutine: *pours the salad dressing onto the salad*. These A-1s are referred to as "cruxes."

> Errors are coded when arguments of the action [task tools or materials] are inappropriate to the task goal (e.g., applying shaving cream to a toothbrush; spreading toothpaste on a razor); or when an A-1 occurs out of sequence (e.g., omission, anticipation, perseveration). Sequence errors are also captured at the A-2 level (e.g., when the entire sugaring routine is omitted) (Schwartz et al., 1993, p. 64).

Errors are also noted when an A-1 is stranded outside an A-2. Such "independent" errors are often associated with exploratory and utilization behavior that results in inefficiency or disorganization of the task performance.

Based on the errors of action described by Schwartz (1995), the occupational therapist might observe the following errors of action (action slips) among persons with or without brain damage, with or without intact executive abilities, who chose to prepare a glass of cranberry juice and a bowl of cereal when performing the AMPS task "cold cereal and beverage":

1. Capture errors (i.e., deviation from expected routine by failure to suppress habitual behavior that commonly occurs in a given context in favor of a required novel behavior): upon opening the refrigerator, takes out the commonly, frequently chosen milk instead of the more novel, less frequently chosen cranberry juice.
2. Omission errors (i.e., deviation from expected routine by the omission of a step): begins to pour the cranberry juice without removing the lid from the jar.
3. Exchange errors (i.e., deviation from expected routine by the transpositioning the objects of two actions but performing the actions in the proper sequence): lifts the glass and attempts to pour into the cranberry juice jar.

4. Substitution (sometimes novel) errors (i.e., deviation from expected routine by replacing the object of the action with another similar or nearby object): putting a spoonful of sugar into the glass of cranberry juice rather than onto the bowl of cereal; putting the cereal away in the refrigerator rather than into the cupboard.

Schwartz (1995) described the following additional errors of action that more specifically characterize the person with brain injury who has decreased executive abilities:

1. Addition errors (i.e., deviation from expected routine by adding an action sequence to those needed or initially intended to complete the task): preparing toast in addition to the cranberry juice and cereal; slicing a banana onto the cereal.
2. Anticipation errors (i.e., deviation from expected routine by performing an action too early in the overall task performance): opening the jar of cranberry juice and then closing it, only to have to reopen it again to pour the juice into the glass.
3. Perseveration errors (i.e., deviation from expected routine by repeating an already completed action sequence): scooping two spoonfuls of sugar onto the cereal, pouring a glass of cranberry juice, and then resugaring the cereal.

Although persons with and without brain injury both demonstrate action slips, a major difference in persons with brain injury is that they demonstrate errors of action even when they are attending closely to the task. The errors seen in persons with brain damage "are more blatant and they may persist for long periods without being corrected. Indeed, patients do not always acknowledge their errors when they are pointed out to them" (Schwartz, 1995, p. 327). Persons with brain damage also are more likely to demonstrate perseverations (i.e., repeating already completed actions) and blatant substitutions; they often use the wrong object for a given action or the wrong action for a given object.

CASE STUDY: CURTIS

BACKGROUND

INTRODUCTION TO THE EXPANDED REHABILITATIVE/COMPENSATORY MODEL OF PRACTICE

In this chapter, the expanded rehabilitative/compensatory model of practice is used to guide the process of planning appropriate intervention for a client with disorders of executive abilities. Although the exact origins of the rehabilitative/compensatory model are unclear (Kielhofner, 1992), Trombly (1989, 1995c, 1995d) was the first to articulate and develop the rehabilitative/compensatory model into an occupational therapy model of practice. The work of Fisher (1997b) extends that of Trombly by (1) articulating more explicitly assumptions made about people within the rehabilitative/compensatory model; (2) generalizing this model beyond persons with physical disabilities to those with developmental, cognitive, or psychosocial disabilities; and (3) adding collaborative consultation to the available strategies used to effect change. That is, Trombly (1995d) indicated that the therapeutic mechanisms or strategies of change within the rehabilitative/compensatory model include providing opportunities for learning through education and promoting competent occupational performance through adaptation. Fisher (1997b) added principles of collaborative consultation as an important strategy of change within the rehabilitative/compensatory model.

In Fisher's expanded rehabilitative/compensatory model (Fig. 6–1), the professional reasoning process of intervention planning begins with a therapist establishing the client-centered performance context. This context is consistent with the top-down approach to assessment (Trombly, 1993) because the therapist begins the assessment process by considering the client's personal characteristics, the environment, and the characteristics of the tasks the client needs and wants to perform. Through chart review, client interview, use of the Canadian Occupational Performance Measure (COPM), and so on, the therapist establishes both the client-centered performance context and a collaborative partnership with the client and together they identify the client's major areas of concern, establish goals, and focus on which ADL tasks to observe.

After the client-centered performance context has been established, the therapist completes a performance analysis. The performance analysis is an observational assessment that occurs in the context of the client's per-

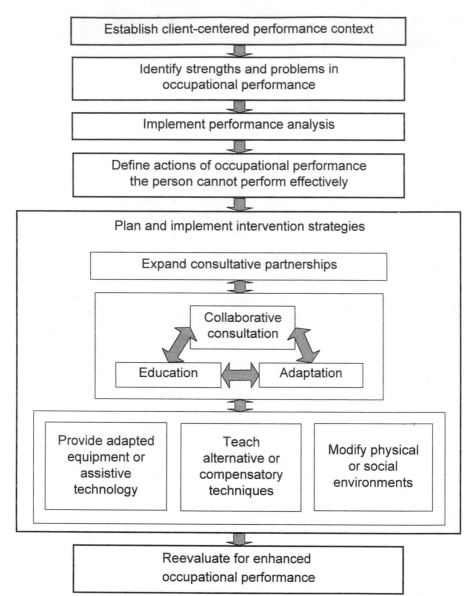

Figure 6–1. Schematic representation of the rehabilitative/compensatory model of practice. (From Fisher [1997a]. *Assessment of motor and process skills* [2nd ed]. Fort Collins, CO: Three Star Press. Reproduced with permission.)

forming familiar and meaningful tasks. While the therapist observes the client, the therapist defines the actions of occupational performance (not performance components) that the client cannot perform effectively. The outcome of the performance analysis is a definition of a client's problems described in terms of occupational performance (e.g., the client is unable to search for and locate plates in the cupboard), not the client's underlying impairments.

Based on the information gathered in the performance analysis, the therapist begins the process of designing and implementing intervention strategies. Because the client, his or her family members, a variety of rehabilitation professionals, and members of the community (e.g., friends, neighbors, church members) may have valuable roles to play in a collaborative intervention process, the therapist and client must identify who should join their existing collaborative partnership. An effective collaborative process requires that the occupational therapist enter into a shared partnership with not only the client but also other members of the consultative partnership (e.g., caregivers, service extenders such as aides and assistants, or other professionals) so that each member of the partnership can communicate the information necessary for shared problem solving. The occupational therapist should let go of his or her own goals for the client while focusing on those of the client; this can be a critical step in the process (Fisher, 1994; Tickle-Degnen, 1995).

Within the collaborative partnership, therapists bring expertise in the following three intervention strategies: collaborative consultation, adaptation, and education. **Collaborative consultation** is a method of building on the collaborative relationships necessary to foster the success of therapeutic interventions using principles of therapeutic rapport (Tickle-Degnen, 1995) to foster openness and trust. Collaborative consultation can be likened to therapeutic rapport because it is based on a mutual and collaborative relationship among equals (Tickle-Degnen, 1995). Consultative partnerships may need to be revised or expanded as intervention progresses.

The steps or principles of the collaborative consultative process are as follows (Fisher, 1997b):

1. Determine which members of the consultative partnership are the most appropriate to implement the intervention—the recipients of the consultative process (e.g., caregiver, service extender, or other professional).
2. Establish the client's baseline level of occupational performance.
3. Establish the expected functional outcomes (set goals).
4. Develop mutually agreed-upon strategies for intervention.

5. Train recipient(s) in implementing the intervention (using principles of education).
6. Reevaluate to verify that the consultative process was effective and the outcome attained.
7. Document effectiveness of intervention.

The second intervention strategy, **adaptation,** is dependent on multiple factors to be successful, including the client's perception of the usefulness of the adaptation and his or her willingness to accept the need for adaptation. Effective adaptation, therefore, requires that we follow the following principles (Fisher, 1997b; Trombly, 1995d):

1. Propose solutions based on knowledge and principles of adaptation.
2. Confirm that proposed solutions will indeed benefit, and are acceptable to, the client.
3. Train the client in safe use of the adaptation (using principles of education).
4. Reevaluate to verify that the adaptation is effective and reliable and document effectiveness of intervention.

The principles of the third intervention strategy, *education*, may be applied to clients, caregivers, service extenders (aides or assistants), or other professionals. Determination of who may be the recipient of the learning process is established using collaborative consultation. The following principles are recommended for the strategy of education to be successful (Fisher, 1997b; Trombly, 1995d):

1. Establish a baseline by determining what the learner knows.
2. Establish the learning objective (the client's goal, not what the learner will know).
3. Choose teaching techniques congruent with what is to be taught.
4. Adapt the presentation to the learner's capabilities.
5. Provide opportunities for practice, considering context and schedule.
6. Offer useful feedback at the right time.
7. Reevaluate the learner in an appropriate context to confirm that learning has occurred and document the effectiveness of the intervention.

The occupational therapist uses the three intervention strategies of collaborative consultation, adaptation, and education simultaneously to develop compensatory or adaptive strategies to improve the client's occupational performance. Such compensatory or adaptive strategies may be developed through providing adaptive equipment, teaching alternative techniques, or modifying physical or social environments (Fisher, 1997b). The strategies are used to enhance the client's occupational performance.

INTRODUCTION TO THE OCCUPATIONAL THERAPIST, HANA

The occupational therapist who we present in this case study, Hana, worked in a rehabilitation setting in a large city. At the time of the case study, Hana was the lead occupational therapist at the facility and was responsible for the supervision of six other occupational therapists and two certified occupational therapy assistants. She had 5 years of clinical experience and a Master of Science degree in occupational therapy. Hana studied executive functions and executive abilities during her masters degree program, and she had completed rater training and calibration for the AMPS. Hana often uses a rehabilitative/compensatory frame of reference when working with clients.

INTRODUCTION TO CURTIS

Curtis is a 66-year-old man who sustained head injuries after a motor vehicle accident. He had been referred to outpatient occupational therapy after acute care hospitalization and 6 weeks of inpatient rehabilitation. In the narrative that follows, Curtis's case is recounted by Hana, his occupational therapist in the outpatient clinic.

INFORMATION GATHERING

ESTABLISHING THE CLIENT-CENTERED CONTEXT: REVIEW OF THE MEDICAL RECORD

Before Curtis's first visit, Hana reviewed his medical chart, which contained some of the paperwork from his inpatient rehabilitation stay. The computed axial tomography (CAT) scan performed in the acute care setting revealed that Curtis sustained diffuse, global brain damage as a result of the accident. In Curtis's discharge summary from inpatient occupational therapy, his therapist documented that Curtis was able to complete all of his personal self-care activities without physical assistance but that he frequently required verbal cueing to initiate these activities. The speech pathologist had developed a day timer that Curtis used in an effort to improve his time-management skills. The neuropsychologist documented that Curtis exhibited behaviors that were consistent with disorders of executive functions. Curtis was discharged home after his inpatient stay. His mother, who had been living with her sister, moved in to Curtis's house before his discharge because the rehabilitation team thought that Curtis required 24-hour supervision at home because of his decreased initiation and poor safety awareness.

ESTABLISHING THE CLIENT-CENTERED CONTEXT: THE INITIAL VISIT

In Box 6–1, Hana describes the first time she met with Curtis.

BOX 6–1. THERAPIST REASONING—THE INITIAL VISIT

On his first visit to the outpatient clinic, Curtis was accompanied by his mother and his son. I believe in using a top-down approach to assessment, so I began the process of Curtis's occupational therapy evaluation with an informal interview to learn about his roles, interests, and values. I prefer the top-down approach (Trombly, 1993) because I believe occupational therapists should not begin the assessment process by evaluating impairments in the capacities of the client's mind, brain, or body and then infer how these impairments may impact that client's occupational performance. I feel that the top-down approach fosters client-centered treatment, clarifies the purpose of occupational therapy for the client, and enhances interactive reasoning and therapeutic rapport. I wanted to learn what was meaningful to Curtis, what activities were part of his typical day before this injury, and what activities he was doing presently at home.

During the interview, Curtis's mother and son answered many of my questions. Curtis did not volunteer unsolicited information, but when I asked him a direct question he would reply in a manner that was matter of fact, albeit polite. I noticed that Curtis had his day timer with him. His affect during the interview was somewhat withdrawn, and he tended to stare straight ahead while people talked around him. He would answer direct questions with short, simple statements. His affect became slightly more animated when he answered questions. It was as if he would "turn on" when specifically spoken to, but "turn off" in between periods of direct interaction.

Through the process of interviewing Curtis and his family, I learned that Curtis had worked for 40 years as an appliance repair man and retired 1 year ago. I also learned that Curtis enjoys watching sports on television, especially basketball. Curtis is presently living in a two-story house, and his bedroom and the home's only bathroom are on the second floor. Before his accident, Curtis was independent in meal preparation, lawn maintenance, and grocery shopping. On Sunday mornings before his accident, Curtis's mother and aunt usually came over, and Curtis would prepare a hot breakfast for the three of them.

(continues)

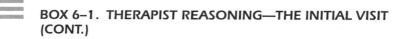

BOX 6–1. THERAPIST REASONING—THE INITIAL VISIT (CONT.)

I asked Curtis about the things he was doing now at home; he replied that he watched a lot of television. I asked him if he would like to be doing more things, and he replied that he would like to because he was quite bored at home. Curtis's mother was doing all of the cooking and housework activities and Curtis's son expressed concern that Curtis's mother was frail and that the demands of caring for Curtis were hard on her. I asked Curtis whether or not he would like to be fixing meals at home. His face lit up, and he said, "Oh, yes, ma'am! If there's one thing I can do, it is cook."

Curtis's mother stated that the hardest thing about caring for Curtis was that he would get upset over "little things," for example, becoming angry if she threw any of her garbage away in his trash can. Curtis's mother also reported that Curtis became angry if she inadvertently rearranged his things, such as his razor, shaving cream, and toothbrush, while she was cleaning the bathroom.

From the interview, I reasoned that if Curtis could participate more fully in meaningful activities of daily living (ADLs) at home, he would be less bored, and some of his mother's caregiver strain would be reduced. Curtis indicated that he was motivated to increase his participation in ADLs. However, I knew from experience that clients with disorders of executive functions often say they are motivated, but they experience difficulty initiating even self-care tasks. As Curtis's occupational dysfunction was impacting not only on himself but also his mother and son, I believed that it was important to involve them in the goal-setting and intervention planning process. I felt that it was also important to include caregiver education in the intervention plan so that Curtis's family members might better understand and manage his unusual behaviors.

IMPLEMENTING THE PERFORMANCE ANALYSIS: EVALUATION OF ADL WITH THE AMPS

After interviewing Curtis and his family, Hana wanted to evaluate Curtis's current level of ADL performance with a standardized, observational assessment. In Box 6–2, Hana discusses her choice of assessment.

Implementing the Performance Analysis: Administration of the AMPS

An AMPS observation begins with a client interview. While interviewing Curtis for the initial occupational therapy evaluation, Hana was

---

BOX 6–2. THERAPIST REASONING—EVALUATION OF ADLs WITH AMPS

I chose to evaluate Curtis using the Assessment of Motor and Process Skills (AMPS) for several reasons. First of all, the AMPS allows for client choice in what tasks he or she performs for the purposes of the assessment. My use of the AMPS, therefore, would enable me to observe Curtis completing tasks that were meaningful to him and that he would like to be doing at home. Secondly, consistent with the top-down approach, I wanted to use an assessment that was at the level of disability (i.e., dysfunction in performance of daily life tasks and executive abilities) rather than a test of cognitive impairments (i.e., dysfunction in underlying capacities and executive functions). I have found that tests of cognitive impairment are inadequate to assess the occupational performance of people with disorders of executive ability.

I wanted to observe Curtis completing tasks that were meaningful to him and that contained open-ended, multiple subgoals. By using the AMPS, I would be able to evaluate Curtis's executive abilities in terms of the specific ADL motor and process skills that were supporting or limiting his occupational performance. This information is extremely useful for planning specific intervention strategies to improve the quality of a client's ADL performance.

Although I used to think otherwise, I now believe that most neuropsychological capacities cannot be remediated. I often use a rehabilitative/compensatory approach for intervention, therefore, one that focuses on adaptations—providing adaptive equipment, teaching alternative strategies for performing ADL tasks, and modifying social and physical environments. The AMPS skill items would help me implement a detailed performance analysis of Curtis's occupational performance. Lastly, by taking advantage of the AMPS computer-scoring software, I would be able to generate objective, quantifiable measures of Curtis's baseline ADL motor ability and ADL process ability. This information is essential for outcomes data (i.e., measuring the effectiveness of my occupational therapy intervention).

---

able to make a natural transition to the "AMPS interview," during which she framed the nature and purpose of the AMPS for Curtis and asked him about specific ADL tasks that he was familiar with and knew how to perform. Box 6–3 provides some of Hana's interactive and procedural reasoning as she negotiates to do the AMPS assessment with Curtis.

BOX 6–3. THERAPIST REASONING—ADMINISTRATION OF AMPS

When I offered a subset of AMPS task options to Curtis, I wanted to be sure to offer only those with which he was familiar and that would provide him with an appropriate challenge. I had already decided not to consider the AMPS personal ADL (PADL) tasks, because they would be too easy for him.

The AMPS interview culminates with an agreement between client and examiner as to which tasks will be done for the purposes of the assessment. This agreement is a critical part of the AMPS. As the examiner, I needed to be sure that Curtis's way of doing a given task was consistent with the standardized task description in the AMPS manual. However, within the standardized AMPS task description, the client is able to choose between certain options, such as which ingredients will be used. The shared agreement between client and examiner as to what task will be done and what ingredients will be used is critical when scoring the AMPS. By ascertaining ahead of time what Curtis intended to do, I could score him based on whether or not his performance deviated in any way from the details of what he said he would do.

Curtis chose to do the following two AMPS tasks:

1. Cook scrambled or fried eggs and meat and boil or brew coffee or tea; and

2. Prepare hot cooked cereal and beverage.

The tasks were familiar to him because he had been completing both of them at home before his accident.

Before each task, I oriented Curtis to the clinic kitchen, and Curtis placed the task objects where he wanted to store them. This is standard practice for any AMPS observation that is done in an unfamiliar setting because it promotes client familiarity with the test environment. I encouraged Curtis to practice turning the stove off and on, opening and closing the refrigerator door, and plugging and unplugging the electric kettle so he would be familiar with how these objects worked. Curtis and I then reviewed the details of what he had agreed to do. For the first task, Curtis stated he would scramble two eggs, cook two pieces of bacon, and brew a pot of tea. For the second task, Curtis stated he would prepare a serving of oatmeal and a glass of orange juice. Then, he completed the tasks while I observed and took notes, which I used later to score his AMPS tasks performances.

Defining Problems of Occupational Performance: AMPS Assessment Findings

After the AMPS observation, Hana reported that Curtis demonstrated several performance difficulties typical of persons with disorders of executive ability. A review of the AMPS skill items, the AMPS rating scale, and an example of the AMPS scoring criteria in Appendixes 6–1, 6–2, and 6–3, respectively, will aid the reader in following Hana's professional reasoning (Box 6–4).

Hana scored Curtis's AMPS observations, entered the scores into her computer using the AMPS scoring software, and printed the following three reports: the AMPS summary report, the AMPS Raw Scores report, and the AMPS Graphic Report.

BOX 6–4. THERAPIST REASONING—AMPS ASSESSMENT FINDINGS

Curtis's occupational performance was impacted by errors of action. For example, at the conclusion of the AMPS interview, Curtis had chosen the two tasks he intended to do and the ingredients he intended to use for both tasks. Curtis stated that he planned to use milk in his scrambled egg mixture, as well as add milk to his oatmeal when he had finished cooking it. We had determined that there was about half a liter of milk, more than enough for both tasks. Knowing this information ahead of time enabled me to identify Curtis's problems; during the performance of the first task, he put all of the milk into his scrambled egg mixture (Terminates = 1) and therefore had none left to put on his oatmeal during the second task. Curtis merely stated that his oatmeal "needs a little milk, but I guess I used it all." Although Curtis later recognized his error, he responded as if the error was of no consequence.

Before performing the first task, Curtis stated that he intended to make scrambled eggs with two eggs, cook two pieces of bacon, and brew and serve a cup of tea. However, during the actual performance, Curtis used all seven of the eggs that were in the carton and all six slices of bacon that were in the package (Chooses = 1, Heeds = 1). This is an example of behavior driven by environmental cues (environmental dependency).

Similar behavior was also apparent in the second task, preparing a serving of oatmeal and a beverage. Before he began, Curtis stated that he intended to serve a glass of orange juice with the oatmeal. During the actual performance, however, he served two glasses of orange juice (Heeds = 2). Lastly, although Curtis gathered a tea bag, he did not initiate heating the water (Initiates = 1) and thus did not effectively complete the stated goal of making tea (Heeds = 1). During the AMPS interview Curtis was able to verbalize what he intended to do, but his actions during the assessment observation did not support attainment of his stated goals.

Curtis demonstrated difficulty terminating task actions and steps at an appropriate time. Besides pouring too much milk into the scrambled egg mixture (Terminates = 1), the bacon was overcooked and almost burnt (Terminates = 2). Curtis hesitated frequently during both tasks (Initiates = 2), and his performance of task actions was discontinuous (Continues = 2).

(continues)

BOX 6–4. THERAPIST REASONING—AMPS ASSESSMENT FINDINGS (CONT.)

In addition to choosing too many eggs, too many slices of bacon, and too much milk, Curtis had other action errors. When Curtis poured one of the glasses of orange juice during the oatmeal task, a small piece of paper fell from the edge of the juice carton into the glass and was floating on top of the orange juice. Curtis did not notice or respond effectively to this problem (Notices/Responds = 2). When he was preparing the oatmeal, Curtis set the burner on high while the water was heating (Adjusts = 1). When the water started to boil, he said, "I'd better turn this down to medium." When he turned the dial, however, he turned the stove off. Curtis did not adjust the stove dial effectively, and the result was undercooked oatmeal (Adjusts = 2, Terminates = 2). Moreover, during the egg task, he left a fork resting with the handle on the stove top and the prongs face down on the edge of the hot pan (Handles = 2). When Curtis later tried to pick the fork up, he immediately dropped it because it had become very hot (Notices/Responds = 1). I felt this behavior presented a safety risk of a burn injury. Finally, he did nothing to modify his behavior when making the eggs (Accommodates = 1), and his problems persisted (Benefits = 1).

At the conclusion of the AMPS observation, I asked Curtis how he felt about his performance. He said, "It went well. I just wish I had some more milk for my oatmeal." This statement indicated to me that Curtis had limited awareness of his performance errors. I thanked Curtis for his participation and told him that I would share the results of the assessment with him at our next session. I also noted that Curtis's mother reminded Curtis to record the date and time of his next occupational therapy session in his day timer.

DOCUMENTING PROBLEMS WITH OCCUPATIONAL PERFORMANCE: WRITING A PROGRESS NOTE

Identifying Curtis's Baseline Level of Instrumental Activities of Daily Living Task Performance

Hana began the process of documenting Curtis's baseline performance in a progress note. The process of writing a progress note to document the results of the AMPS is typically done in three steps (Park, Duran, & Fisher, 1997). The first step is to write a global summary statement of the client's overall task performance. The second step is to describe in more detail the specific ADL motor and process skills that support or limit the task performance. The final step is to document the client's potential to benefit from occupational therapy intervention. In Box 6–5, Hana describes her professional reasoning during the writing of each part of the

> ### BOX 6–5. THERAPIST REASONING—BASELINE LEVEL OF ADL PERFORMANCE
>
> In order to begin to think about Curtis's baseline level of ADL performance, I examined the AMPS summary report (Figs. 6–2 and 6–3). This report lists Curtis's demographic information, the tasks he performed, and a ranking of his ADL motor and ADL process skills according to whether they were adequate (scores of 3 or 4), caused him difficulty (scores of 2), or were markedly deficient (scores of 1). If a client's score on a given item differed across the tasks, the lower score is reported.
>
> By examining the AMPS summary report of Curtis's ADL motor skills (see Fig. 6–2), I could see that he had adequate skill on most of the AMPS motor items and that he experienced difficulty on only a few ADL motor skills. None of Curtis's ADL motor skills was markedly deficient. When I examined the summary report of Curtis's ADL process skills (Fig. 6–3), I could see that although Curtis had a few ADL process skills that were adequate in the context of the tasks that he performed, the majority of his ADL process skills were causing difficulty or were markedly deficient.
>
> Based on my global interpretation of these summary profiles, I reflected that Curtis's main problems were his disorganization of actions over time toward effective completion of a specified task. I concluded that he was moderately inefficient and demonstrated marked difficulty adapting to his ADL process skill deficits. Curtis's behavior was moderately unsafe when he picked up the fork that had been resting against the edge of the hot pan. Overall, I was not concerned about the motor aspects of his ADL performance because he demonstrated no increase in physical difficulty beyond that which might be seen in persons without disabilities.

progress note. Although the progress note has been divided into three parts in this chapter (each with a section on Hana's professional reasoning), in reality these three parts would be written as one note.

Progress Note, Part 1: Global Summary Statement

Curtis was moderately inefficient in organizing the actions of task performance and markedly inefficient in self-correcting errors during the performance of two stovetop meal preparation tasks (preparing eggs, meat, and tea; preparing hot cereal and juice). His performance was moderately unsafe because he was at modest risk of burning himself. Curtis did not receive any verbal or physical assistance during the tasks, and he experienced no increase in physical difficulty.

ASSESSMENT OF MOTOR AND PROCESS SKILLS

Client:	CURTIS	Therapist:	
Id:		Gender:	
Age:		Evaluation Date:	

The Assessment of Motor and Process Skills (AMPS) was used to determine how CURTIS's MOTOR and ORGANIZATIONAL/ADAPTIVE (process) capabilities affect CURTIS's ability to perform functional DAILY LIVING TASKS necessary for COMMUNITY LIVING. The tasks were chosen from a list of standard functional activities rated according to their level of complexity. CURTIS chose to perform the following tasks which CURTIS considered to be meaningful and necessary for functional independence in the community:

Task 1: D-3 Scrambled or fried eggs, meat, and brewed coffee

Task 2: C-2 Hot cooked cereal and beverage

The level of complexity of the tasks chosen was average to harder than average. Overall performance in each skill area is summarized below using the following scale: ADEQUATE SKILL: no apparent disruption was observed; DIFFICULTY: ineffective skill was observed; or MARKEDLY DEFICIENT SKILL: observed problems were severe enough to be unsafe or require therapist intervention.

The following strengths and problems were observed during the administration of the AMPS:

Adequate = A   Difficulty = D   Markedly Deficient = MD

MOTOR SKILLS:

Skills needed to move self and objects.

	A	D	MD
Posture:			
STABILIZING the body for balance.	X		
ALIGNING the body in a vertical position.	X		
POSITIONING the body or arms appropriate to the task.		X	
Mobility:			
WALKING: moving about the task environment (level surface).	X		
REACHING for task objects.	X		
BENDING or rotating the body appropriate to the task.	X		
Coordination:			
COORDINATING two body parts to securely stabilize task objects.	X		
MANIPULATING task objects.		X	
FLOWS: executing smooth and fluid arm and hand movements.	X		
Strength and Effort:			
MOVES: pushing and pulling task objects on level surfaces or opening and closing doors or drawers.	X		
TRANSPORTING task objects from one place to another.	X		
LIFTING objects used during the task.	X		
CALIBRATES: regulating the force and extent of movements.		X	
GRIPS: maintaining a secure grasp on task objects.	X		
Energy:			
ENDURING for the duration of the task performance.	X		
Maintaining an even and appropriate PACE during task performance.		X	

Figure 6–2. Curtis's computer-generated AMPS summary report—motor.

ASSESSMENT OF MOTOR AND PROCESS SKILLS

Client: CURTIS   Therapist:
Id: Gender:
Age: Evaluation Date:

Adequate = A   Difficulty = D   Markedly Deficient = MD

PROCESS SKILLS:

Skills needed to organize and adapt actions to complete a task.

	A	D	MD
Energy:			
Maintaining an even and appropriate PACE during task performance.		X	
Maintaining focused ATTENTION throughout the task performance.	X		
Using Knowledge:			
CHOOSING appropriate tools and materials needed for task performance.			X
USING task objects according to their intended purposes.	X		
Knowing when and how to stabilize and support or HANDLE task objects.		X	
HEEDING the goal of the specified task.			X
INQUIRES: asking for needed information.	X		
Temporal Organization:			
INITIATING actions or steps of task without hesitation.			X
CONTINUING actions through to completion.		X	
Logically SEQUENCING the steps of the task.		X	
TERMINATING actions or steps at the appropriate time.			X
Space and Objects:			
SEARCHING for AND LOCATING tools and materials.	X		
GATHERING tools and materials into the task workspace.		X	
ORGANIZING tools and materials in an orderly, logical, and spatially appropriate fashion.		X	
RESTORES: putting away tools and materials or straightening the workspace.			X
NAVIGATES: maneuvering the hand and body around obstacles.	X		
Adaptation:			
NOTICING AND RESPONDING appropriately to nonverbal task-related environmental cues.			X
ACCOMMODATES: modifying ones actions to overcome problems.			X
ADJUSTS: changing the workspace to overcome problems.			X
BENEFITS: preventing problems from reoccuring or persisting.			X

Figure 6–3. Curtis's computer-generated AMPS summary report—process.

Specifying the Motor and Process Skills That Support or Limit Curtis's Instrumental Activities of Daily Living Task Performance

Box 6–6 outlines Hana's reflections on the reasons Curtis's performance was inefficient and unsafe.

Defining Actions of Occupational Performance the Person Cannot Perform Effectively: Hana's Observations of Curtis's Performance

Posture: Curtis stabilized his body (Stabilizes) effectively during the task performance; however, he tended to lean to one side (Aligns). He had

---

BOX 6–6. THERAPIST REASONING—SPECIFYING MOTOR AND PROCESS SKILLS

Having documented Curtis's global baseline performance, I next wanted to consider in more detail why Curtis's performance was inefficient and unsafe. I turned to Curtis's AMPS Raw Scores reports (Figs. 6–4 and 6–5). Because these reports list the raw scores Curtis received for each task he completed, I was able to use them to compare his performance on individual ADL motor and process skill items across both tasks. Items that are consistently rated as 4s or 3s are considered to be relative strengths; items that are consistently rated as 2 are ineffective; and items with any score of 1 are of particular concern because a score of 1 indicates that something happened that was unacceptable, presented an imminent safety risk, or required therapist intervention.

Using the AMPS Raw Scores reports, I jotted down some informal notes to help me summarize in more detail what I had seen during Curtis's AMPS task performances. These notes enabled me to document Curtis's strengths and problems more descriptively, which in turn assisted my process of planning intervention. I considered what I had observed in Curtis's performances across each ADL motor and ADL process skill domain.

---

minimal difficulty positioning himself appropriately, often using awkward arm movements and being too far away from the counters he was working at (Positions).

Mobility: Curtis had no observable difficulty walking around the kitchen during his task performance and reaching for task objects (Walks, Reaches). This domain on the whole is an area of strength for Curtis.

Coordination: Curtis used two body parts together effectively toward a single action, such as pouring milk into a bowl (Coordinates), and his arm and hand movements were smooth and fluid as he interacted with tools and materials during the tasks (Flows). Separating two halves of an eggshell (Manipulates) was minimally difficult, but on the whole, this domain was an area of strength for Curtis.

Strength and effort: Curtis had no observable difficulty pushing, pulling, and transporting task objects (Moves, Transports) in the kitchen environment. When he attempted to crack eggs or shake oatmeal into a pan (Calibrates), he experienced minimal difficulty regulating the force of his movements. He had no apparent difficulty gripping or lifting task objects (Grips, Lifts).

Energy: Curtis was able to complete both tasks without visible evidence of fatigue (Endures), but his pace was moderately slow (Paces).

Client:　　　　CURTIS　　　　　　　　Therapist:

Id:　　　　　　　　　　　　　　　　　Gender:

Age:　　　　　　　　　　　　　　　　Evaluation Date:

Task 1:　　　　D-3 Scrambled or fried eggs, meat, and brewed coffee

Task 2:　　　　C-2 Hot cooked cereal and beverage

MOTOR SKILLS

Posture:	Task 1	Task 2
Stabilizes:	4	4
Aligns:	3	3
Positions:	2	2

Mobility:	Task 1	Task 2
Walks:	4	4
Reaches:	4	4
Bends:	3	4

Coordination:	Task 1	Task 2
Coordinates:	4	4
Manipulates:	2	4
Flows:	4	4

Strength and Effort:	Task 1	Task 2
Moves:	4	4
Transports:	4	4
Lifts:	4	4
Calibrates:	2	2
Grips:	4	4

Energy:	Task 1	Task 2
Endures:	4	4
Paces:	2	2

Figure 6–4. Curtis's computer-generated AMPS Raw Scores report—motor.

Client:	CURTIS	Therapist:
Id:		Gender:
Age:		Evaluation Date:

PROCESS SKILLS

Energy:	Task 1	Task 2
Paces:	2	2
Attends:	3	4

Using Knowledge:	Task 1	Task 2
Chooses:	1	2
Uses:	4	4
Handles:	2	2
Heeds:	1	2
Inquires:	4	4

Temporal Organization:	Task 1	Task 2
Initiates:	1	2
Continues:	2	2
Sequences:	2	2
Terminates:	1	2

Space and Objects:	Task 1	Task 2
Searches/Locates:	4	4
Gathers:	4	2
Organizes:	2	2
Restores:	2	1
Navigates:	4	4

Adaptation:	Task 1	Task 2
Notices/Responds:	1	1
Accommodates:	1	1
Adjusts:	1	2
Benefits:	1	1

Figure 6–5. Curtis's computer-generated AMPS Raw Scores report—process.

He was not distracted from his task performance by irrelevant environmental stimuli (Attends).

Using knowledge: Curtis chose too many of some objects (e.g., slices of bacon, eggs), and did not choose other items that he needed (e.g., hot water for tea) (Chooses). His marked inefficiency choosing resulted in his failure to heed his intended task goals (Heeds). He demonstrated minimal delay when opening packages, and he supported a fork on a hot pan (Handles) in an unsafe manner. He did use tools and materials according to their intended purpose (Uses), and no problems were observed with his ability to inquire for information (Inquires).

Temporal organization: Curtis failed to initiate major task steps (e.g., making a kettle of tea), indicating markedly inefficient performance. There were many hesitations when initiating actions during both task performances, and these hesitations indicated minimal difficulty in continuing task actions until completion (Initiates, Continues). During the more complex task of making eggs, bacon, and tea, his ability to sequence task steps was minimally inefficient because he inappropriately repeated steps of the task (Sequences). His food was under- or overcooked and he added too many eggs and too much bacon and milk (Terminates). These problems indicated poor **temporal organization**.

Space and objects: Curtis was able to logically search for and locate task objects in the kitchen (Searches, Locates). He did not regather oatmeal that had spilled on the counter (Gathers). He placed task objects very close together (Organizes), which was moderately inefficient. His restoration of the workspace (Restores) was moderately inefficient because he did not wipe dirty counters or put the oatmeal and beverage containers away in their storage places. He navigated around objects in the environment (Navigates) competently.

Adaptation: Curtis did not effectively change his methods of doing to accommodate for his process skill deficits (Accommodates). His failure to notice and respond to certain details of task progression, such as resting the fork against the hot pan and then trying to pick the fork up (Notices, Responds) resulted in a safety risk (i.e., risk of burning himself). When he attempted to adjust the heat on the stove (Adjusts), the outcome was unacceptable (i.e., the oatmeal was undercooked). His motor and process skill problems persisted throughout the task performances, and he did not benefit from previous mistakes (Benefits). Box 6–7 explores and evaluates the motor and process skills that delimited Curtis's task performance.

In summary, Hana added the following descriptive statements to Curtis's progress note:

Progress Note, Part 2: Descriptive Statement

BOX 6–7. THERAPIST REASONING—DELIMITING MOTOR AND PROCESS SKILLS

I now wanted to find out which motor and process skills most delimited Curtis's task performance. Looking again at the AMPS Raw Scores reports (see Figs. 6–2 and 6–3) and my own notes, I compared the ADL motor and ADL process skill items that were difficult or markedly deficient for Curtis with the ADL motor and process skill item hierarchies in the AMPS manual. These hierarchies give insight as to which ADL motor and process skill items most people experience as being easier and which most people experience as harder. On the ADL motor scale, Curtis experienced minimal difficulty with some items. The three items (Positions, Paces, and Calibrates) that Curtis received consistent scores of 2 on are three of the four hardest AMPS motor items. These ADL motor items are hard even for people without motor disability. Because Curtis had only minimal difficulty with these items, I concluded that his motor skills were adequate for performance of ADL tasks and not a priority for his intervention plan.

On the ADL process scale, Curtis consistently experienced problems with the easier-than-average items Chooses and Handles. Curtis's problems with handling task objects contributed to his lack of safety when he supported the fork against the hot pan, although the larger problem was that he did not self-correct this handling problem in a safe manner. That he chose far more than the prespecified number of task materials led to an unacceptable task outcome, so I reasoned that the ADL process item Chooses was one of the skill items that most delimited Curtis's ADL process ability.

Curtis received scores of 2s or 1s on the temporal organization items (Initiates, Sequences, Continues, and Terminates) and frequently 1s (indicative of unacceptable or unsafe performance) on the adaptation items (Notices/Responds, Accommodates, Adjusts, and Benefits). I reasoned that if Curtis could better organize his actions over time and adapt his actions to prevent problems from occurring or recurring, the quality of his occupational performance would improve. I reasoned, therefore, that I would need to address the ADL process skill domains of temporal organization and adaptation when planning intervention strategies. Curtis's lack of self-awareness indicated that his performance was most likely to improve through an intervention plan that focused on environmental modification and caregiver education.

- Motor Ability: Although Curtis experienced minimal difficulty with some motor skills (i.e., positioning his body to promote efficient arm movements during task performance and calibrating the force of his arm and hand movements), his motor ability is adequate and supports his performance of daily life tasks.
- Process Ability: Curtis demonstrated markedly deficient skill in choosing the prespecified number of task tools and materials, initiating

major task steps, and appropriately terminating task actions and steps. These problems impacted his ability to heed the specified goal of the task and resulted in undesirable task outcomes. The overall pace of his task performance was slow. His markedly deficient skill in adapting to problems encountered during the task performance persisted throughout both tasks. At present, his ability to overcome these ADL motor and ADL process deficits is markedly inefficient, which results in unsafe task performance.

Establishing Curtis's Potential to Benefit from Occupational Therapy Intervention

Box 6–8 reflects on the benefit of intervention to improve Curtis's occupational performance.

BOX 6–8. THERAPIST REASONING—BENEFIT OF INTERVENTION

I believed that Curtis had the potential to benefit from intervention to enhance the quality of his occupational performance. To confirm my intuition, I looked at the Graphic Report of Curtis's AMPS Results (Fig. 6–6). His motor ability measure was 2.6 logits, which is above the motor cut-off ability measure of 2.0 logits. This ability measure supported my professional judgment that Curtis's ADL motor skills were adequate because persons who score above 2.0 logits on the ADL motor scale do not experience undue physical effort during completion of ADL tasks.

Curtis's ADL process ability measure was 0.3 logits, which is below the cut-off ability measure of 1.0 logit. This measure was not surprising. The process cut-off ability measure indicates a point below which 93% of people require some sort of assistance to live in the community (Fisher, 1997a).

Curtis's relatively high ADL motor, low ADL process ability measure profile on the AMPS Graphic Report indicated that he was most likely to benefit from interventions targeted at environmental modification and caregiver training. Curtis was willing to participate in ADL tasks for the AMPS assessment, and he had stated that he would like to get back to doing more such tasks around his home. Curtis's mother and son were very supportive of him, and they had expressed an interest in being involved in his occupational therapy sessions. I reasoned that Curtis might be willing to explore environmental modifications that would make it easier for him to perform ADL tasks safely and more efficiently.

At the end of Curtis's progress note, I added the following statement regarding his potential to benefit from therapy.

GRAPHIC REPORT OF CURTIS'S AMPS RESULTS

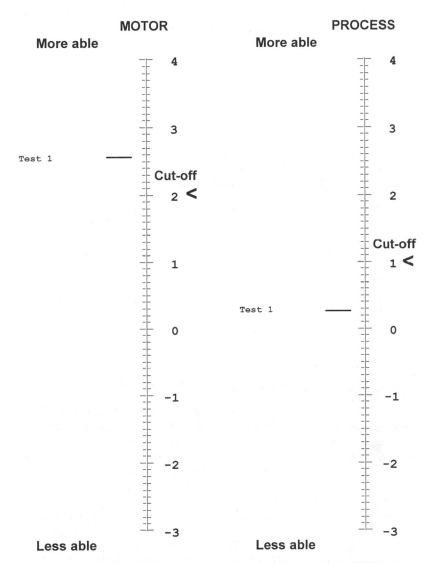

CURTIS'S AMPS motor and process ability measures plotted in reference to AMPS scale cut-off measures indicative of evidence of problems that impact on performance.

	MOTOR	PROCESS
Test 1	2.6	0.3

Figure 6–6. Curtis's computer-generated AMPS Graphic Report—Test 1.

Progress Note, Part 3: Documenting Potential to Benefit from Occupational Therapy

Although currently Curtis is experiencing difficulty adapting to his process skill deficits, his willingness to participate in ADLs and the support of his family indicate that Curtis has good potential to benefit from intervention targeted at environmental modification and caregiver training.

SETTING GOALS

During the goal-setting process, Hana elicited the input of Curtis, his mother, and his son to ensure that Curtis's occupational therapy goals were client centered (Box 6–9). The process of setting client-centered goals combines procedural, interactive, and conditional reasoning. Hana used procedural reasoning to interpret assessment results, analyze Curtis's performance, and consider which gains in his occupational performance would be realistic to expect. Hana also used conditional reasoning to consider Curtis's life in a larger context, including the environment to which he would be returning and what the future might hold for him there. Throughout the evaluation and the goal-setting process, Hana relied on interactive reasoning to learn what was important to Curtis and to ascertain his goals for occupational therapy.

BOX 6–9. THERAPIST REASONING—SETTING GOALS

Curtis, his mother, his son, and I developed a collaborative partnership as we developed Curtis's goals for occupational therapy. I shared the results of my assessment with Curtis, his mother, and his son, and they in turn shared more deeply with me what they hoped to accomplish by the time of Curtis's discharge from outpatient occupational therapy. Curtis wanted to be able to prepare his own breakfast, lunch, and snacks; to watch basketball games with friends; and to prepare a hot breakfast for his mother and aunt on the weekends. His mother was willing to do light housekeeping, laundry, and the majority of the evening food preparation activities. Curtis's son was available to come by for short periods of time several evenings a week, if needed, and was willing to do lawn maintenance and repairs around the home. Based on this information and on my observations of Curtis's ADL performance, I documented the mutually agreed-upon goals and objectives for Curtis's occupational performance after occupational therapy intervention. Two sample long-term goals and their related short-term objectives are included here.

Goal: Curtis will prepare a simple breakfast or cold lunch safely and independently with minimal inefficiency.
Objectives:

- Curtis will readily choose the appropriate number of items needed for task completion.
- Curtis will initiate all necessary steps of the performance without hesitation.
- Curtis will terminate task action sequences at the appropriate time.

Goal: Curtis will prepare a hot breakfast (e.g., eggs, oatmeal, bacon) safely with minimal cueing, experiencing only minimal inefficiency.
Objectives:

- Curtis will heat foods in a safe and efficient manner.
- Curtis will readily notice and make effective responses to environmental cues regarding task progression.

INTERVENTION

DESIGNING INTERVENTION STRATEGIES

Box 6–10 outlines the reasoning behind Hana's intervention planning.

IMPLEMENTING INTERVENTION FOCUSING ON ADLs

Intervention implementation is discussed in Box 6–11.

IMPLEMENTING INTERVENTION FOCUSING ON SITUATIONAL RESPONSE

During one treatment session, Hana wanted to focus on Curtis's ability to generate appropriate responses to unfamiliar situations. A portion of our conversation during this session follows:

> Hana: Curtis, I am going to describe a couple of different situations and I'd like for you to tell me what you think you might do in each one. Okay?
>
> Curtis: (nods)
>
> Hana: Okay, here's an example. If I asked you, "Curtis, what would you do if your car was stolen?" you might tell me that you would call the police department and report it, and then you would call your insurance agent. Does that make sense?

BOX 6–10. THERAPIST REASONING—INTERVENTION STRATEGIES

Having worked with Curtis and his family to set goals, I was now ready to begin to work with them to plan specific intervention strategies. Because of Curtis's high motor, low process ability profile on the AMPS Graphic Report, I felt that Curtis was most likely to benefit from intervention targeted at environmental modification and caregiver training. Furthermore, I knew that if such intervention was to be effective, I would need to collaborate with Curtis and members of his family not just during the goal setting process, but to ensure that the intervention strategies were acceptable to Curtis and his family. To guide the intervention process, therefore, I chose to use the expanded rehabilitative/compensatory model of practice (Fisher, 1997b), in which the principles of adaptation, education, and collaborative consultation are used to develop strategies that enable the client to compensate for his or her problems with completing occupational performance. The focus of the rehabilitative/compensatory model of practice is on adaptation or compensation and does not address remediation of impairments (Trombly, 1995c). The process of providing adaptations that promote competence in occupational performance, however, can indirectly lead to some degree of remediation of impairments or the prevention of potential for decline (Fisher, 1997b).

I had already completed a performance analysis of Curtis's ability to complete ADL tasks by analyzing his performance in terms of the specific ADL motor and process skill items. I had already begun to incorporate principles of collaborative consultation when I entered into a shared partnership with Curtis and his family to set goals and discuss potential intervention strategies. The collaborative nature of this process fostered interactive reasoning and therapeutic rapport. I contributed knowledge I gathered during the performance analysis, and Curtis and his family contributed knowledge of their goals and the types of potential intervention strategies that would be acceptable to them.

As Curtis, his family, and I discussed and experimented with adaptation through various environmental modifications, I used principles of education to instruct Curtis in the use of those modifications. When the modification was to the social environment (i.e., caregiver training), I used principles of education to teach Curtis's family members specific strategies for assisting him at home. I also used education to teach Curtis and his family about the nature of executive ability disorder and specifically, how the disorder was manifested in Curtis's behavior.

BOX 6–11. THERAPIST REASONING—INTERVENTION IMPLEMENTATION

Based on my interpretation of Curtis's AMPS results, I began to think about specific intervention strategies that would enhance his occupational performance of ADL tasks, including compensatory strategies for specific ADL process skills that were difficult or markedly deficient for Curtis. I had identified the skill item Chooses, the temporal organization items (Initiates, Continues, Sequences, and Terminates), and the adaptation items (Notices/Responds, Accommodates, Adjusts, and Benefits) as the skill items that were most limiting Curtis's ADL process ability. I was also concerned about Curtis's safety in the kitchen, particularly around the hot stove. Curtis wanted to be able to prepare a hot breakfast for his mother and his aunt; therefore, I wanted to explore environmental modifications that might make it possible for Curtis to prepare hot foods more safely.

I asked Curtis if he owns a microwave oven. He said that he did and that he used it once in a while. I asked him if he might be willing to use it to cook hot breakfast items such as scrambled eggs, tea, oatmeal, and bacon. He said that he would be willing to try. I felt that, to be successful, Curtis would need repeated practice using the microwave so that using it became a part of his cooking routine. I also believed that the intervention would generalize more easily if Curtis could practice using the same microwave that he would be using at home. I asked Curtis's son to bring in Curtis's microwave from home so that Curtis and I could begin to practice using it to prepare different kinds of hot foods. Initially, we started with a limited number of easy tasks (e.g., heating water for tea, heating up a piece of pie). As Curtis acquired skill with these select tasks, I introduced new, harder tasks (e.g., cooking oatmeal, preparing scrambled eggs) for him to practice.

I used the AMPS task process hierarchy to educate Curtis and his family about which tasks might be easier for Curtis to complete independently. This hierarchy lists the AMPS tasks in order from easiest to most difficult. Using this list, I can consider the difficulty of the tasks that he completed for the assessment to predict how well he would do on tasks of differing challenges. I cautioned Curtis's family that Curtis would likely need supervision when completing harder tasks, such as making scrambled eggs, that required the use of the stove.

I explained to Curtis and his family that one of the things that was hard for Curtis was choosing an appropriate number of objects needed for task performance. I explained to them that one possible strategy to compensate for this problem was to reduce as much clutter as possible in the kitchen. Another compensatory strategy was to rearrange the kitchen so that similar objects would be grouped together. I also educated Curtis's mother about how to provide Curtis with specific cues when he encountered difficulty

(continues)

BOX 6–11. THERAPIST REASONING—INTERVENTION IMPLEMENTATION (CONT.)

choosing an appropriate number of items needed for task completion (e.g., "take two eggs"). Thus, we discussed modification of the physical as well as the social environment to compensate for Curtis's problem with choosing.

To compensate for Curtis's difficulty with temporal organization, Curtis and I agreed to try an alternative strategy that built on his existing day timer. We developed step-by-step task cards for certain familiar kitchen activities (e.g., preparing juice and cold cereal, preparing soup and crackers). The cards were laminated so that Curtis could use an erasable marker to check off each step of the task as he completed it. This compensatory strategy helped Curtis to more easily initiate, continue, and sequence the steps of the task in an efficient manner. The strategy also had an element of familiarity because it built on Curtis's existing day timer. The step-by-step task cards were also beneficial in that they provided structure to the tasks and promoted development of new routines and habits.

I spent some treatment time educating Curtis's family regarding the importance of routine and habit to support Curtis's occupational functioning. Familiar organization of the environment ("a place for everything and everything in its place") made it easier for Curtis to efficiently complete meaningful activity. I explained to Curtis's mother that lack of flexibility and environmental dependency were the reasons Curtis became so upset when she threw garbage away in a trash can that Curtis viewed as "his" or rearranged his toiletries in the bathroom. In this instance, I used my knowledge of impairment of executive function to explain the reason behind Curtis's behavior (executive ability).

Curtis: Yeah—call the police department and report it.

Hana: Here's the first one. What would you do if you locked your keys in your car?

Curtis: I'd call the police department and report it.

Hana: Is there anything else you'd do?

Curtis: (pause) Get angry.

Hana: Here's another one. What do you think you would do if your son told you that he was going to come over to your house after work, but 2 hours after you expected him to come he still wasn't there? What would you do in that situation?

Curtis: I would call the police department and report it.

Hana: Is there anyone you might call before you called the police?

Curtis: (long pause) Call my son.

Hana: Yeah, that would be a good idea. What are two different places that you might try to reach him?

Curtis: His house. . .

Hana: Yes, his house is one place. Where else might you try? (Waits for a reply, but none is given.) If he told you he was going to come straight over from work, where else might you try to call him?

Curtis: Work.

Hana: That's right, you could try calling him at work and also at his house. (At this point, Curtis wrote down in his day timer, "Home and call work," a self-initiated, but incomplete, reminder.) Okay, Curtis, let's talk about one more situation. What would you do if your mother fell down on the floor and was not able to get back up?

Curtis: I would call the police department and report it.

Hana: Is there anyone else you could call? (pause) What if you thought she needed medical attention?

Curtis: Call the doctor.

Hana: Well, you'd probably want to make sure she got to see the doctor, but the doctor wouldn't be able to come to the house. Who could you call if you wanted someone to come over to your house right away?

Curtis: Call the . . . ambulance.

Hana: That's right, an ambulance would be able to come fast. What number would you call if you needed an ambulance?

Curtis: (long pause) I guess that'd be 9-1-1.

Hana: Yes, that's the number to call in an emergency. So if your mother fell and couldn't get up by herself, who would you call?

Curtis: The ambulance.

Hana: That's right, and what number would you dial for the ambulance?

Curtis: 9-1-1 (writes, "Ambulance 911" in his day timer).

Hana's reflections on this conversation are provided in Box 6–12.

BOX 6–12. THERAPIST REASONING—SITUATIONAL RESPONSES

During this conversation, Curtis demonstrated several behaviors that are typical of people with disorders of executive ability. For example, his perseveration on my statement "Call the police department and report it" is an example of difficulty generating alternate solutions to problems. I realized that clear, specific cues helped him. When I said his son was "at work," for example, Curtis knew the place to try to call was "work." With structure and specific cues, Curtis was able to generate more appropriate responses for the specific situations; he also was familiar with the 911 emergency telephone number. This information was useful for me clinically because I could then think about environmental modifications that would build on his ability to benefit from cues to compensate for his difficulties.

Curtis and I worked on creating an emergency phone number list that he would be able to put in his day timer and also by his phone at home. On the list, in large, clear print we wrote "Emergency: Dial 9-1-1." We also listed the work and home phone numbers of Curtis's son. Curtis's mother suggested that we also include the home phone number of her sister who lives nearby, so we added that number to the list. Curtis practiced using the list to find his family members' numbers and dial them.

Although this exercise was in the clinic and, therefore, removed from a natural setting, it gave me a chance to observe Curtis using the environmental modification of the phone list to dial. By involving Curtis's mother in the session, we were able to get additional input about phone numbers to include and discuss the optimal places to post the phone list at home. By providing time to practice using the list, we moved the session from the abstract discussion of "what would you do in this situation?" to hands-on opportunities to practice doing it. It was important for me to observe Curtis as he used the phone list so that he and I could problem solve as to how to make it as effective an adaptation as possible. I encouraged Curtis and his family to practice using the phone list at home.

REEVALUATION FOR ENHANCED ADL TASK PERFORMANCE: RE-ADMINISTERING THE AMPS

As Curtis progressed, Hana re-administered the AMPS to determine if Curtis's occupational performance had improved. For the second AMPS observation, Curtis chose to prepare the following: (1) toast and instant tea and (2) oatmeal and a beverage. He had his day timer and task cards with him during the tasks, and Hana told him to refer to them if needed during the course of the evaluation (Box 6–13).

BOX 6–13. THERAPIST REASONING—RE-EVALUATION AND RE-ADMINISTRATION OF AMPS

For the first task, Curtis chose to toast two slices of bread, apply butter to the toast, and prepare a cup of tea. Curtis used the microwave oven to heat the water for the tea. He heated the cup of water appropriately in the microwave oven, then added a tea bag. There were some hesitations in his performance, and his pace was slow. He removed the toast from the toaster, spread both butter and strawberry jam on the bread, and served the toast on a napkin. During the task performance, I did not feel that he was at imminent risk of injury.

For the second task, Curtis chose to prepare oatmeal and a glass of orange juice. During the task performance, he chose a glass of milk instead of the orange juice he had originally agreed upon. He cooked the oatmeal in the microwave oven. He restored the oatmeal, milk, and utensils, but he put the oatmeal in a different cupboard than where it was originally. Although the outcome of the task was slightly different than we had agreed upon (milk instead of orange juice), it was not unacceptable, and I did not question his safety during the task performance.

After the task performance, I scored Curtis's AMPS task performances. Many of Curtis's ADL process scores for the second observation were higher. The most dramatic example of this was in his adaptation scores, which were consistently scores of 2 during the second observation instead of the frequent scores of 1 he had been given during the initial evaluation. His performance was safe, although he did experience minimal inefficiency and the outcome of both tasks was slightly different than originally agreed upon. I entered the scores from Curtis's second observation into the AMPS computer-scoring program and generated the AMPS Graphic Report (Fig. 6–7) that showed Curtis's baseline ADL motor and process ability measures, as well as his current ADL ability measures. An improvement of 0.5 or greater between the two measures is considered to be a clinically meaningful change (Park, Duran, & Fisher, 1997).

Subjectively, Curtis's current ADL performance appeared safer and more efficient than it had been at admission. I was pleased, therefore, to see on the AMPS Graphic Report that Curtis's ADL ability measures had improved on the process scale by 0.6 logits. This report gave quantitative evidence to support my qualitative observations. Curtis's ADL process ability measure was still below the cut-off ADL process ability measure, indicating that although he had made a clinically meaningful improvement, he would still probably need supervision to live in the community. It was also interesting to note that although I had not specifically targeted ADL motor skills in my intervention plan, Curtis's ADL motor ability had improved slightly but not enough to be clinically meaningful.

(continues on page 249)

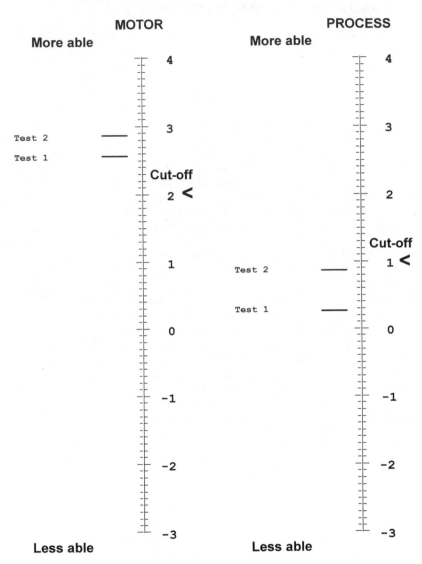

GRAPHIC REPORT OF CURTIS'S AMPS RESULTS

CURTIS'S AMPS motor and process ability measures plotted in reference to AMPS scale cut-off measures indicative of evidence of problems that impact on performance.

	MOTOR	PROCESS
Test 1	2.6	0.3
Test 2	2.9	0.9

Figure 6–7. Curtis's computer-generated AMPS Graphic Report—Test 1 and Test 2.

BOX 6–13. THERAPIST REASONING—RE-EVALUATION AND RE-ADMINISTRATION OF AMPS (CONT.)

After reviewing the computer-generated reports from his second AMPS assessment, I wrote a note in Curtis's chart, in which I documented the following progress toward his ADL goals:

● Curtis is now able to prepare a simple meal (e.g., toast and tea) safely and independently, experiencing only minimal inefficiency.

● Curtis is now able to prepare a hot breakfast (e.g., oatmeal and a beverage) safely, experiencing only minimal inefficiency.

DISCHARGE

At the time of Curtis's discharge from outpatient occupational therapy, he was preparing his own breakfasts, lunches, and snacks daily with supervision and occasional verbal cues from his mother. Curtis reported that it was good to be doing more things around his home and his mother reported that she felt better able to understand his behavior and structure his environment accordingly so that he could continue to do more things around the house.

SUMMARY

This chapter presented information regarding the professional reasoning process of evaluating and planning intervention for a client who has disorders of executive abilities. Detailed information was provided that describes the expanded rehabilitative/compensatory model (Fisher, 1997b), including the use of the principles of education, adaptation, and collaborative consultation to plan intervention strategies. An introduction to disorders of executive functions and executive abilities was presented, including a summary of current literature related to assessment and treatment methodologies, research trends, and neuroanatomical substrates. The case study of Curtis was then presented with a brief introduction to the occupational therapist and the client. The processes of gathering information about the client using a top-down approach (including interviewing the client and his family, administrating the AMPS, and interpreting the assessment results); the process of setting goals; and using the rehabilitative/compensatory model to guide intervention planning were described in detail. Lastly, an additional client case was presented followed by questions posed for the reader to answer.

≡ REVIEW CASE STUDY: KEVIN

Kevin is a 40-year-old man who was involved in an automobile accident and sustained diffuse head injuries. After 5 days in an acute care setting, he was admitted to the inpatient rehabilitation unit of a long-term care center. He was referred to occupational therapy for evaluation and treatment to improve functioning in daily life tasks.

Kevin's occupational therapist reviewed his chart before meeting him. From the chart, the therapist learned that Kevin lives on the second floor of a house and rents the lower floor out to a tenant. He has a sister who lives in the same city. His parents also live in the same city and are in poor health, especially his mother, who is severely disabled and spends much of her time in a wheelchair or in bed.

The occupational therapist went in to introduce herself to Kevin. During the initial interview, Kevin told the therapist that everything was fine, that he did not have any problems, and that he wanted to go home. He was quite insistent about his desire to return home, and the therapist had difficulty getting much more verbal information from him. The therapist noted that he looked a bit unclean and had not shaved for several days. After a long talk, Kevin agreed to participate in a performance evaluation of PADLs and IADLs the next day.

When the occupational therapist arrived the next morning, Kevin was sitting on the edge of his bed with his clothes on. He told the therapist that he had taken a shower and dressed himself earlier that morning. The therapist could tell by looking at him that this was not the case. Kevin's roommate whispered to the occupational therapist that Kevin had been sleeping in his clothes the past two nights.

Kevin agreed to do the AMPS PADL task *Upper body grooming* as a part of his assessment. As a part of this task, he agreed to shave his face with his electric razor. Kevin became upset because his electric razor did not work. He had started to "shave" but had not plugged in the razor or taken the plastic cover off. Verbal cues did not help, and the therapist had to guide his hands to remove the cover and to put the razor to Kevin's face. Without this hand-over-hand guidance, the razor did not meet his face.

That afternoon Kevin agreed to complete the AMPS IADL task *Sweeping the floor*. Kevin and his therapist agreed that for this task, Kevin would use a broom to sweep a designated section of the occupational therapy clinic floor and put away the broom when he was finished. Kevin had difficulty getting the broom out of the cleaning closet. Once he got the broom out, he swept the floor in a circle around his feet, then said, "Now I'm going to do this properly." He put away the broom and started to get the vacuum cleaner out. It was difficult for him to get the vacuum hoses together, but he managed to do it. He started to vacuum but did not plug the vacuum in. He did not notice that the vacuum cleaner was silent and he "vacuumed" the same area of the floor around his feet before he started to restore the vacuum to the closet. Kevin was very satisfied with himself and the great job he had done.

≡ REVIEW QUESTIONS

1. What methods did the therapist use to assess Kevin? Did the therapist follow a bottom-up or a top-down approach to Kevin's assessment?
2. What behaviors did Kevin demonstrate during his PADL task performance that are typical of persons with disorders of executive ability?
3. What behaviors did Kevin demonstrate during his IADL tasks performance that are typical of persons with disorders of executive ability?
4. Kevin's therapist decided to use the rehabilitative/compensatory model to guide the process of intervention planning. Who besides Kevin and the occupational therapist might be the critical members of the collaborative consultative partnership? What contributing role would each member play?
5. What are some adaptations the occupational therapist might suggest to enhance Kevin's occupational performance? Consider modification of the social and physical environment as well as teaching compensatory strategies.

≡ ACKNOWLEDGMENTS

The authors gratefully acknowledge the following individuals for their critical feedback on earlier versions of this chapter: Doug Agne, Birgitta Bernspång, Barbara Borg, Steven Duke, Lisa Stauffer, and Kerstin Tham. We also extend our appreciation to Monica Widman-Lundmark for her contributions to the development of the Kevin case study.

APPENDIX 6–1

AMPS SKILL ITEMS

ADL MOTOR SKILLS

Stabilizes
Aligns
Positions
Walks
Reaches
Bends
Coordinates
Manipulates
Flows
Moves
Transports
Lifts
Calibrates
Grips
Endures
Paces

ADL PROCESS SKILLS

Paces
Attends
Chooses
Uses
Handles
Heeds
Inquires
Initiates
Continues
Sequences
Terminates
Searches/locates
Gathers
Organizes
Restores
Navigates
Notices/responds
Accommodates
Adjusts
Benefits

≡ APPENDIX 6–2

AMPS RATING SCALE

The quality of performance of each motor and process skill item is rated based on the quality of the person/environment interaction and not on judgments of underlying capacities. The rating scale for each item is as follows:

4 = Action performance is *competent* and supports the action progression and outcome. When performing the skill item, the client demonstrates no evidence of increased effort, inefficiency, lack of safety, or need for assistance. There is no doubt in the examiner's mind that the client's performance is competent.

3 = Action performance is *questionable.* The examiner questions the quality of the performance and may have a vague sense of uncertainty as to whether or not the client demonstrates evidence of increased effort, inefficiency, lack of safety, or need for assistance during the performance of the skill item.

2 = Action performance disrupts or interferes with the action progression and yields undesirable outcomes. The client demonstrates at least minimal evidence of increased effort, inefficiency, or potential for future safety risk during the performance of the skill item.

1 = Action performance is *deficient.* The examiner observes an unacceptable delay, an unacceptable level of difficulty, an imminent risk of damage or danger, breakdown of task performance, or a need for the examiner to intervene.

From Fisher 1997a. Assessment of Motor and Process Skills (2nd ed). Fort Collins, CO: Three Star Press. Reproduced with permission.

≣ APPENDIX 6–3

EXAMPLE OF AMPS SCORING CRITERIA

TERMINATES: Finishes or brings to completion *single actions or single steps* without perseveration, inappropriate persistence, or premature cessation; implies stopping action or step at the right time in preparation for beginning the next action or step

Key Concepts: too long, too little; enough, but not too much (actions or steps)

The examiner observes the client to:

4 = *Readily and consistently* bring to completion an action or step at an appropriate time.

Mixes the mayonnaise into the tuna and stops mixing once they are thoroughly combined

Thoroughly buffs the shoes to bring them to a shine but stops buffing once the entire shoe is shined

3 = Have questionable terminating skill that *does not lead to apparent disruption* of action item or task performance or have an impact on other skill items.

Possibly hesitates or is slow to terminate an action

Possibly stops an action too soon

2 = Have ineffective terminating skill that *disrupts* action item or task performance or results in inefficient use of time or energy.

Continuing to mix mayonnaise and tuna beyond when they are thoroughly combined delays task progression

Stops buffing before entire shoe is polished

Stops vacuuming before entire rug is clean (e.g., some visible dirt remains)

Fills the coffee cup to the brim, with a little possibly spilling over

Tearing up enough lettuce for four people instead of the two specified delays task progression

Stops toasting bread before it browns, or toasts it until it is extremely brown but not burned

1 = Have severe terminating skill deficits that clearly *impede* action item or task performance such that the results are unacceptable, or damage or danger is imminent.

(continues)

(continued)

Premature cessation of vacuuming results in an unacceptable outcome
(e.g., a large area of the rug remains unvacuumed)

Continues pouring coffee until there is marked spillage, or spillage
results in imminent risk that the client will get burned

Puts bread in the toaster but does not toast it or cooks toast until it
burns

Peeling and cutting up three cucumbers for a salad for two people
results in an unacceptable delay in task progression

Examiner intervention required because severity of terminating skill
deficit results in unacceptable delay, task breakdown, or imminent
risk of damage or danger

From Fisher 1997a. Assessment of Motor and Process Skills (2nd ed). Fort Collins, CO: Three
Star Press. Reproduced with permission.

7

Evaluation and Intervention with Apraxia

JENNIFER A. BUTLER, BScHons, Dip COT, T Cert (HE), PhD

- Aphasia
- Apraxia
- Buccofacial Apraxia
- Ideational Apraxia

- Ideomotor Apraxia
- Post-Traumatic Amnesia
- Praxis

On completion of this chapter, the reader will be able to:

- Define apraxia and discuss the two main forms of apraxia identified in the literature
- Describe the anatomical basis for apraxia
- List at least three standardized assessments to screen for this disorder
- List at least three intervention techniques that a therapist can use to treat a client who has apraxia
- Successfully work through the Review Questions

≡ INTRODUCTION

This chapter introduces apraxia and presents the case of Amanda, a young woman who experiences ideomotor apraxia as a result of a severe closed-head injury. The chapter demonstrates the reasoning behind the evaluations and interventions carried out with this client. There is a brief review of both ideational and ideomotor apraxia that provides the features of these disorders and assessment protocols used in research. A synopsis of current thinking in apraxia and research trends concerning neuroanatomical correlates of apraxic disorders is presented. The case of Amanda starts with her admission into the rehabilitation center 6 months after her head injury and shows the planning and reasoning behind the overall intervention program. Specific illustrations of therapy sessions are provided. Some of the results from case study research are also presented to show the efficacy of intervention.

WHAT IS APRAXIA?

Adult-onset **apraxia** is an impairment of the capacity to perform purposeful movement not due to any primary motor or sensory deficit nor attributable to lack of comprehension, attention, or willingness to perform the movement (Croce, 1993; Geschwind, 1975; Heilman & Valenstein, 1993; Kirshner, 1991; Tate & McDonald, 1995). Many people with apraxia also have coexisting language deficits, motor and sensory deficits, or both. The clinician must try to determine to what extent such impairments contribute to the dysfunction.

Most clinicians and clinical researchers identify two main varieties of apraxia, ideomotor and ideational. People with **ideational apraxia** do not have the idea of what to do; that is, they have lost the concept of how to carry out a required series of actions toward a set goal. They perform badly when the activity is composed of a series of movements. Bizarre errors can often be seen during everyday activities (e.g., putting clothes onto the wrong body part, drinking from an empty cup, eating food with knife, using a lid as a spoon, buttering hot coffee, putting custard on bread, putting toothpaste on a razor) (Mayer et al., 1990). Clearly the types of errors made by these clients include the misuse or mislocation of objects, and sequence and omission errors (DeRenzi & Luccelli, 1988).

Ideomotor apraxia involves the incorrect execution of the movement required. Individuals with ideomotor apraxia do know what to do, but they are unable to implement the required action successfully. The kinds of errors authors associate with ideomotor apraxia are described in detail later in the chapter (Mozaz et al., 1990; Raade et al., 1991). Generally the movements are observed to be clumsy and awkward, with impairment in the timing, sequencing, and spatial organization of movement (Tate & McDonald, 1995).

Buccofacial apraxia is the same kind of disorder as ideomotor apraxia but relates to the execution of purposeful movements of the face and lips for language production and emotional expression. Rehabilitation texts often describe two other "types" of apraxia, namely *constructional apraxia* and *dressing apraxia*. It is thought that these are not true apraxias in terms of the disruption to motor organization and planning but are compounded by perceptual and cognitive dysfunction. Both "types" are often associated with right hemisphere lesions and are essentially descriptive terms used when there is evidence of poor drawing and constructional capacities or poor dressing performance.

NEUROANATOMICAL CORRELATES AND MECHANISMS

The exploration of the neuroanatomical correlates and the mechanisms underlying apraxia as a route to understanding the organization of motor control has been a focus of research for several decades. Particular interest has centered around the location of lesions that lead to apraxia (Basso et al., 1980; Berthier et al., 1987; Buxbaum et al., 1995; Classen et al., 1995; Faglioni & Basso, 1985; Halsband et al., 1993; Kertesz & Ferro, 1984; Papagno et al., 1993; Selnes et al., 1991). Authors agree that apraxia results most frequently from lesions in the left, dominant hemisphere. There is evidence from research that both frontal lesions and posterior parietal lesions can result in apraxia, as can a disruption of pathways between the two lobes (i.e., subcortical lesions). Some research indicates that lesions in the corpus callosum or right hemisphere may also result in apraxia in certain cases, but they are less common (Archibald, 1987; Buxbaum et al., 1995; Graff-Radford et al., 1987; Mozaz et al., 1990).

Other research has explored the relationship between **aphasia** and apraxia, which frequently coexist (Papagno et al., 1993; Selnes et al., 1991). There has been some recent interest in analyzing kinematic limb actions in individuals with ideomotor apraxia using accurate quantitative measures of movement (e.g., acceleration and velocity patterns, trajectory of movement, joint angles, and hand position) to determine differences in apraxia rather than relying on observer judgment (Hermsdorfer et al., 1996; Poizner et al., 1990). Such research projects have shown impairments in the control of the timing of movements, disruption to the spatial-temporal dimensions of movement and the overuse of proximal musculature to compensate for impairment of distal musculature control in individuals with apraxia.

Much of the research in this field has concentrated on the things both ideational and ideomotor apraxias can teach us about the organization of motor control within the brain. A theoretical concept of apraxia is now established as a multistep, multimodal model of impaired sensory and motor processing. Research concerning the effectiveness of rehabilitation for apraxia is sparse but suggests that compensatory strategies may be the most effective approach (Pilgrim & Humphreys, 1994; Wilson, 1988). Others (Ayres, 1985; Croce, 1993; Goodgold-Edwards & Cermak, 1990) suggest that a visual and verbal mediation strategy combined with appropriate tactile and kinesthetic input provides the multimodal stimulation needed to facilitate movement in apraxia. In practice, this involves cueing people with apraxia to look at what they are doing and where they are going, as well as demonstrating activities or movements to give a visual model of how the activity or movement is to be performed. This strategy is accompanied by encouraging individuals to verbalize what they want to do and what they have done (e.g., "I want to open my hand," "I want to reach for a cup," "I am stretching my fingers out," "I am closing my fingers around a cup"). Croce (1993) suggests that such visual and verbal mediations should be linked with additional tactile and proprioceptive stimulation to afford individuals with apraxia the opportunities to use a maximum amount of available information for planning and producing motor actions despite limitations in sensory-motor processing and integration.

A combination of both strategies is, in practice, usually the most practicable because the client often needs a "quick result" in some areas of independence that can be achieved by compensatory and adaptive strategies. The client may also see the need for more long-term mediation rehabilitation strategies that will improve quality of movement and task performance.

EVALUATION PROTOCOLS

Some brief notes are provided here on assessment in apraxia since this information is not readily available in other texts. Standardized clinical test items for the diagnosis of both ideational and ideomotor apraxia are usually encased within larger test batteries such as the Rivermead Perceptual Assessment Battery (RPAB) (Whiting et al., 1985) or the Loewenstein Occupational Therapy Cognitive Assessment (LOTCA) (Itzkovich et al., 1990) (both of these assessments are reviewed in Chapter 3) and are mostly useful only as screening tests. Two apraxia assessments devised by occupational therapists are the Praxis Test—Santa Clara Valley Medical Center (Zoltan et al., 1983) and the Solet Test for Apraxia (Solet, 1974). The Solet Test for Apraxia is not standardized. Research test batteries such as those devised by De Renzi et al. (1980), York-Haaland and Flaherty (1984), and De Renzi and Lucchelli (1988) are lengthy, thorough, and reliable assessments of apraxia. They have reasonable scoring guidelines and adequate normative data specific to apraxia to make the testing and diagnostic procedures more meaningful (Tate & McDonald, 1995). It should be kept in mind that such tests take **praxis** out of context and are carried out in an artificial environment. Occupational therapists are concerned with the functional implications resulting from impairments such as apraxia and, therefore, any diagnostic assessments should include those that use functional tasks within an appropriate context (Árnadóttir, 1990).

There are four main types of test batteries in common use within published research for assessing elements of ideomotor apraxia and ideational apraxia. They are identified only by the authors who devised them and are not standardized. In this section, details of the testing and scoring of these assessments together with suggested assessment and scoring forms are provided because they are scattered throughout the research literature and are not contained neatly and accessibly elsewhere.

The most comprehensive test for eliciting ideomotor apraxia involves imitating gestures (De Renzi et al., 1980). This test contains 24 movements that are carried out in front of the client, who is then required to reproduce these movements immediately afterward from memory using the limb ipsilateral to the side of the lesion (to avoid the confounding variables associated with hemiparetic limb performance). The test involves finger and hand movements, single postures, carrying out a sequence of movements, and meaningful and nonmeaningful gestures (see Table 7–1). Three trials are given for each item if necessary. Scoring is given as 3, 2, 1, or 0 points depending on whether the performance is correct on the first, second, or third presentation or if all trials are unsatisfactory. A total of 72 is therefore possible. Neurologically intact individuals do not normally score lower than 65 and usually score between 70 and 72.

Another test battery described by York Haaland and Flaherty (1984) uses meaningful and nonmeaningful gestures to both verbal command and a

Table 7–1. Ideomotor apraxia test items: Gesture and movement copying (De Renzi et al., 1980)

Note: Put a check (√) in the correct column to score for accurate performance:
3 = correct performance at first trial; 2 = correct at second trial; 1 = correct at third trial; 0 = incorrect performance.
Maximum score = 72

FINGER MOVEMENTS	TRIAL 1 SCORE 3	TRIAL 2 SCORE 2	TRIAL 3 SCORE 1	UNABLE SCORE 0
1 Index finger and middle finger extended and abducted (sign of victory)				
2 Thumb and index finger together in a ring (sign of OK)				
3 Index finger and little finger extended; other fingers flexed (sign of cuckold)				
4 Index finger extended; other fingers flexed				
5 Middle finger arched over the dorsal aspect of top joint of index finger; other fingers flexed				
6 Thumb imprisoned between the flexed index finger and middle finger; other fingers flexed				

(continues)

(continued)

Table 7–1. Ideomotor apraxia test items: Gesture and movement copying (De Renzi et al., 1980)

FINGER MOVEMENTS	TRIAL 1 SCORE 3	TRIAL 2 SCORE 2	TRIAL 3 SCORE 1	UNABLE SCORE 0
7 Flick middle finger three times over top of thumb				
8 Click middle finger three times with the thumb				
9 "Walk" index finger and middle finger on the table				
10 Make scissor movement with index finger and middle finger; other fingers flexed				
11 Tap the table top with four fingers in succession starting with index finger (drum fingers)				
12 Back of the hand on the tabletop; index finger and middle finger extended; other fingers flexed; flex the index finger and straighten, flex the middle finger and straighten, in turn, three times				
HAND AND ARM MOVEMENTS	TRIAL 3	TRIAL 2	TRIAL 1	TRIAL 0
1 Open palm of the hand onto the opposite shoulder				
2 Open palm of the hand onto the back of the neck				
3 Open hand on the chin				
4 Salute				
5 Hand circled as a tube, place to mouth and blow				
6 Halt somebody—arm forward, elbow extended, open hand vertical				

(continues)

(continued)

Table 7–1. Ideomotor apraxia test items: Gesture and movement copying (De Renzi et al., 1980)

HAND AND ARM MOVEMENTS	TRIAL 3	TRIAL 2	TRIAL 1	TRIAL 0
7 Sequence: Closed fist—thump sideways on the tabletop; open hand—slap palm on table top, in turn, three times				
8 Sequence: Fist on forehead, open palm to mouth, in turn, three times				
9 Movement: Open hand forward on one side perpendicular to body; sweep slowly across front of body to opposite shoulder, extended fingers moving from spaced apart (abducted) to touching each other (adducted) as the hand moves				
10 Make the sign of the cross (touch forehead, chest, opposite shoulder, other shoulder)				
11 Extended fingers, closed together; touch forehead three times with fingernails (palmar surface of hand facing forward)				
12 Send a kiss—fingertips and thumb together; touch mouth, extend and abduct arm, spacing the fingers as you do so, three times				

copying instruction (Table 7–2). Scoring of these tests are 2, 1, or 0, respectively, for correct performance, incorrect but recognizable performance, and incorrect and unrecognizable performance. There is published research using similar tests (Poeck, 1986; Agostoni et al., 1983; Alexander et al., 1992; Riddock et al., 1989). Each of these studies uses a variety of meaningful and nonmeaningful gestures for eliciting apraxic errors with similar scoring systems.

Table 7–2. Ideomotor apraxia test: Meaningful and meaningless movements (York Haaland & Flaherty, 1988)

Note: Items to be tested to verbal command, then repeated by copying tester gesture. Check (√) the correct box for: 2 = accurate performance; 1 = inaccurate but recognizable performance; 0 = unrecognizable performance. Maximum score = 40

	VERBAL			COPY		
	2	1	0	2	1	0
MEANINGFUL GESTURES						
1 Salute like a soldier						
2 Wave good-bye						
3 Scratch your head						
4 Throw or blow a kiss						
5 Snap or click your fingers						
MEANINGLESS GESTURES						
1 Hand on your nose						
2 Hand under your chin						
3 Index finger on your ear						
4 Thumb on your forehead						
5 Hand behind your head						

Most clinicians and researchers also use a test for pantomiming the use of objects (Table 7–3). These tests vary in the type of objects used but are generally presented in three conditions:

● Verbal instruction: "Pretend to hold an [item] and show me how you would use it."
● Visual presentation of the object to the client without touching it: "Show me how you would hold and use one of these."
● Giving the object to the client: "Show me how you would use this." Examples of objects used in these tests include a hammer, razor, comb, pen, key, toothbrush (Alexander et al., 1992; Riddock et al., 1989; York Haaland and Flaherty, 1984).

Errors in movement performance elicited during these assessment procedures typical of those made by people with ideomotor apraxia have been identified and classified by a number of researchers (Cicerone & Tupper, 1991; Mayer et al., 1990; Mozaz, 1992). These errors are not individually di-

Table 7–3. Pantomimed use of objects (Alexander et al., 1992; Riddock et al., 1989; York Haaland & Flaherty, 1984)

Note: Place tick in correct box for scoring: 2 = correct performance; 1 = incorrect but identifiable performance; 0 = unidentifiable performance or body part used as object.
Maximum score = 36

	VERBAL			VISUAL			REAL		
	2	1	0	2	1	0	2	1	0
1 Hammer									
2 Razor									
3 Comb									
4 Pen									
5 Toothbrush									
6 Key									

agnostic of ideomotor apraxia but can help the clinician to identify where the difficulties lie for particular clients. Raade et al. (1991) present particularly clear categories of error types (Table 7–4). Tate and McDonald (1995) suggest the need to develop a qualitative, standardized, reliable system of error analysis to aid in the diagnosis of apraxia. In practice, there is an element of clinical judgment and experience, and the novice clinician is strongly advised to practice and carry out these tests for apraxia on a number of normal individuals of all ages in order to obtain a baseline concept of the ways people without impairment react to and perform the tests.

Table 7–4. Error type categories in ideomotor apraxia (Raade et al., 1991)

ERROR TYPE	DESCRIPTION OF ERRORS
CONTENT	
Perseverative	The subject produces a response that includes all or part of a previously produced movement
Related	The movement is an accurately produced movement associated in content to the target
Nonrelated	The movement is an accurately produced movement that is not associated in content to the target

(continues)

(continued)

Table 7–4. Error type categories in ideomotor apraxia (Raade et al., 1991)	
ERROR TYPE	**DESCRIPTION OF ERRORS**
TEMPORAL	
Sequencing	Some movements require multiple positionings that are performed in a characteristic sequence; sequencing errors involve any perturbation of this sequence, including addition, deletion, or transposition of movement elements, as long as the overall movement structure remains recognizable
Timing	This error reflects any alterations from the typical timing or speed of a movement and may include abnormally increased, decreased, or irregular rate of production
Occurrence	Movements may involve either single or repetitive movement cycles; this error type reflects any multiplication of single cycles or reduction of a repetitive cycle to a single event
Delay	Delay in the initiation of a movement with no intervening facilitative movement
SPATIAL	
Internal configuration (limb only)	When performing a movement, the fingers and hand must be in a specific spatial relation to one another to reflect recognition and respect for the imagined tool; this error type reflects any abnormality of the required finger or hand posture and its relationship to the target tool
Amplitude	Any amplification, reduction, or irregularity of the characteristic amplitude of a target movement
External configuration or orientation (limb only)	When performing a movement, the fingers/hand/arm and the imagined tool must be in a specific relationship to the "object" receiving the action; errors of this type involve difficulties in orienting to the "object" or in placing the "object" in space
Body-part-as-object (limb only)	The client used the finger/hand/arm as the imagined tool of movement

(continues)

(continued)

Table 7–4. Error type categories in ideomotor apraxia (Raade et al., 1991)	
ERROR TYPE	**DESCRIPTION OF ERRORS**
SPATIAL (continued)	
Movement	When acting on an object with a tool, a movement characteristic of the action and necessary to accomplishing the goal is required; any disturbance of the characteristic movement reflects a movement error
Extraneous	Recognizable production of a movement with additional or extra movement or movements involved of nontarget articulators or body parts
Place of articulation (buccofacial)	An inappropriate point or place of articulation employed in production of a movement
OTHER	
No response	Subject may conclude his response with verbalization such as, "I can't" or, "No"
Unrecognizable response	A response that is not recognizable and shares no temporal or spatial features of the target
Verbalization	The subject produces a verbalization or written output instead of a movement; it should be recognized and semantically related

(Reprinted with permission from the authors and publisher.)

The testing for ideational apraxia generally involves using several objects in a sequence (De Renzi & Lucchelli, 1988). Examples used in many tests are locking a box (using a box, padlock, and key), lighting a candle (using a candle, candlestick, and matches), putting paper into a file (using a sheet of paper, file, and hole punch), polishing shoes (using shoes, polish, brush, and cloth), sending a letter (using paper, envelope, and stamp), and making a cup of tea (using teapot, kettle, cup, saucer, spoon, teabag, milk jug, and sugar bowl). The client is scored according to his or her capacity to sequence and correctly use the objects to carry out each task. Scores of 2, 1, 0 are awarded for correct, partially correct, and noncompletion of task, respectively (Table 7–5).

Table 7–5. Ideational apraxia scoring sheet

Note: Put a tick in the box to score performance: 2 = correct execution of task sequence; 1 = incorrect but identifiable completion of task goal; 0 = incorrect and unidentifiable use of objects to complete task.

ACTIVITY AND MATERIALS	SCORE 2	1	0	COMMENTS OR ERRORS MADE
1 Lock a box (box, padlock and key)				
2 Put paper into a file (sheet of paper, file, hole punch)				
3 Polish shoes (shoes, polish, brush, cloth)				
4 Send a letter (paper, envelope, stamp)				
5 Light a candle (candle, candlestick, matches)				
6 Make a cup of tea (teapot, kettle, cup, saucer, spoon, teabag, milk jug, sugar bowl)				

≡ CASE STUDY: AMANDA

BACKGROUND

THE REHABILITATION SETTING

The rehabilitation center where Amanda was admitted caters to both inpatients and outpatients with severe, usually complex neurologically based impairments and disabilities (usually after stroke or head injury). Clients' ages range from 20 to 70 years. There is a physiotherapy department with a hydrotherapy pool, occupational therapy department, speech and language therapy services, social work department, and psychology department. There is also specialist disability information and advice services, an independent living unit, facilities for reestablishing leisure activities and skills, and an inpatient ward. Clients are referred to the center by primary care physicians and hospitals and sometimes by social workers, families, or clients themselves. There is a recognition of the need for specialist, prolonged, and intensive rehabilitation services after the initial medical or emergency care is completed or after the initial rehabilitation programs have been completed. The center is part of the National Health Service (British public health system).

As a guiding philosophy, the center has a client-centered approach to rehabilitation with a focus on the needs and desires of client and their families. The main objectives are to concentrate on the aspirations of client and their families and to ensure that all interventions relate to their desires. The ultimate aim is to enable each client to lead the best life he can within the limits of any permanent damage he may have. Most clients are discharged from inpatient status within 9 months. Some clients remain involved with the rehabilitation center on an outpatient basis for several years. Some attend for a limited evaluation period of a few weeks long after their initial injury or illness to be advised on final placement or on work or occupation.

INTRODUCTION TO AMANDA

Amanda, a 25-year-old right-handed woman, arrived at the rehabilitation center 6 months after sustaining a severe head injury in a motor vehicle accident. She had **post-traumatic amnesia** (PTA) for 6 weeks, which is an indicator of the severity of her injury. Before the initial interview with Amanda, several sources of information were accessed. First, a brief description outlining her medical background and case management to date was given by the physiatrist in charge of the rehabilitation center. Second, the case notes were read for more detailed medical and social information. This led to discovery of contact names for the previous occupational therapists involved early in her recovery and rehabilitation and the name of the home care occupational therapist. These individuals were contacted and verbal reports were received regarding the previous intervention procedures and the client's home circumstances. From all these sources, it was established that Amanda was fully mobile but was dependent in all personal activities, including eating and drinking, because she was unable to use her upper limbs in any sustained, coordinated way. Power of grip in both hands was deemed to be good, but no useful functional grasp was possible. Amanda was also reported as being mute because of a buccofacial apraxia. She used an alphabet board to communicate, managing to point with reasonable accuracy to the letters she wanted. Her understanding of spoken and written language was said to be largely unimpaired, as was her memory. No formal neuropsychological testing had been carried out to determine the details of her cognitive functioning. This was partly due to her language and communication difficulties and partly because Amanda was resistant to the idea of formal tests and unwilling to cooperate. She lived at home with her mother in a two-story house and returned there after her discharge from the hospital. No adaptations had been carried out in the home, but her mother had given up work to care for Amanda. Before her head injury, Amanda was working as a teaching assistant in a local school and had been accepted to a training course for teaching.

Medical information indicated that she had recovered from the severe internal injuries sustained at the time of the accident with no long-term effects apart from pronounced scarring on her torso and legs. Some dental repair was necessary to replace lost front teeth. The magnetic resonance imaging and computed tomography scan reports noted widespread and extensive bi-hemispheric cortical damage, especially in the right posterior parietal lobe, left inferior parietal lobule, left frontal lobe (these are the motor and premotor areas). In addition, there was extensive subcortical white matter destruction, especially in the right hemisphere, and a small area of damage to the right caudate nucleus.

INITIAL INTERVIEW: INTERACTIVE REASONING

Box 7–1 outlines the therapist's description of her first encounter with Amanda.

INITIAL FINDINGS AND PLAN OF ACTION: PROCEDURAL REASONING

Amanda presented as a calm individual able to concentrate for the duration of an initial interview lasting 45 minutes. She answered questions appropriately through an alphabet board, head nods and shakes, and facial expression and was able to express a variety of emotions and feelings by such means. She applied herself well to the questioning and gave the appearance of being interested and engaged in the task.

A nonstandardized role and activity checklist (created by the rehabilitation staff at the center) indicated a drastic reduction in Amanda's current functioning compared with her premorbid roles and activities. There was

BOX 7–1. THERAPIST REASONING—INTERACTIVE REASONING

At our first meeting, Amanda walked into the room with ease and at a good pace. She was able to seat herself appropriately in the chair. Because Amanda was mute, it was important to conduct the interview in a manner that would give her the maximum opportunity to express her views and wishes, yet not tire her by prolonged periods of spelling out the words she wanted to say. I introduced myself and told her about my role within the rehabilitation center. I suggested that I try to ask her things in a way that would require a yes or no response given by nodding or shaking her head, but that at times she would have to spell out certain things and I would try to interpret what she wished to say. She could then agree or disagree with my interpretation. At this point I was attempting to establish a partnership between us and agree to some ground rules that would form the basis of this relationship. I wondered if she would tell me if I got things wrong when interpreting her words. She did agree to this system, and I in return stated my intention to be open and straightforward in my communications with her. I wanted her to think that she could always say what she wanted to me without worry or anxiety.

The second point I wanted to make concerned the need to establish that she was in control of her rehabilitation program. I explained to her that I would be guided by her through her expressing her needs and desires. I would suggest ways of achieving her desires, but she was able to disagree and to say no to anything she was uncomfortable with. This would only be achievable by our open communication already agreed upon. I was trying to establish right from the start that she was the one with the control. Although she was dependent on others for all her personal and practical activities, this was an area that she could have independence and control over. I believed that my role in the partnership was to aid her through the process of getting as much physical control and independence as she could, but I was not there to dictate that process. Having agreed to the nature of the partnership we were about to engage in, I suggested that to set goals for her rehabilitation it was necessary to ask her things about herself in the past, about how she was now, and about the future as she saw it. I used the Canadian Occupational Performance Measure (COPM) (Law et al., 1994) for this, together with a role and activities checklist. The next stage involved asking her about how important or valuable she considered each of those roles and activities. From the COPM and checklist we determined that her problems lay in all areas (i.e., self-care, productivity, and leisure) and that her current activities were reduced to watching TV, listening to the radio, and walking. When discussing areas of her self-care, Amanda confirmed that she was dependent for all activities, including eating, drinking, dressing, washing,

(continues)

BOX 7–1. THERAPIST REASONING—INTERACTIVE REASONING (CONT.)

toileting, and grooming. It became clear that Amanda was puzzled by her inability to successfully carry out any activity at all. After all, she was not paralyzed, and she could feel her hands. There was some considerable degree of fear expressed because she could not understand why she could not do things. In addition, she "said" that trying and failing in all these activities made her feel "like a berk" (sic). Her embarrassment at her performances was acute. Areas of dissatisfaction for her were focused on all aspects of self-care, her socialization (she previously socialized at clubs and pubs with others), and her active recreation (prior activities, such as cycling, swimming, walking, clothes, hair styling, shopping, cooking and baking, dancing, listening to pop music, vacations, movies, dog walking, reading, drawing, and playing cards, were all aspired to).

Talking about friends and socializing activities also opened up opportunities to talk about relationships in general. She volunteered that her boyfriend still came around to see her, although her facial expression and shoulder shrugs gave an impression of her not being too happy about this relationship. I did not, at this stage, pursue this line of inquiry because it seemed too intrusive for a first meeting. I did, however, say that if at any time she wanted to talk about her friends or relationships or how she was managing them, I would be very pleased to listen and respond. I wanted to give a clear message to Amanda that this was a legitimate area in her life for us to discuss, should she wish to do so. I was giving her "permission" to talk about this part of her life with me. Given the slow nature of our conversation, the completion of the COPM and the role and activity checklist comprised the entire first interview.

Discussing roles and activities in her life in such a way enabled me to get a picture of her past way of life, where her interests lay, and the anticipation of how her future life might turn out. It was also an ideal way to establish the aim of her occupational therapy by looking at ways of achieving such roles and activities. Clearly such a role and activity checklist could also open up other avenues for discussion as they arise. In Amanda's case, for instance, I asked her why she did not go out and socialize with her friends on weekends when this was a normal activity for her before her accident. Her reply indicated a deep embarrassment at her present condition and disability. She thought that everyone would look at her. To me, this indicated an area that we would have to address in the future: her acceptance of herself in her post-accident state, whatever that might ultimately become. I later learned that before her accident, Amanda and her friends had rather despised people with disabilities, and her need to appear "normal" now stemmed from these premorbid ideas and attitudes.

(continues)

BOX 7–1. THERAPIST REASONING—INTERACTIVE REASONING (CONT.)

At the end of this first interview, Amanda independently asked about our next meeting, indicating an interest in the process and a recall of the nature of the timetabled program of the rehabilitation center. I suggested the aim for the next session was, with her agreement, to look at her physical capabilities in a more formal way. I knew, from information given to me by her previous therapist at the hospital, that she disliked formal testing. However, I considered it essential to let Amanda know why such tests of physical capabilities and functions were carried out, their importance in planning and monitoring intervention, and that ultimately they would be useful to both of us in working out the rehabilitation program that she wanted. I also wanted her to know that I acknowledged, and was very aware of, how she might feel during such procedures. I told her that I realized that such assessments could be very difficult and dispiriting because they emphasized losses, but that I would try to make the encounters as easy as I could for her. With these explanations and reassurances, Amanda agreed to the content of the next session. We parted from a first meeting that had been informal, relaxed, and informative for both of us, with the start of a therapeutic relationship founded on stated ground rules and the potential for our work and collaboration in her future rehabilitation all stated clearly.

During the interview I was also observing and considering Amanda's reactions to and behavior in the situation she found herself. I wanted to determine if she was engaged in what we were doing and interested in that process. I judged her responses to questions to determine if she had understood and rephrased the questions when it seemed that she had difficulty.

---

an indication that Amanda was embarrassed and self-conscious about her difficulties and that this might be causing Amanda to avoid social and public interactions. She was fully ambulant, but she was reported to be unable to use her hands in any functional way and was dependent for all her self-care activities.

The areas to investigate in the plan of action for Amanda's occupational therapy were:

- Amanda's needs and desires for rehabilitation
- Amanda's physical functioning, particularly of her upper limbs (motor and sensory assessment) to determine the extent of physical capabilities and losses
- The possible presence of limb apraxia (given her buccofacial apraxia, this is a likely contributor to her disability)

- Amanda's self-care skills and possible compensatory strategies
- Amanda's perceptual or cognitive difficulties (functional tasks would be used to determine them)
- Amanda's home and social circumstances
- Amanda's hopes and aspirations for the future

EVALUATION SELECTION AND RATIONALE

The Canadian Occupational Performance Measure (COPM) (Law et al., 1994) was the first assessment tool used with Amanda. This tool is useful for establishing rehabilitation priorities from the client's perspective. It is also a way of measuring change and the effectiveness of intervention. An example of Amanda's COPM form can be found in Figure 7–1. Secondly, a systematic physical assessment of Amanda's capacities and losses was essential in order to understand the nature of her difficulties and then be able to formulate the best strategy for facilitating functional activity. Testing active and passive ranges of movement, particularly in the upper limbs, would be the first step, with sensory testing in all modalities (i.e., temperature, light touch, deep pressure, sharp touch, proprioception) completing the assessment.

The third assessment used arose from the knowledge that the speech and language therapists had diagnosed a buccofacial apraxia in Amanda. Therefore, it seemed likely that some of Amanda's physical disabilities would be due to some degree of limb apraxia. It seemed appropriate to make use of the more lengthy research batteries for testing apraxia to ensure a thorough exploration of her difficulties in this area. The apraxia assessment procedures would also highlight any subtle deficits in performance that could help formulate an intervention strategy. Finally, additional information regarding Amanda's physical abilities would be achieved through observation of her performance in functional tasks in an appropriate context, for example, self-care activities at the start of the day or eating skills during mealtimes (Árnadóttir, 1990).

In the initial interview, Amanda reported disliking formal assessments because they showed her very clearly the extent of her deficits and difficulties. It was therefore important to do only the most important assessments formally; these were the tests for apraxia. Cognitive function and perceptual capacities could be assessed through observation during normal functional self-care activities rather than through the formal assessments such as the Rivermead Behavioral Memory Test (Wilson et al., 1985) or the RPAB (Whiting et al., 1985) (both reviewed in Chapter 3).

Scoring:

Occupational performance problems	Initial assessment performance	Initial assessment satisfaction	Reassessment performance	Reassessment satisfaction
Eating	1	1	5	3
Drinking	1	1	7	4
Watching TV	1	1	10	10
Toileting	1	1	7	6
Dressing	1	1	6	5

Scoring Summary:

	Initial assessment performance score	Initial assessment satisfaction score	Reassessment performance score	Reassessment satisfaction score
Total Score	5/5 = 1	5/5 = 1	35/7 = 7	28/5 = 5.6

Change in performance = 7 - 1 = 6

Figure 7–1. Amanda's completed assessment form from the Canadian Occupational Performance Measure (Law, Baptiste, Carswell-Opzoomer, McColl, Polatakjo, & Pollok, 1994, CAOT Publications).

Identification of occupational performance issues.

Occupational Performance Issues		Importance Rating
Self-care	Eating	10
	Drinking	10
	Dressing	10
	Toileting	10
	Grooming—teeth	10
	Grooming—hair	10
	Driving a car	6
	Shopping	8
Productivity	Train as a teacher	7
	Making own meals/baking	8
	Look after clothes/laundry	6
Leisure	Drawing	6
	Watching TV	9
	Playing cards	5
	Swimming	6
	Movies	6
	Vacations with friend	7
	Clubs and bars with friends	8
	Phone calls	8
	Parties	7

Figure 7–1. (continued)

Scoring:

Occupational performance problems	Initial assessment performance	Initial assessment satisfaction	Reassessment performance	Reassessment satisfaction
Eating	1	1	5	3
Drinking	1	1	7	4
Watching TV	1	1	10	10
Toileting	1	1	7	6
Dressing	1	1	6	5

Scoring Summary:

	Initial assessment performance score	Initial assessment satisfaction score	Reassessment performance score	Reassessment satisfaction score
Total Score	5/5 = 1	5/5 = 1	35/7 = 7	28/5 = 5.6

Change in performance = 7 - 1 = 6

Change in satisfaction = 5.6 - 1 = 4.6

Summary of assessment information using the COPM 2nd Edition forms, 1994. Reprinted with permission from the authors.

Figure 7–1. (continued)

BOX 7–2. THERAPIST REASONING—CONDITIONAL REASONING

I want Amanda to be independent enough in the future to live with her mother and yet not be dependent on her. I imagine a future time when Amanda can take care of her own personal needs and have some social life at home. Using the COPM helps me to make sure that Amanda's hopes and aspirations for the future are also incorporated into the rehabilitation team's goals. All our interventions are aimed toward achieving those stated goals and aspirations. In the future, I also see my role as helping Amanda to re-adjust and modify those goals and aspirations to achieve satisfaction with life within the limitations imposed by the residual disabilities with which she will inevitably have to live.

Box 7–2 outlines the process of conditional reasoning used by the therapist as she tells her story of her own, and Amanda's, hopes for Amanda's future.

EVALUATION FINDINGS

PRIORITY LIST FOR REHABILITATION TARGETS

As presented in Figure 7–1 on the COPM, Amanda's five most important problems listed in priority order were eating, drinking, switching the TV on and off and changing channels independently, managing the toilet, and dressing. Other areas she identified for the future as being important were brushing her hair, taking a shower, putting on her face cream, cleaning her teeth, and putting on lip balm. All of her concerns were focused in the area of self-care. It would be expected that as rehabilitation progressed, other areas of her life would assume a more important focus, such as socialization, recreation, household management, and work. These would be established through a system of reassessment and review.

PHYSICAL FUNCTION

When apraxia is suspected, it is essential to have an accurate and detailed assessment of physical function to be able to distinguish which parts of the client's motor performance can be attributed to purely physical difficulties and which might be attributable to the dysfunction of underlying mechanisms of cognitive motor-sensory programming and planning capacities. An assessment of Amanda's physical function is outlined in Table 7–6.

SENSORY CAPACITIES

Assessment in this area with Amanda indicated considerable sensory mislocation in all modalities in the distal portion of both upper limbs (i.e., stimulation of the fingers was perceived as coming from the hands; stimulation of the hands was perceived on the lower part of the forearms). Sensation in the upper arm and proximal part of the forearm was intact. Proprioception was intact for the shoulder and elbow but was diminished in the wrist and fingers in both the right and left upper limbs.

VISUAL AGNOSIA ASSESSMENT

A screening test for visual agnosia was carried out with Amanda. Her score was 19 out of a possible 20. It was concluded that she had no difficulties with recognition of objects. Again, if apraxia is suspected, it is essential to be able to distinguish that any difficulties with object use cannot be attributable to a nonrecognition of the objects themselves but rather to the inability to be able to use the objects in a purposeful way. In attempting to explain the problems that Amanda experienced, other alternative explanations must be discounted or, alternatively, recognized as contributing to the complexity of the difficulties. This process was described as "hypothesis testing" in Chapter 3.

PRAXIC CAPACITIES

Four assessments were used to investigate Amanda's praxic capacities. Each assessment and the findings are:

1. Ideomotor apraxia test (De Renzi et al., 1980) (see Table 7–1). Score = 6 out of a possible 72 for both the left and right hands. Complex finger and hand gesture copying were all performed inaccurately. Errors made included timing of movements, mispositioning of fingers, sequencing errors, and inaccurate plane of movement or hand posture, with gross overuse of the elbow and shoulder during all gesture and

Table 7–6. Assessment of Amanda's physical functioning

AREA INVESTIGATED	THERAPIST COMMENTS
Lower limbs	Full, active range of movement in right and left hip, knee, ankle
Sitting posture and balance	Good, symmetrical
Walking	Independent; good pace; good balance
Shoulder, elbow, forearm	Full, active range of movement, right and left; some scarring on dorsal aspect both forearms
Wrist	• Flexion: full, active. Right and left • Extension: 60° active (left), 45° active (right); full passive movement, right and left • Abduction (radial deviation): minimal active; full passive movement, right and left • Adduction (ulnar deviation): full active and passive movement, right and left
Hands	Appearance: some scarring on both dorsal surfaces; at rest, both right and left thumbs held to the side of the palm but had no loss of thenar bulk; MCP joints held in hyperextension in both hands
MCP joints	• Flexion: full active movement, right and left • Extension: joints held in hyperextension • Abduction: slight active movement; full passive movement, right and left • Adduction: no active movement when fingers held abducted, right and left
IP joints	• Flexion: active movement in all joints; not full range, right and left • Extension: active movement in all joints, right and left
Thumb	• Opposition: none • Other movements: some abduction and adduction possible; some weak flexion and extension of the thumb IP joint possible • Observation: effort at producing the movements resulted in associated reactions of hyperextension in MCP joints

IP = interphalangeal; MCP = metacarpophalangeal.

movement copying. She had a marked difficulty with placing her hands in the correct plane and orientation to her face.

2. Test for apraxia using meaningful and nonmeaningful gestures to both verbal command and a copying instruction (York Haaland & Flaherty, 1984) (see Table 7–2). Score = 16 (left hand) and 17 (right hand) out of a possible 40. All movements for both verbal command and copying were recognizable but incorrect, showing errors of timing, speed, plane of movement, and orientation of the hands. Elbow and shoulder movements were used extensively and inappropriately. Again, evidence of particular difficulty in positioning the hands near the face was shown.

3. Tests for pantomiming the use of objects were presented in three conditions: verbal instruction, visual presentation, and using the real object. Objects used in these tests were a hammer, razor, comb, pen, key, and toothbrush (Alexander et al., 1992; Riddock et al., 1989; York Haaland & Flaherty, 1984) (see Table 7–3). Score=18 (left hand) and 14 (right hand) out of a possible 36. Pantomimed use of objects was recognizable but inaccurate, showing errors similar to those in gesture-copying tests, especially in the plane of movement for using the object.

4. Ideational apraxia test using several objects in a sequence (De Renzi & Lucchelli, 1988). No score was possible because Amanda was unable to manipulate the objects sufficiently to complete the test. However, she was able to indicate where, how, and in what sequence each should be used. It was considered unlikely, therefore, that she had an ideational apraxia because such awareness of objects is not apparent in a person who has lost the idea of movements and object use. If Amanda had displayed a sense of not knowing in what order to pick up, position, and use the objects in front of her; had made errors in her instructions to the therapist in the object use; or had shown any air of bewilderment about the requirements of the tasks, the therapist would (in the absence of her capacity to actually demonstrate the actions for herself) be only able to report that ideational apraxia could not be discounted.

In conclusion, performance on all tests for apraxia was compounded by Amanda's motor and sensory impairments. Object use was particularly affected by her inability to oppose her thumbs. Despite these confounding variables, the errors made by Amanda were of the type and quality recognized and identified as apraxic in origin. The accumulation of evidence from the tests suggests a severe ideomotor apraxia in both upper limbs. There was no evidence of ideational apraxia or visual agnosia.

ACTIVITIES OF DAILY LIVING: OBSERVATIONAL EVALUATION

Eating

With therapist help in positioning her right hand around a large-handled spoon, Amanda was able to sustain a grip while bending her elbow. She was not able to obtain a correct position and orientation of the spoon in relation to the dish of food, nor could she retrieve food from the dish. When food was placed on the spoon by the therapist, Amanda could not adjust her movement to achieve the correct position of the spoon in relation to her mouth, which resulted in spills. Some finger foods were retrieved from a plate and moved toward her mouth, but both the method and results were haphazard, very messy, and unacceptable to Amanda, who preferred to be passively fed in these circumstances.

Drinking

Amanda was unable to position her hands correctly in relation to a glass of liquid before gripping and lifting the glass. If a glass was passively placed in her hands, she was able to sustain a grip but was unable to lift and position the glass in correct orientation to her mouth for drinking. This resulted in her spilling the drink. At the time of assessment, Amanda was drinking using a straw, lowering her head toward the table to suck on the straw.

Dressing

Amanda correctly identified underwear and clothes from a drawer and selected those she wished to wear. Throughout the entire dressing process, Amanda was unable to manipulate any items of clothing sufficiently to place them onto her body. She was able to cooperate in her dressing by inserting her arms into bra straps or sleeve holes. She could step into panties and slacks if they were placed on the floor, but she was unable to pull them up. All difficulties in this area of self-care could be attributed to an inability to adjust her grasp or alter the position of her hands as required. This was over and above what might be expected from the motor and sensory loss. The ideomotor apraxia identified in formal testing accounted for the errors and difficulties being experienced. No evidence of any perceptual problem such as hemi-neglect was observed during the dressing activity.

Home Environment

Home and social circumstances were investigated using a variety of sources, including interviews with Amanda, her mother, and the home care occupational therapist. She lived in a two-story house near the center of a town. At this stage of the evaluation process, no adaptations had been carried out on the house; Amanda was managing at home but was totally dependent on the help of her mother. It was anticipated that a home visit would be carried out with Amanda later in her rehabilitation program to discuss any changes or adaptations to her environment that might aid in her independence. Further information regarding social and family relationships emerged over time through informal conversations during therapy with her and her family.

PRIORITIZED PROBLEM LIST

After the formal and informal evaluations, Amanda and the therapist set a prioritized problem list. The four broad areas of difficulty were:

1. Loss of all self-care independence mainly due to severe ideomotor apraxia,
2. Loss of activities: work, leisure and social; all of these were attributable, either directly or indirectly, to her inability to use her hands in a purposeful and functional way,
3. Loss of roles resulting from loss of independence and loss of activities, and
4. Disruption of social and emotional relationships because of her loss of spoken communication.

GOALS AND OBJECTIVES

A goal-planning meeting was held with Amanda, her mother, and the rehabilitation team involved in the initial assessments. Amanda's own priority list as expressed in the COPM was instrumental in formulating aims, objectives, and targeted interventions.

Long-term goals:

1. To return to live independently with her mother
2. To return to an occupation similar to teaching

To achieve these aims, objectives were formulated with Amanda and her mother as the controlling focus of discussions.

Objectives: Six objectives were devised. These objectives, the interventions planned to achieve these, and the therapist's reasoning are presented in Table 7–7.

SELECTION OF INTERVENTION STRATEGIES AND ACTIVITIES

Box 7–3 indicates the therapist's acknowledgment of the need to have some success in therapy and to work on an activity with which Amanda could make fast progress.

Outline of steps for working with a client who has ideomotor apraxia:

1. Therapist talks client through the tasks section by section
2. Client says the same instructions in her head or out loud (because Amanda cannot say them out loud, she will do this in her head)
3. Client has written or diagrammatic instructions to follow when therapist is not available (e.g., during breakfast, evening meals, or on weekends)
4. Client is instructed to look at her limbs and be aware of what she is doing during each task

Together Amanda and the therapist set up the program of her rehabilitation in occupational therapy with a task priority order and target dates for achievement. For the first 2 weeks, the areas we agreed to concentrate on were:

1. To take a drink independently, lifting a cup
2. To eat independently using a large-handled spoon and adapted plate with a lip
3. To turn the TV on and off and change channels independently

All therapy sessions would be devoted to achieving these aims either through the use of facilitatory techniques or by practicing the functional tasks herself.

OUTLINE OF THERAPY SESSIONS OVER A FOUR-DAY PERIOD

Aim: to practice components of the drinking activity.
    Seated at a table, Amanda was instructed:

1. To try to always be aware of where her elbows were positioned

Table 7-7. Occupational therapy objectives and interventions for Amanda

OBJECTIVE	INTERVENTION PLANNED	THERAPIST REASONING
To achieve selective control over hand movements	Facilitation techniques used in both physical and occupational therapy sessions using specific hand exercises and functional tasks	Given the motor and sensory losses in Amanda's hands in addition to the apraxia, we thought the use of facilitation techniques in a movement-specific program would have the potential for enabling Amanda to regain some of her lost movement control. We thought that for this particular objective, a visual and verbal mediation strategy would be most appropriate. We cued Amanda to look at what she was doing and demonstrated movements to give a visual model of how the movement was to be performed. In addition, we verbalized the description of the movement being facilitated and encouraged Amanda to verbalize sub-vocally (given her buccofacial apraxia) what she was trying to do. Use of such movements in functional tasks were practical alongside the pure hand exercises using the same visual and verbal mediation strategies alongside task breakdown to ensure a purposeful, functional outcome.
To achieve independence in personal ADLs with priority for	Breakdown of functional tasks and practice of those components using verbal and visual mediation. Taken in priority order (as given by Amanda), each of the ADL tasks were broken down into the	I thought that Amanda needed to regain some aspects of her independence rapidly. The combination of task breakdown, compensatory techniques, and adaptive equipment would all help in this objective.

(continues)

(continued)

Table 7-7. Occupational therapy objectives and interventions for Amanda

OBJECTIVE	INTERVENTION PLANNED	THERAPIST REASONING
eating, drinking, managing the toilet, and dressing (taken from the COPM)	smallest component parts, and Amanda practiced those component parts. Particular focus concerned regaining the control and decreasing the overactivity of shoulder and elbow movements during tasks.	
To achieve spoken communication	Speech and language therapist to facilitate production of individual sounds and automatic language	Encouraging spoken communication in all therapy sessions and general activities was considered a natural and relaxed way to facilitate Amanda's use of the sounds available to her. In addition, her embarrassment at the sound of her voice would need to be overcome if she were to achieve any normal social communication. The more she practiced, it was hoped the more she would become used to the new timbre and sound of this voice that was alien to her, not "hers" as she knew it before the accident.
To explore need for communication aids	Instruction in basic computer skills	Amanda was not interested in using a portable electronic communication aid because this seemed to be, for her, an overt expression of her disability and she wanted to look "normal" at all times. However, she did think that learning to use a computer would be a useful skill for her and could help her general communication such as keeping

(continues)

(continued)

Table 7-7. Occupational therapy objectives and interventions for Amanda

OBJECTIVE	INTERVENTION PLANNED	THERAPIST REASONING
		in touch with friends through letter writing. It also had the potential to give her a vehicle to express her emotions and feelings about her experiences through the written word, given that extensive verbal expression was not possible.
To participate in some leisure activities	To facilitate independent use of TV, as identified by the COPM, by using task breakdown strategies. To encourage Amanda to participate in the leisure projects available at the rehabilitation center; painting activities were identified by her as being of particular interest because she enjoyed drawing prior to her accident. To encourage Amanda into the world outside the protective environment of her home and the rehabilitation center by dog-walking at home with her mother because this was an activity she used to enjoy before her accident. For similar reasons, it was agreed that she would try shopping trips locally with the occupational therapist and with her mother. Amanda also agreed to think about participating in some social trips with her mother or friends on weekends. Discussion about potential leisure interests led again to the possibility of basic computer skills,	Amanda could, potentially, become very isolated unless she was encouraged to develop and resume some social and leisure activities. It was considered important to encourage her to explore the outside world and regain her confidence in being able to cope in the normal social environment. The shopping trips would enable her to look at clothes and fashions that she was interested in and get used to being in the world again. Hopefully these trips would gradually reduce her self-consciousness and embarrassment, give an extra dimension to her conversations, and be a point of contact with her friends on weekends. The therapy sessions devoted to the pursuit of leisure and social activities were, therefore, given a high priority, especially later on as the months of her rehabilitation program went by.

(continues)

(continued)

Table 7-7. Occupational therapy objectives and interventions for Amanda

OBJECTIVE	INTERVENTION PLANNED	THERAPIST REASONING
	and this was an area that Amanda thought she might find interesting and enjoyable.	
To start assessing work potential	Cognitive assessment	Although it was very early in her rehabilitation program, discussion about work potential in relation to Amanda's long-term aims was important. Amanda agreed that the therapists were able to make professional judgments about her abilities and potential for work during therapy sessions but that a formal neuropsychological assessment was of use too. She agreed to have that formal assessment.
To counsel and support Amanda and her mother as needed	Formal and informal support was available from all the rehabilitation team if and when Amanda and her mother needed or requested it.	Discussion and support frequently occur informally and opportunistically with whoever the patient or family member feels most comfortable with. We considered it important, therefore, that Amanda and her mother knew that discussion of problems and anxieties, feelings and fears, were a daily part of the rehabilitationist's job. They should feel free to avail themselves of that support. Formal counseling was also available should either of them feel it to be necessary at any time.

BOX 7–3. THERAPIST REASONING—SELECTION OF INTERVENTIONS

Amanda needed to become more independent quickly. Her feelings of dependence and vulnerability and the fear she expressed concerning her inability to care for her own body were acute. I explained to Amanda that she would need to do specific exercises with me in order to reach her goal of independence, and she indicated that she was willing to cooperate and participate as fully as possible. Amanda had already expressed that her priority was to be able to eat and drink without help. We started work in this area. At this early stage of the rehabilitation process, Amanda's future vision of herself was of "normality" and complete recovery from her difficulties, although she accepted the idea that it could be a very long process. I was more reserved in my opinion about how much recovery Amanda would make, but I knew that she was not ready to face this vision of the future yet.

Amanda appeared to have a good understanding of ideas and concepts explained to her. I therefore explained the need for task breakdown and the reasons special concentration would be placed on stabilizing her shoulder and elbow to gain more control over her upper limb movements. I then explained the process we would go through, which is outlined below. In this way we would achieve the verbal and visual mediation strategies combined with the compensatory task breakdown suggested as being possibly the most effective remediation for ideomotor apraxia (Ayres, 1985; Croce, 1993; Goodgold-Edwards & Cernak, 1990; Pilgrim & Humphreys, 1994; Wilson, 1988). I like to use this task breakdown and a "bottom-up" approach in treating ideomotor apraxia because:

- In my clinical experience it quickly achieves good results in many of the basic tasks of self-care.
- The client can see very clearly the objective he or she is working toward.
- The client can have a sense of rapid improvement in his or her functional abilities.
- Research evidence (Wilson, 1988) suggests this may be the best approach for clients with apraxia.

---

2. That the activity would aim to minimize or eliminate shoulder and elbow activity because they were interfering with function
3. That although her arm and hand movements were unreliable at present, her capacity to move her head was unimpaired and we would make use of this skill

The drinking task was then started. The therapist gave the movement instructions, asking Amanda to repeat them in her head. Amanda would then attempt to carry out the individual movement described, with the therapist facilitating or adjusting the movement as required. Amanda was asked to look at her arms as she was moving and to try to make the adjustment herself in light of that information. The first movement component was taken in isolation and practiced (a bottom-up approach rather than top-down). When achieved, the next component was to be added, and then both were completed together. When these had been achieved, the third component was added, and so on until all movement components had been mastered in sequence.

The following sequence was used to help Amanda lift a tall, empty glass *(note: asterisk denotes later additions to the sequence):*

- I put my hands flat on the table.
- I slide my hands forward at a level with the cup.
- I look to see that my elbows are on the tabletop.
- I turn my hands onto their sides.
- I slide my hands toward each other until they touch the cup.
- I close my hands together tightly around the cup.
- I look to see that my hands are in the right place.*
- I keep my elbows on the table.*
- I bend my elbows slightly, slowly lifting the cup halfway to my mouth.
- I stop moving my arms but still grasp the cup.*
- I bend my head down to the cup.
- I put my mouth on the cup.
- I use my head to tip the cup and drink.
- I lift my head.
- I straighten my elbows.
- I put the cup onto the table.
- I open my hands and straighten my fingers.
- I slide my hands sideways away from the cup.
- I slide my hands toward me and off the table.*

The later additions were made to this sequence in light of errors made during trials. Generally, Amanda achieved each movement component within three attempts, and only minor physical adjustments to the positions were required by the therapist. She learned the entire sequence very quickly and could reliably carry it out after two therapy sessions. Amanda concentrated very hard during these sessions, trying her utmost to carry out the movements required. She was able to follow the instructions and carry out the itemized movements. When we both felt confident in her ability to manage the sequence to verbal instruction, water was placed in the glass and Amanda managed to take a drink successfully. This was practiced several times. Her rapid progress during

---

BOX 7–4. THERAPIST REASONING—REALISTIC PACING

I could see that Amanda was delighted to find a way of getting around her difficulties. I, too, was extremely pleased that this compensatory strategy had worked so well. My only concern at this point was that Amanda should not assume that *all* tasks would be completed successfully so quickly. Therefore, although I did not wish to take away any sense of her pleasure, I gently introduced the idea that we would try this technique with other aspects of her self care but that more complicated tasks such as dressing could take considerably longer. Amanda seemed to accept this.

---

each session encouraged her a great deal. The therapist's thoughts at this time are shown in Box 7–4.

In session three, after successful completion of the task with verbal instructions, the written instructions of the drinking sequence were introduced. This was a more lengthy operation because Amanda had to read each item in the sequence before carrying out the instruction. Amanda was not allowed to progress to the next step unless the movement or position was correct. Again, minor adjustments were necessary to verbal prompting (e.g., "Look again at where your hands are" or, "Are your elbows in the right position?"). A fourth therapy session was needed to consolidate the successful completion of the drinking task using written instructions, with five or six repetitions of the complete sequence being the maximum possible in the 45 minutes allocated in the rehabilitation timetable. We celebrated with a hot cup of tea using an insulated cup when we were both confident that no spills would occur. Amanda had her own written copy of the sequence to follow and to say subvocally whenever she wanted to take a drink outside the therapy sessions. Nursing and other staff, as well as Amanda's mother, were informed of this program and were instructed on how to use verbal prompting if necessary.

Amanda continued to use these written instructions for several weeks. Eventually she learned the sequence by heart and would say all the items to herself as she performed the task without using the external aid. After a while, she was making shortcuts in the sequence. She knew where the "danger spots" were and simply checked at those points that her hands were in the correct position or that her elbows were placed correctly. Full recitation of the instructions became redundant. Similar procedures and strategies were carried out for eating and all other self-care tasks.

PROGRESS AND DISCHARGE

The task breakdown approach was continued throughout Amanda's rehabilitation program in the area of self-care, taken in priority order as suggested by her at the outset and adjusting and modifying goals as she wished. Managing the toilet, dressing (taking each separate item in turn and doing a task breakdown for removing and putting on the clothes), brushing her hair, taking a shower, putting on her face cream, cleaning her teeth, and putting on lip balm were all dealt with during the rehabilitation process. The dressing aspect of Amanda's self-care was a long-term goal. Items were taken in turn as she deemed appropriate (e.g., taking pants off and on would clearly be a priority because it would help in her first goal of managing the toilet independently; taking her robe off would be incorporated into showering independently). Other self-care activities were tackled alongside the dressing program because they could be practiced out of context in therapy sessions (e.g., brushing hair, putting on face cream, cleaning teeth, and putting on lip balm).

A home visit was carried out with Amanda after she had been attending the rehabilitation center for 8 weeks. She had been going home each weekend and was coping well but was dependent on the help of her mother. Amanda was reluctant to "advertise" her disability by having changes made to her home. She wanted minimal home adaptations but did agree to the following adaptations:

● Change taps and door handles to lever style
● Change light switches to push on and off buttons to enable her to use them independently and easily
● Provide an adapted telephone with large keys so that she would be able to call friends, emergency services, and so on
● Install an alarm system to alert neighbors if she was in difficulty

Leisure skills were pursued through a local gym to reestablish her swimming, jogging, and aerobics activities. Social contacts were encouraged but proved to be somewhat difficult to maintain because her friends were drifting away to other jobs and different parts of the country. In addition, Amanda felt she no longer had things in common with them to talk about or to do together. Her relationship with her boyfriend also ceased. Establishing new friendships was an unresolved difficulty. Her spoken communication skills improved so that although speech was effortful and breathy, it was intelligible. Amanda continued to dislike her "new" voice and although she was reluctant to volunteer speech, she was gradually increasing her vocal output.

Work potential was explored through colleges for people with disabilities. The first one did not suit Amanda because she considered herself not "belonging." Everyone there had seemed so obviously disabled, most being in wheelchairs; Amanda had much more of a hidden disability. It continued to be of great concern to Amanda that she look and be as "normal" as possible. She did not want to belong to such a disabled group of students. A second college that catered for people with special needs better suited her. She considered trying a computer course that could provide her with skills for future employment.

One year after first attending the rehabilitation center and 18 months after her accident, Amanda decided that she had achieved what she wanted to as an inpatient. She was becoming bored with the process of therapy and of the rehabilitation environment. At this point she was independent in drinking, eating with a spoon (but not cutting up food), and in managing the toilet (but not her menstruation). She was largely independent in dressing but still needed assistance in such tasks as putting on her bra, tying laces on tennis shoes, and coping with tight clothing or small buttons (she was unwilling to have any clothing adaptations or modifications). Amanda was also independent in showering, brushing her hair, cleaning her teeth, and applying face cream and lip balm. She was dependent on her mother for all food preparation and most domestic activities. Her social activities remained reduced, but she was participating in swimming, dog walking, and shopping with her mother.

Amanda's discharge to outpatient status at this time was not wholly satisfactory from the rehabilitation team's perspective. Everyone thought that she would continue to benefit from the daily program of activities offered by the center, especially because her physical and functional abilities were still showing improvement. In addition, many issues had yet to be resolved, especially in regard to her social functioning and long-term vision for a future role in society. Leisure roles were not well established, and a program of education and training for her future work role was not in place. A second COPM was administered, revealing a significant change in both her performance and satisfaction with her performance (see Fig. 7–1).

Discussions with Amanda concluded that she was determined to leave the center but would participate in a specially designed home program and would return for monthly reassessment. She was, therefore, given exercises and an activity program to continue at home with follow-up and review appointments. At these reviews, Amanda would ask for and get new goals to work toward over the next 4 weeks. She continued in this way for a little over 12 months, always showing some degree of improvement at each reassessment and a gradual increase in her skills and levels of activity.

One year after discharge from the inpatient to the outpatient service of the rehabilitation center and 2.5 years after her accident, Amanda was functioning relatively independently despite her continuing physical difficulties. She was able to use a knife and fork to eat, make a sandwich, peel a banana and orange, shave her legs, write legibly, assist in baking and other household tasks, polish her nails, and apply her make-up. Social work involvement continued, and further education and work possibilities were explored.

SINGLE-CASE RESEARCH

Amanda agreed to participate in some research evaluating the effectiveness of sensory input within the inpatient rehabilitation program. Research on the effectiveness of different therapeutic interventions is sparse. Croce (1993) suggests that verbal and visual mediation should be linked with additional tactile and proprioceptive stimulation. This case study investigation aimed to test the hypothesis that tactile and proprioceptive input enhances motor performance in individuals with ideomotor apraxia.

A case study protocol was devised with measures taken daily immediately before, and immediately after, every therapy session in physical and occupational therapy. This was to determine if there were any immediate effects of or changes that might occur over time. The baseline phase consisted of the normal rehabilitation program that Amanda had been participating in with the inclusion of the research measurements. The baseline was extended for 6 weeks because her performance on all measures was extremely variable depending on many factors, including the weather, her menstrual cycle, her mood, and the anniversary of her accident.

The intervention phase also lasted 6 weeks and was composed of the normal rehabilitation program plus a specific protocol involving sensory stimulation to the hands and forearms for a total of 20 minutes. The sensory stimulation program used all modalities and consisted of deep-pressure massage, soft touch, sharp touch, and proprioceptive input from the therapist plus self-stimulation of the hands and forearms by Amanda herself.

Only a short postintervention stage was possible because Amanda discontinued her inpatient attendance at the rehabilitation center.

ABA Single-Case Design:

Baseline phase (A): Verbal and visual mediation strategies with task breakdown and specific hand exercises; measurements taken before and after each therapy session

Intervention phase (B): The baseline program **plus** sensory stimulation protocol (i.e., tactile and proprioceptive input); measurements taken before and after each therapy session.

Postintervention phase (A): A return to the baseline protocol (i.e., without sensory input); measurements taken before and after each therapy session.

Results indicated significant differences between the baseline (normal therapy), intervention (additional sensory input), and postintervention phases on a range of quantitative movement measures. For example, differences between these three phases were found in Amanda's performance of a timed task (nine-hole peg test) with her right, dominant hand, $F(2,16) = 6.03$ ($p<0.01$) with the post-hoc analysis using Bonferroni and Student-Newman-Keuls procedures showing significant differences at $p<0.05$ between baseline and intervention phases. This provided evidence that the addition of sensory input during the intervention phase improved motor performance on this particular task, and such improvement was maintained in the postintervention phase.

Differences were also shown in Amanda's ability to selectively control specified hand movements. Opposition in the right hand improved significantly in the intervention phase, $F(2,35) = 32.216$ ($p<0.001$), and in the left hand, $F(2,35) = 9.402$ ($p<0.001$). The post-hoc analysis using Bonferroni and Student-Newman-Keuls procedures indicated significant differences at $p<0.05$ between the baseline phase and the intervention and postintervention phases. This again provides evidence that the strategies used in the intervention phase had a significant effect on motor performance in this case.

Where data points were minimal in the postintervention phase, only the baseline and intervention phases could be compared. T tests indicated significant differences in such measures as wrist extension and radial deviation. Variability of motor performance was a feature of this case study, and linear regression analysis was shown to be inappropriate, accounting for very little of the variance of the data in each phase of the experiment. Serial dependency of the data was analyzed using autocorrelation statistics and was demonstrated not to be present. The data could, therefore, be treated as independent data points and conventional t and F tests used for analysis (Barlow & Hersen, 1984).

General conclusions from this single-case research are that the addition of a sensory stimulation protocol to the verbal and visual mediation rehabilitation program enhanced motor performance in a variety of tasks. This enhanced performance was maintained as a long-term effect even when the sensory input was withdrawn in the postintervention phase (Butler, 1996a, 1996b).

SUMMARY

This chapter has presented the reasoning behind assessing and treating a client with apraxia. It opened with a review of apraxia and the latest research in this field. The case study client, Amanda, was then introduced. The chapter traced Amanda's progress over her 12-month inpatient and 12-month outpatient rehabilitation programs. Finally, some research supporting the intervention techniques used with Amanda were presented.

≡ REVIEW QUESTIONS

1. Devise a breakdown of movement sequences similar to the one given for drinking. How would you enable Amanda to:

- Eat using a large handled spoon and an adapted plate with a lip?
- Manage to pull down her pants for using the bathroom?
- Take off her dressing gown before a shower?
- Put on face cream?

2. Consider the following four scenarios. In each of these different scenarios, think about:

- How might the therapeutic intervention be changed?
- How might the priorities change?
- What impact would there be on the effects on lifestyle and performance (roles and activities)?

A. What if Amanda were more cognitively impaired and unable to remember activity sequences so readily?
B. What if Amanda was more distractible and more behaviorally impaired and perhaps had some challenging behavior?

C. What if Amanda had a hemiplegia and was not so competent in her walking abilities?

D. What if Amanda was married and had small children?

≡ ACKNOWLEDGMENTS

I would like to thank Jenny Carter, Rosie Laking, Nicky Proffitt, and Lindsey Smith, therapists at the Rehabilitation Centre, Oxford, England, and Dr. Derick Wade for help in compiling this chapter. I am also very grateful to Amanda for sharing her insights into the therapeutic process.

8

Evaluation and Intervention with Simple Perceptual Impairment (Agnosias)

ALISON LAVER, PhD, OT (L), Dip COT, SROT, and
CAROLYN UNSWORTH, PhD, OTR

- Achromatopsia
- Agnosia
- Alexia
- Anosognosia
- Astereognosis
- Auditory Agnosia
- Color Agnosia

- Form Discrimination
- Perception
- Prosopagnosia
- Simultanagnosia
- Somatoagnosia
- Tactile Agnosia
- Visual Object Agnosia

On completion of this chapter, the reader will be able to:

- Define what disorders of simple perception are and provide examples of several kinds of agnosias
- Describe the anatomical basis for simple perceptual problems (agnosias)
- List at least three assessments that an occupational therapist may use to screen for the presence of simple perceptual problems
- Understand the procedural, interactive, and conditional reasoning behind assessment of and intervention planning for clients with simple perceptual problems
- Be more familiar with the Structured Observational Test of Function
- Successfully work through the Review Questions

≡ INTRODUCTION

The purpose of this chapter is to present the reasoning behind the assessment of and intervention with a client who is experiencing simple perceptual problems after a stroke. An individual with intact simple perceptual capacities is able to name objects and have an understanding of them through the senses (i.e., sight, sound, taste, smell, touch, and movement), able to recognize people by face, identify colors, and understand written material. Damage to the brain can cause disruption in any or all of these capacities. This chapter opens with a brief review of the features of this disorder and a neuroanatomical basis for the problems experienced. The case study of Sam follows. The therapist's reasoning behind the overall intervention program for Sam is presented and details for a treatment session are provided.

WHAT ARE DISORDERS OF SIMPLE PERCEPTION (AGNOSIAS)?

Definitions

Perception was defined in Chapter 1 as being the dynamic process of receiving the environment through sensory impulses (e.g., visual, auditory, tactile) and translating those impulses into meaning based on previous environmental experience or learning (Grieve, 1993; Árnadóttir, 1990). More specifically, disorders of perception are often classified as either simple or complex. Whereas Chapter 9 deals with complex disorders of perception such as spatial relations syndrome, the purpose of this chapter is to examine the reasoning behind the assessment of and intervention approaches used to overcome simple perceptual problems, or agnosias. Clients with **agnosia** generally have an inability to recognize or make sense of incoming information despite intact sensory capacities (Bauer & Rubens, 1993). Although this condition is relatively rare, it can affect any modality (e.g., vision, audition, touch, taste) and any thing (e.g., faces, sounds, colors, familiar or less familiar objects). When agnosia only affects one modality, it may not be detected in a functional setting because other senses may compensate. Agnosias are often classified according to the sensory modality that is affected. The main types of agnosias are **alexia, auditory agnosia, color agnosia** and **achromatopsia, prosopagnosia, simultanagnosia, tactile agnosia** (also called **astereognosis**), and **visual object agnosia**. Each of these problems is defined in Table 8–1. Although **anosognosia** and **somatoagnosia** can be included as problems of recognition (the former being lack of recognition or denial of paresis and the latter being difficulty recognizing body parts or their relation to each other), these problem are also associated with disturbances in body scheme and are therefore discussed in Chapters 9 (under body scheme disorders) and 10.

Anatomical Basis and Mechanisms of Simple Perceptual Problems

According to Luria (1966), three units are responsible for all brain functioning (these were briefly described in Chapter 1). The second unit of this system allows the processing of sensory information and is composed of three areas. The primary projection areas are responsible for elementary-level processing. They process basic sensory information and are responsible for senses such as sight and hearing. Lesions in the primary areas of the sensory unit lead to sensory disorders. The secondary areas are known as the

Table 8–1. Types of simple perceptual problems

TYPE	DESCRIPTION AND POSSIBLE LESION SITES
Alexia	This may be defined as an acquired inability to comprehend written language (Friedman, Ween, & Albert, 1993) and is commonly known as *word blindness*. There may also be an impairment in the ability to read. Alexia may be accompanied by agraphia (i.e., the inability to write), acalculia (i.e., the inability to calculate numbers), and color anomia (i.e., the inability to name colors) (Friedman, Ween, & Albert, 1993). Usually clients with this disorder have no difficulty with oral (spoken) language. Alexia usually follows a lesion in the dominant angular gyrus. For a detailed discussion on this disorder, the reader is referred to Friedman, Ween, & Albert (1993).
Anosognosia and somatoagnosia	Anosognosia is a lack of awareness, or denial, of a paretic extremity as belonging to the person, or a lack of insight concerning, or denial of, paralysis. This problem has most often been associated with frontal lobe damage. Somatoagnosia is a failure to recognize one's own body parts and their relationship to each other and is often seen after damage in the dominant parietal lobe. Somatoagnosia is also referred to as *autopagnosia* or simply *body agnosia* (Walsh, 1994). Although somatoagnosia and anosognosia may be classified as simple perceptual problems, many clinicians classify and deal with these problems as disorders of body scheme (i.e., unilateral neglect). Unilateral neglect can follow damage to the inferior-posterior regions of the right parietal lobe (Vallar, 1993) and subcortical structures such as the thalamus, basal ganglia, and internal capsule. Both anosognosia and somatoagnosia are also discussed in Chapters 9 and 10.
Auditory agnosia	Auditory agnosia is the inability to distinguish between sounds or to recognize familiar sounds. When using the telephone, a client with this problem may not be able to recognize the voice of the speaker until he identifies himself. Clients may not recognize sirens or horns when driving and may not realize that the radio has been left on. Amusia is the inability to recognize melodies. Auditory agnosias may follow lesions in the temporal lobe (Árnadóttir, 1990).

(continues)

(continued)

Table 8–1. Types of simple perceptual problems	
TYPE	**DESCRIPTION AND POSSIBLE LESION SITES**
Color perception disturbances	Impaired color perception presents in two forms: color agnosia and achromatopsia. Achromatopsia is difficulty with recognizing or matching colors or sorting different shades of the same color. All colors appear less bright. Meadows (1974) reported that after cerebral lesions, some loss of color discrimination is common, particularly toward the blue end of the spectrum. In severe cases of achromatopsia, the world may be viewed in shades of grey and white. However, this is unusual and generally follows bilateral inferior occipitotemporal lesions (Bauer & Rubens, 1993). Achromatopsia is generally thought to result from a lesion in the inferomesial occipitotemporal cortex (Bradshaw & Mattingley, 1995). On the other hand, color agnosia is the inability to associate objects with particular colors. For example, a client may declare that the ducks in a picture are pink. The client is unable to name a color shown or point to a color named by the examiner. However, correct color associations, such as matching color chips, can be made. This indicates that color vision is still intact. Color agnosia is thought to result from a lesion in the angular gyrus (Bradshaw & Mattingley, 1995). Difficulties with color perception can cause clients problems when shopping (e.g., recognizing foods quickly and in money handling in countries where notes and coins are different colors), dressing and grooming (e.g., selecting clothes and make-up), and in a variety of jobs that require color discrimination.
Prosopagnosia	Prosopagnosia is the inability to recognize familiar faces despite intact sensory abilities (Bauer & Rubens, 1993). Clients with this condition know that faces are different but cannot tell who the person is. Rather, people are recognized through their voices, smell, mannerisms, or sometimes their facial expressions. This problem is thought to be caused by lesions in the occipito-temporal junction, right occipital lobe (Árnadóttir, 1990; Grieve, 1993; Parker, 1990), or anterior portion of the infero-temporal cortex (Bradshaw & Mattingley, 1995), and is often seen in conjunction with visual object agnosia.

(continues)

(continued)

Table 8–1. Types of simple perceptual problems

TYPE	DESCRIPTION AND POSSIBLE LESION SITES
Simultanagnosia	Simultanagnosia is difficulty in recognizing the elements of a visual array (Ellis & Young, 1988). This term was coined by Wolpert in 1924, and the problem is generally regarded as a component of visual agnosia (Benton, 1993). Although the elements of such an array may be correctly perceived, clients with this form of agnosia have difficulty in recognizing the meaning of the total picture. The kinds of brain damage that produce this disorder are not yet well understood. Whereas some researchers suggest that this problem may be produced by left-sided or bilateral problems in the occipital lobe, others suggest that it is produced by lesions in diverse areas (Fogel, 1967; Kinsbourne & Warrington, 1962).
Tactile agnosia or astereognosis	Tactile agnosia, which is also called *astereognosis*, is the inability to recognize objects by touch alone (with vision occluded) despite intact sensory abilities. This problem may be seen after patients acquire lesions in either hemisphere involving the somatosensory areas posterior to the postcentral gyrus. Tactile agnosia involves impaired perception of shape, texture, temperature, weight, density, and therefore identity (Bradshaw & Mattingley, 1995). Generally, clients can compensate for this problem by watching what they are doing. However, in cases in which vision may be occluded (e.g., searching for an object in a pocket or handbag), clients may have considerable difficulty. It is important to distinguish between tactile anomia (i.e., inability to name an object by touch despite recognizing what the object is) and tactile agnosia (i.e., inability to recognize an object by touch).
Visual object agnosia	Visual object agnosia is the inability to recognize objects by looking at them despite intact vision. People who experience visual object agnosia are usually able to compensate by using information from other senses, such as touch, audition, and smell to recognize the object. However, this problem produces difficulties in carrying out all daily living activities; choosing objects for cooking, selecting clothing for dressing, shopping, and home

(continues)

(continued)

Table 8–1. Types of simple perceptual problems	
TYPE	DESCRIPTION AND POSSIBLE LESION SITES
	maintenance are just a few areas in which difficulties may arise. Lesion sites associated with this problem include the right parietal lobe and the anterior portion of the inferotemporal cortex (Bradshaw & Mattingley, 1995). Cases of pure visual object agnosia are rare and are usually seen in conjunction with other forms of agnosias.

projection-association cortex; in these areas, incoming sensory information is interpreted so that meaning is attached to the information. For example, noises or sounds may be perceived as a dog barking or a woman singing, and the object in our hand that we are drinking from is recognized as a glass. Lesions in the secondary area of the sensory unit tend to produce agnosias. Finally, the tertiary areas in the sensory unit enable interpretation of information from all sources to produce appropriate interactions with the environment. Lesions in these areas produce complex perceptual dysfunctions such as spatial relations disorders. These problems are discussed in Chapter 10.

Most agnosia-related research to date has focused on identifying the brain regions where lesions have produced agnosias. In addition to providing definitions for the main types of simple perceptual problems, Table 8–1 also provides a summary of possible lesion sites for these impairments. It is only quite recently that attention has shifted from identification of brain regions where lesions produce agnosias to determination of the processes that underlie simple perception and possible modes of disruption (Bradshaw & Mattingley, 1995). The focus of this work has been in the area of visual object recognition. Current attempts to understand visual object recognition draw on an information-processing approach. Bradshaw and Mattingley (1995) describe the adoption of this as being particularly useful given that recognition is a multistage process. Object recognition involves components such as:

● Coding of lines, depth, color, angles of an object, and light intensity
● Integrating relationships between objects, overall form, and possible movement

- Drawing on past memories and associations
- Output including how the object is used, described, or identified (Bradshaw & Mattingley, 1995)

Most researchers in this area view these components as occurring in parallel or cascading (i.e., updating each other continually) to produce recognition of an object. Despite this ongoing research to determine how objects are recognized and how brain damage may disrupt it, the taxonomies and classification systems used today to describe agnosias are clearly derived from those mapped out more than 100 years ago (Bradshaw & Mattingley, 1995). There is still a great deal of research required to assist us to understand all the forms of agnosia and the disrupted mechanisms that produce these complex disorders.

CASE STUDY: SAM

BACKGROUND

INTRODUCTION TO THE OCCUPATIONAL THERAPIST, EVA

Eva has been working as an occupational therapist for 11 years. She has worked in a variety of treatment settings, including inpatient and day hospital rehabilitation for older adults and adults with mental illness and in a long-term residential setting for adults with learning and physical disabilities. Eva currently works in the outpatient clinic of an occupational therapy department at a local hospital, treating clients with a variety of neurological problems. Eva has worked extensively with the Structured Observational Test of Function (SOTOF) (Laver & Powell, 1995) to assess her clients and has conducted research on this assessment. Eva often uses the Model of Human Occupation (MOHO) (Kielhofner, 1995a) frame of reference and draws on the work of Toglia (1989b) to provide a framework for intervention with clients who have cognitive and perceptual deficits.

Box 8–1 provides some of Eva's reflections on her choice of orientation to therapy using a mixture of "top-down" and "bottom-up" approaches to therapy, including some of the models that guide her practice.

BOX 8–1. THERAPIST REASONING—SELECTION OF THERAPEUTIC APPROACHES

In terms of my overall approach to working with clients who have cognitive and perceptual problems, I don't take a rigid "top-down" or "bottom-up" approach because I think you have to be more flexible than that. Certainly I start with more of a "top-down" approach and try to understand who the client is, beginning with a sense of his or her life story, roles, values, and interests; then I move to activities linked to those roles, interests, and values. I observe the client's performance of tasks nested within these activities to evaluate underlying performance component deficits. I then use that understanding to hypothesize the impact of the performance component deficits on other tasks, activities, and roles. For the intervention phase I move up and down the spectrum of compensatory ("top-down") and remedial ("bottom-up") approaches and believe in trying to capture different levels of function simultaneously. Therefore, I like to use assessments that simultaneously explore aspects of the disability level (i.e., activities of daily living), aspects of the functional limitation level (i.e., the specific tasks observed and the skill components of those tasks), the impairment level (i.e., the broad performance component areas), and the pathophysiology level (i.e., the specific neurological deficits), for example the SOTOF or A-ONE (both described later). Although these assessments don't explore the societal limitation level that addresses roles and the physical and social environment, they are very different from traditional "bottom-up" assessments, which test performance component functioning out of the context of the performance of every day tasks.

In terms of therapy models, I find the Model of Human Occupation (MOHO) (Kielhofner, 1995a) useful in guiding my overall approach with a client. Specifically, in the area of assessment, I like to adopt a client-centered approach (CAOT, 1991) and use an assessment such as the Canadian Occupational Performance Measure (COPM) (Law et al., 1994). For intervention, I find Toglia's work (1989b) on a multicontext approach particularly useful when working with clients who have simple perceptual problems. I also like to spend time educating the client about my role as his or her occupational therapist. I also like to build good rapport and form an image of the client as a person in order to understand his or her lifestyle and goals (using interactive reasoning) before selecting performance component measures.

INTRODUCTION TO THE REHABILITATION SETTING

The hospital where Eva works has a large supportive occupational therapy department. This department shares assessment and treatment environments with a multidisciplinary team including physiotherapists, speech language therapists, and social workers. The hospital has an EASY

STREET ENVIRONMENTS (Habitat Inc., 6031 S. Maple Ave., Tempe, AZ 85283; phone [800] 733-8442) and a separate activities of daily living (ADL) apartment. The ADL apartment includes a living room, kitchen, bathroom, and bedroom. The EASY STREET ENVIRONMENTS at the hospital includes transportation, which includes a car for practicing car transfers and educating caregivers about transfers and lifting equipment, such as wheelchairs in and out of the car; and part of a bus that moves on springs to provide realistic movement and can be used to assess and train clients in skills such as mobility, climbing up a large step, balance, communicating with the driver, assertiveness, and money management; a bank and automated teller machine (ATM); a cinema; a grocery shop; a clothes shop; a coffee shop; a kitchen area; sidewalks and steps; different entrances and doors; and a treatment area.

The EASY STREET ENVIRONMENTS has been constructed to replicate streetscapes from the local community in which the hospital is based. It has been built to incorporate relevant city codes (e.g., gradients at the curb on sidewalks are the same as those that clients encounter in the community). Effort has been made to provide a functional, realistic treatment environment and to create a rehabilitation environment that exposes clients to a variety of realistic daily living situations in order to assess their ability to function in the community. The EASY STREET ENVIRONMENTS also provides a normalizing environment for clients involved in long-term care. A simple example is that each of the doors within EASY STREET ENVIRONMENTS has a different type of door handle, locking mechanism, and key to provide a variety of opening mechanisms (e.g., pull and push, double and single doors). The EASY STREET ENVIRONMENTS is a maximum-barrier environment; therefore, clients are assessed and treated in a setting in which they can prepare for realistic task demands. For example, the floor tiling in the grocery store part of EASY STREET ENVIRONMENTS has been patterned in a way that might be confusing for a client with perceptual impairments such as figure/ground discrimination or spatial relations problems. Another example is that there is a step down from a raised sidewalk that is hard to perceive because the area of stone is the same color as the sidewalk. This area can be useful for assessing figure/ground discrimination as well as clients' attention to safety hazards.

INTRODUCTION TO SAM

Sam is a 29-year-old man who had been experiencing severe headaches for several months, which he attributed to stress. He had experienced some blurred vision and slight right-side weakness but had not mentioned it to his family or doctor. One evening he collapsed at home and was admitted to his local hospital. A computed tomography scan revealed several bleeds with lesions in diverse areas of the brain, predominantly in the left hemisphere and including lesions in the motor cortex and the visual association cortex; several parietal lobe lesions, including small bleeds in the superior and inferior parietal association cortex; and a lesion around the occipital-temporal junction. A diagnosis of stroke was made, and assessment revealed that Sam experienced weakness on his right side, receptive and expressive language problems, simple perceptual problems, and visual perceptual problems (i.e., spatial relations syndrome). Sam remained in the hospital for 3 months and was discharged home after making a good motor recovery and gaining independence with most of his self-care tasks, indoor mobility, and basic transfers. After discharge, he was referred for outpatient rehabilitation twice a week to focus on instrumental activities of daily living (IADLs) and work rehabilitation. This case study presents Sam during his outpatient rehabilitation.

DATA GATHERING

REFERRAL

Eva received the referral from the neurology consultant at the hospital and was asked to conduct an initial assessment. Box 8–2 provides some of Eva's reflections after receiving the referral information.

INITIAL OUTPATIENT APPOINTMENT

Two weeks after inpatient hospital discharge, Sam attended his first outpatient occupational therapy appointment. He was accompanied to this appointment by his 27-year-old girlfriend, Lisa, who drove him to the appointment. Sam has been unable to drive since his stroke. The therapist asked Sam if he would like Lisa to stay for his first interview. Sam stated that he wanted her to stay because he said that sometimes he had difficulty explaining things. Box 8–3 provides a description of Eva's first session with the couple.

REPORT OF INITIAL FINDINGS

Evaluation of Upper Limbs

The brief evaluation of Sam's upper limb function revealed normal control of his left arm. Sam's right arm demonstrated full passive and active

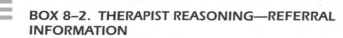

BOX 8–2. THERAPIST REASONING—REFERRAL INFORMATION

When I read the referral, including the client's diagnosis and age, I was struck by how young this man was, a very similar age to myself and much younger than my usual case load of clients with stroke who range from about 55 to 80 years old. I noted that the similarity of our ages might impact the client–therapist relationship in a way that was qualitatively different from working with older adults and that I should be aware of this. I also thought that he would probably have different issues and goals compared with those of my older clients because he was at a different life stage; many of my older clients are retired, and their occupational performance goals are mainly oriented to self-care, IADLs, and leisure tasks. I hypothesized that Sam would be concerned with productivity and return to work.

I chose to conduct an initial interview with Sam to:

- Informally assess Sam's orientation, language, and insight through observation of his responses to questioning
- Build rapport and explain the occupational therapy process
- Get background information about his previous pre-stroke ability, lifestyle, and environment, including his roles, interests, and values.

I find the Model of Human Occupation (MOHO) (Kielhofner, 1995a) a useful approach for framing my initial interactions with clients; sometimes I use the Role-Checklist (Oakley, Kielhofner, & Barris, 1986) and the Interest Checklist (Kielhofner & Neville, 1983), but this can be time consuming. Therefore with Sam I decided not to administer any formal measures but to use MOHO to frame a semistructured interview.

If my client has good expressive language, I generally use the Canadian Occupational Performance Measure (COPM) (Law et al., 1994) early on in the assessment process, either in the first interview (if the client had sufficient stamina) or during the second meeting. I like the COPM because it:

- Encourages the client's voice
- Covers the occupational performance domains of self-care, productivity, and leisure
- Involves the rating of the importance of an occupational performance area to the client and his or her satisfaction with performance as well as his or her actual ability to perform in an area

BOX 8–3. THERAPIST REASONING—INITIAL SESSION

SETTING THE SCENE

I suggested we conduct the interview at a round table in the EASY STREET ENVIRONMENTS coffee shop–simulated area because it was a quiet and informal area conducive to conversation. I noticed that Sam walked slowly and dragged his right foot a little. He negotiated the step carefully, and Lisa hovered behind him anxiously as if she thought he might fall. They both looked very tired; in particular, Lisa had dark circles under her eyes and looked pale. As they sat and talked, I observed that they sat close to each other and held hands under the table. Sam told me that he had an occupational therapist before and had a good idea of my role. I asked Sam and Lisa to tell me about their lifestyle before Sam's stroke and then describe how they had been coping since Sam had been discharged home from the hospital 2 weeks earlier.

Sam spoke slowly and hesitated over some words. At times he seemed frustrated and sighed but was motivated to continue. Sam told me that before his stroke he had been working for 9 months as an animator for a firm in the nearby city. He said this work was hard to find and he and Lisa had been delighted when he got the job. He had loved this work, but it was very intense. That's why he thought his headaches were stress-related, due to the long hours, tight deadlines, and his desire to do well at his new job. It was clear that Sam's career had been really important to him. Sam explained that he had premorbid dyslexia and had found reading and writing tough at school but that he had always been good at art. He had undertaken undergraduate and graduate studies in fine arts, design, and animation. He had been a teaching assistant at the university while in graduate study and had been doing some sessional teaching at the university. He had also been teaching an evening class at the local art school for the past 2 years.

DESCRIPTION OF SAM AND LISA'S LIFE TOGETHER

I asked Sam and Lisa to tell me a little about their life together. Sam reported that he and Lisa had known each other for 3 years. Lisa said she was currently a secretary and they had met at the university. Lisa described that she was also an artist but that she couldn't live off her art work and had taken a secretarial course and then found a job in this field to pay the bills. Before Sam's stroke, they had been planning to get married and buy a house the next year and had talked about wanting children. They had planned to announce their engagement at a family party on the holiday weekend 2 weeks after the date that Sam had had his stroke. His hospitalization had not made this possible. At this point Lisa interrupted and said she would have gotten engaged anyway but that Sam wouldn't hear of it. I sensed some strain as

(continues)

BOX 8–3. THERAPIST REASONING—INITIAL SESSION (CONT.)

they talked about this; Lisa looked tense and close to tears. I hypothesized that there were some important issues in their relationship that they might need support to resolve, and I thought they might benefit from some counseling and would need a referral to a social worker. I acknowledged their feelings and mentioned that there was a social worker on our team who could talk to them about their relationship if they would find it helpful. They said they would think about it. I refocused the conversation and asked them to continue describing their lifestyle and tell me about leisure interests. They had both been very active and had gone on a few cycling and camping holidays together and used to go rollerblading along the promenade by the lake several evenings a week during the summer. They loved going to the cinema and renting videos. I asked them to talk about their current lifestyle and living arrangements. They described living in a ground floor rented apartment that Lisa had gotten for them after Sam's stroke. After the stroke, Lisa had also taken responsibility for most of the decision making, finances, and household tasks. I suggested that, in order to discuss their current goals and problems and to focus on areas for us work on together during Sam's outpatient visits, we work through the COPM.

ADMINISTRATION OF THE COPM

The next 30 minutes was spent on the COPM interview. Sam answered the questions but initially had trouble grasping the 10-point scoring scales for importance, performance, and satisfaction. I had to explain the scoring system several times. When he was rating performance, Lisa's body language suggested that she disagreed with some of his ratings, so I thought I would give Lisa a caregiver performance checklist in the next session to elicit her viewpoints. I chose to end with a brief physical assessment; however, after examining his upper limbs Sam appeared to be getting tired so I suggested that we stop. We agreed to conduct some ADL tasks and assess Sam's current cognitive-perceptual functioning at the next session.

range of motion; however, he had decreased strength and increased tone in his shoulder, wrist, and fingers. Sam reported that he found it hard to pick up small things with his right hand and he was "really clumsy and kept dropping stuff." Sensation for light touch and deep pressure was intact bilaterally.

Summary of Canadian Occupational Performance Measure Results

Sam identified 15 problem areas, each on a 10-point scale (where 10 represents very important and 1 represents not at all important) on the Canadian Occupational Performance Measure (COPM) (Law et al., 1994). Sam rated 7 of 15 problems as very important, and from these he chose his five most important areas for his initial therapy goals. Sam then rated each of these five areas in terms of his current performance and his level of satisfaction with his performance. His ratings were as follows:

- Self-care (personal ADLs [PADLs]): Sam wanted to focus on fine motor tasks such as buttoning shirts and learning not to spill food and liquids when eating and preparing snacks (performance, 8/10; satisfaction, 6/10).
- Simple meal preparation: Sam wanted to make his own snacks and lunch while Lisa was at work; his long-term goal was to make supper for them both (performance, 4/10; satisfaction, 5/10).
- Work: Sam desperately wanted to get back to drawing and animation; his job was going to be held for him for 1 year, and he had 7 months left to get back to this job (performance, 2/10; satisfaction, 1/10).
- Reading: Sam reported that reading had always been hard because he had dyslexia but that it had gotten worse since his stroke (performance, 3/10; satisfaction, 1/10).
- Computer use: Before his stroke, Sam had used a computer at home and work for some of his animation tasks (performance, 5/10; satisfaction, 5/10).

His overall performance score was 4.4 and his satisfaction score was 3.6. (The COPM score forms are not presented here but are presented in full in Chapter 7.)

Formulation of Possible Problem Areas to Assess

Eva decided that several areas required further assessment. In addition to these assessments, Eva decided to refer Sam to the team's speech-language

BOX 8–4. THERAPIST REASONING—REFERRAL TO OTHER PROFESSIONALS

I think it's important to get an idea of Sam's current receptive and expressive language, especially his reading. Language problems were noted in Sam's history, and I think they may continue to be a problem in relation to his work. Given that Sam experienced dyslexia before his stroke, I think it is a priority to assess him in this area. In addition, I think it would be useful for Sam and Lisa to talk to the social worker about recent events. Sam's stroke has produced many significant changes in their lives, and they may need additional support to manage at this time.

pathologist for assessment and the social worker for counseling. Eva's assessments and rationales are presented in Box 8–4.

SELECTION OF STANDARDIZED AND NONSTANDARDIZED ASSESSMENTS

The focus for assessment in this chapter is agnosias. A range of standardized functional and tabletop evaluations are available to screen for agnosias (Table 8–2). In this chapter, the therapist chose to use the functionally based SOTOF (Laver & Powell, 1995) as the main assessment; however, the A-ONE (Occupational Therapy Activities of Daily Living Neurobehavioral Evaluation) (Árnadóttir, 1990) could also have been used. Table 8–3 describes the five main areas Eva wanted to assess further after her initial data gathering, together with the rationale for each. Listed below are some of the evaluations Eva could use to assess these areas and the reasoning behind her assessment selection.

However, before assessing a client when disorders of simple perception are suspected, it is important to establish that the client has a reliable form of verbal or gestural response. It is also important to determine the integrity of the client's somatosensory abilities, particularly of the visual, tactile, and auditory systems. For example, an individual may appear to be having difficulty recognizing or finding objects such as toothpaste and a toothbrush while grooming, but the primary problem may be a homonymous hemianopia or diminished visual acuity rather than a visual object agnosia. In addition to sensory capabilities, deficits in other cognitive areas may result in what appears to be a perceptual problem, for example, a deficit in selective attention, a severe memory problem, or language processing difficulties.

Table 8–2. Evaluations used to detect agnosias

TYPE OF AGNOSIA	EVALUATION OR ASSESSMENT	ITEM AND NAME
Astereognosis	COTNAB (Tyerman et al., 1986)	Section 3, Test I
Color agnosia	RPAB (Whiting et al., 1985)	Item 3, color matching
	Ishihara Color Plates (Kanehura & Co., 1977)	Entire assessment
Prosopagnosia	Test of Facial Recognision (Benton & Allen, 1968)	Entire assessment
Tactile agnosia	Southern California Sensory Integration Test (Ayres, 1972)	Subtest: Ayres' Manual Form Perception
Visual object agnosia	LOTCA (Itzkovich et al., 1990)	Visual identification of objects
	RPAB (Whiting et al., 1985)	Item 6, animal halves

COTNAB = Chessington Occupational Therapy Neurological Assessment Battery; LOTCA = Lowenstein Occupational Therapy Cognitive Assessment; RPAB = Rivermead Perceptual Assessment Battery.

Performance of Personal Activities of Daily Living

Eva decided to use a combination of standardized and nonstandardized observational assessments to evaluate Sam's occupational performance and performance component functioning. Eva chose to use the SOTOF (Laver & Powell, 1995; Laver, 1996, 1994b, 1991, 1990) to assess Sam's performance component functioning within a functional context (see Chapter 3 for a full description of this assessment). Therapists often choose to use this assessment because of its functional base and because it has been found to have good ecological validity, clinical utility, and face validity (Laver & Powell, 1995). The SOTOF comprises a screening assessment and four self-care subscales. It involves the structured observation of feeding, pouring, and drinking (which Eva thought would be good to assess because Sam had said that he spilled things when eating and drinking), washing and drying hands, and putting on an upper limb garment (which Eva wanted to assess because Sam had reported difficulty with fine motor bilateral tasks such as buttoning). Using the SOTOF, the therapist works through a structured diagnostic reasoning process to identify the motor, sensory, cognitive, and perceptual deficits that are impacting self-care performance. In this way, the therapist can understand

---

Table 8–3. Areas to assess further and reasoning

AREA TO ASSESS	REASONING
Performance of PADLs	Determine Sam's current ability to care for himself and determine any further interventions required to assist in this area
Performance of IADLs	Determine Sam's current ability to manage in the community and determine any further interventions required to assist in this area
Assessment of underlying neuropsychological functioning that may be impacting performance	I like to use both "top-down" and "bottom-up" approaches when working with clients. Therefore it's useful to have knowledge of their underlying impairments and the ways they impact performance.
Computer use	In his work as an animator, Sam spends considerable time working on a computer. I want to get an idea of what his skills are like now so that I know if we need to do specific computer retraining. I also want to be able to use the computer in general to work on Sam's cognitive and perceptual problems.
Survey Lisa about her perception of Sam's functioning and possible physical and emotional caregiver burden	I'm worried about Lisa. She looks tired and anxious and has assumed most responsibilities for the couple. I would like to get an idea about how much burden she thinks she is experiencing. I can then follow this up by organizing extra supports or referring Lisa for professional support.

---

the direct influence of performance component deficits on occupational performance functioning.

Given the location of Sam's stroke, one of the areas in which he may be having difficulty is object recognition. The effect of environmental context on the ability to recognize objects has been discussed by Toglia (1989b) and Palmer (1975), who both found that recognition of objects was significantly better when the objects tested were appropriate to their normal contextual scenes. Grieve (1993), therefore, stresses the importance of "functional assessment of patients being carried out in a familiar environment with objects previously known to them" (p. 30). The SOTOF (Laver and Powell, 1995) provides such a functional assessment and helps the therapist to specify the task conditions and demands, environmental context, prompts, and cues that influence the client's visual perception.

Performance of Instrumental Activities of Daily Living

Therapists often use an assessment such as the SOTOF (Laver and Powell, 1995) or the A-ONE (Árnadóttir, 1990) (presented in detail in Chapter 10) to gain a comprehensive profile of a client's self-care performance and neuropsychological deficits. Many therapists then use observation to determine IADL performance (including financial and transport management and shopping). The EASY STREET ENVIRONMENTS provides an ideal setting to gain more information about a client's IADL abilities. However, several assessments are available to assist the therapist in examining particular components of IADLs. For example, when undertaking an assessment of a client's ability to prepare a meal, three standardized assessments are usually considered. These are the Assessment of Motor Process Skills (AMPS) (Fisher, 1997a), the Kitchen Task Assessment (KTA) (Baum & Edwards, 1993), and the Rabideau Kitchen Assessment (Neistadt, 1994b). When assessing financial management, therapists have the choice of observation during simulated tasks or the financial management subtest from the Cognitive Competency test (Wang & Ennis, 1986). Eva chose to use observations in the EASY STREET ENVIRONMENTS with Sam to gain an understanding of his IADL abilities and not undertake any of the other assessments mentioned given. This decision was based on economy of time and a desire to limit the number of standardized instruments used in Sam's assessment process.

Assessment of Underlying Neuropsychological Functioning

As mentioned previously, if a therapist is working from a bottom-up perspective, then there are a selection of standardized cognitive and perceptual assessments, such as the Chessington Neurological Assessment Battery (COTNAB) (Tyerman et al., 1986) or the Rivermead Perceptual Assessment Battery (RPAB) (Whiting et al., 1985) that a therapist can use to identify a client's underlying impairments. Items from these assessments that can be used to identify particular types of agnosias were presented in Table 8–2. Eva chose not to use any of these assessments with Sam because she felt she would gain enough information about his problems from the other standardized and informal methods of assessment.

Computer Use

Computer use had been an important part of Sam's employment. To gain an understanding of Sam's current ability to manage using the computer, Eva set up a simple game to observe Sam's computer skills both in terms of general computer skills and his ability to transfer past knowledge of computers to the computer available in the occupational therapy department. Eva thought this would be a good way to assess Sam's computer skills in a simple way before investigating this area more fully regarding Sam's return to work.

Assessment of Caregiver's Perceptions of Client Ability and Caregiver Burden

To gain information about Sam's girlfriend's perception of his functional ability and related problems, Eva chose to give the Memory and Behaviour Problems Checklist (MBPC) (Zarit, Orr, & Zarit, 1985, revised by Zarit & Zarit, 1990) to Lisa to complete. This is a quick, comprehensive, standardized assessment, one of only a few assessments in this area. The therapist also wanted to assess whether Lisa was experiencing any caregiver burden, and she chose to use the Burden Interview (Zarit, Orr, & Zarit, 1985) for this purpose. Another assessment frequently used to determine caregiver burden is the Caregiver Strain Index (Robinson, 1983). However, the Burden Interview was chosen because it is quick to administer and easy to score.

EVALUATION RESULTS AND PRIORITIZED PROBLEM LIST

During Sam's second session, the therapist gave Lisa the two surveys (MBPC and Burden Interview) to complete on her own in the coffee shop area (see Figs. 8–1 and 8–2) while Eva and Sam completed the SOTOF (see Fig. 8–3) in the treatment area. This also gave her the opportunity to interview Sam on his own. Sam revealed that he was very concerned about being a burden on Lisa and not being able to fulfill his desired future roles of husband, worker and provider, and father.

Eva referred to Sam's COPM importance ratings to help prioritize the problem list for planning intervention. She then discussed the problem list with Sam and Lisa, and they negotiated the type of intervention activities that would be developed. Table 8–4 outlines Sam's areas of

(text continues on page 337)

Instructions to caregiver:

"I am going to read you a list of common problems that people with dementia can have. Tell me if your relative has had any of these problems. If so, how often has the problem occurred during the past week."

Read through the choices for the first problem which is reported as having occurred. For each subsequent item, ask if the problem has occurred and then how often.

Reaction ratings: For each problem that the caregiver reports as having occurred (codes 1 through 4), ask: "How much has this problem bothered or upset you when it happened?"

Frequency Ratings	Reaction Ratings
0 = never occurred	0 = not at all
1 = not in past week	1 = a little
2 = 1 to 2 times in the past week	2 = moderately
3 = 3 to 6 times in the past week	3 = very much
4 = daily or more often	4 = extremely
9 = don't know/not applicable	

Behaviors	Frequency	Reaction
1. Asks the same question over and over again	0 ① 2 3 4 9	0 ① 2 3 4
2. Mixes up past and present (eg., thinking a deceased parent is alive)	0 1 ② 3 4 9	0 ① 2 3 4
3. Loses, misplaces, or hides things	0 1 ② 3 4 9	0 ① 2 3 4
4. Wanders or gets lost	⓪ 1 2 3 4 9	⓪ 1 2 3 4
5. Does not recognize familiar people	⓪ 1 2 3 4 9	⓪ 1 2 3 4

Figure 8–1. Memory and Behavior Problems Checklist (MBPC). (Modified by the authors in 1990, from the original in Zarit, Orr, and Zarit, 1985. Reprinted with permission of the authors.)

6. Forgets what day it is	⓪ 1 2 3 4 9	⓪ 1 2 3 4
7. Unable to keep occupied or busy by self	0 ① 2 3 4 9	0 ① 2 3 4
8. Follows you around	⓪ 1 2 3 4 9	⓪ 1 2 3 4
9. Constantly restless or agitated	⓪ 1 2 3 4 9	⓪ 1 2 3 4
10. Interrupts you when you are busy	0 ① 2 3 4 9	⓪ 1 2 3 4
11. Spends long periods of time inactive	0 1 2 3 ④ 9	0 1 2 ③ 4
12. Talks constantly	⓪ 1 2 3 4 9	⓪ 1 2 3 4
13. Talks little or not at all	0 1 ② 3 4 9	⓪ 1 2 3 4
14. Is suspicious or makes accusations	⓪ 1 2 3 4 9	⓪ 1 2 3 4
15. Wakes you up at night	⓪ 1 2 3 4 9	⓪ 1 2 3 4
16. Appears sad or depressed	⓪ 1 2 3 4 9	⓪ 1 2 3 4
17. Becomes angry	⓪ 1 2 3 4 9	⓪ 1 2 3 4
18. Strikes out or tries to hit	⓪ 1 2 3 4 9	⓪ 1 2 3 4
19. Engages in behavior that is potentially dangerous to others or self	0 ① 2 3 4 9	0 1 ② 3 4
20. Sees or hears things that are not there (hallucinations or illusions)	⓪ 1 2 3 4 9	⓪ 1 2 3 4
21. Talks in an aggressive or threatening manner	⓪ 1 2 3 4 9	⓪ 1 2 3 4
22. Cries or becomes tearful	0 ① 2 3 4 9	0 ① 2 3 4
23. Problems eating: Eats excessively or not at all	⓪ 1 2 3 4 9	⓪ 1 2 3 4
24. Incontinent of bowel or bladder	⓪ 1 2 3 4 9	⓪ 1 2 3 4
25. Is uncooperative when I want him/her to do something	⓪ 1 2 3 4 9	⓪ 1 2 3 4
26. Any other problems (specify):	⓪ 1 2 3 4 9	⓪ 1 2 3 4

Figure 8–1. (continued)

Instructions:

The following is a list of statements, which reflect how people sometimes feel when taking care of another person. After each statement, indicate how often you feel that way: never, rarely, sometimes, quite frequently, or nearly always. There are no right or wrong answers.

Scoring:

0= Never   1= Rarely   2= Sometimes   3= Quite frequently   4= Nearly always

1. Do you feel that your relative asks for more help than he/she needs?	⓪	1	2	3	4
2. Do you feel that because of the time you spend with your relative that you don't have enough time for yourself?	⓪	1	2	3	4
3. Do you feel stressed between caring for your relative and trying to meet other responsibilities for your family or work?	⓪	1	2	3	4
4. Do you feel embarrassed over your relative's behavior?	0	①	2	3	4
5. Do you feel angry when you are around your relative?	0	①	2	3	4
6. Do you feel that your relative currently affects your relationship with other family members or friends in a negative way?	0	①	2	3	4
7. Are you afraid of what the future holds for your relative?	0	1	2	3	④
8. Do you feel your relative is dependent upon you?	0	1	2	3	④
9. Do you feel strained when you are around your relative?	0	①	2	3	4
10. Do you feel your health has suffered because of your involvement with your relative?	0	1	②	3	4

Figure 8–2. Zarit Caregiver Burden Survey (Zarit, Todd, and Zarit, 1986).

11. Do you feel that you don't have as much privacy as you would like, because of your relative?	0	1	2	③	4
12. Do you feel that your social life has suffered because you are caring for your relative?	0	1	2	③	4
13. Do you feel uncomfortable about having friends over, because of your relative?	0	1	②	3	4
14. Do you feel that your relative seems to expect you to take care of him/her as if you were the only one he/she could depend on?	0	1	2	③	4
15. Do you feel that you don't have enough money to care for your relative, in addition to the rest of your expenses?	0	1	2	3	④
16. Do you feel that you will be unable to take care of your relative much longer?	0	①	2	3	4
17. Do you feel you have lost control of your life since your relative's illness?	0	1	2	③	4
18. Do you wish you could just leave the care of your relative to someone else?	0	1	②	3	4
19. Do you feel uncertain about what to do about your relative?	0	①	2	3	4
20. Do you feel you should be doing more for your relative?	0	①	2	3	4
21. Do you feel you could do a better job in caring for your relative?	0	①	2	3	4
22. Overall, how burdened do you feel in caring for your relative?	0	1	2	③	4

Figure 8–2. (continued)

The Structured Observational Test of Function
Alison J. Laver with Graham E. Powell

Screening Assessment Record Form

Client's name: Sam

Tester's name: **Date:**

ITEM	ABLE (YES)	UNABLE (NO)	FURTHER PROMPTS OR ASSESSMENTS REQUIRED	HYPOTHESES, CUES AND COMMENTS
1 Name	*			
2 Vision	*		Check for expressive language, or object recognition deficits.	Hesitated before naming cup. Query word finding. Reached and touched it.
3 Sitting balance	*			
4 Upper limb	[*] Right [*] Left	[ ] Right [ ] Left		Decreased pronation on right. Increased tone in right shoulder, wrist and fingers.
5 Hand grip	[ ] Right [*] Left	[*] Right [ ] Left	Conduct full upper limb motor-assessment, ROM, strength, tone.	Problems releasing grip on right. Decreased co-ordination on right.
6 Dominant hand Right.				
7 Equipment required Client wears glasses.				

Summary: Observations/hypotheses

Time: 1'50"

Client was orientated for person.
Wears glasses to correct vision.
Was able to see and name the cup – but was hesitant.
Query an expressive language deficit – word-finding problems.
Able to perform gross upper limb movements. Some decreased pronation and increased tone on right upper limb.
Decreased strength on right. Was able to pick up cup in right hand but had difficulty releasing grasp and had
decreased fine co-ordination in right hand.

Good static sitting balance.

Signature: **Date:**

Figure 8–3. Structured Observational Test of Function (SOTOF) (Laver and Powell, 1995).

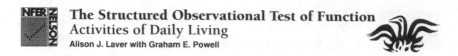

The Structured Observational Test of Function
Activities of Daily Living
Alison J. Laver with Graham E. Powell

Combined ADL and Neuropsychological Record Form

Client's name: Sam

Tester's name:	**Task 1**	**Date:**
	Task 2	**Date:** Tested in one sitting.
	Task 3	**Date:**
	Task 4	**Date:**

Diagnosis: Stroke - diffuse bleeds in several locations.

<u>Occupational performance dysfunction</u>: independent feeding from bowl; needed prompt to initiate washing; needed physical assistance with button fastening. Worker role as artist limited by right upper limb function and agnosia.

<u>Performance component deficits</u>: expressive and receptive language; motor: increased tone, decreased strength, decreased dexterity on right and decreased bilateral integration.

Spatial relations: right/left discrimination and position in space deficits.

Problems with object, colour, taste, temperature and tactile recognition. Consistent colour agnosia deficit exhibited.

Visual object and tactile recognition more variable - responds better to both visual and tactile stimuli.

Equipment: Client wears glasses.
(glasses, etc.)

Figure 8–3. (continued)

Task 1: Eating

Key: (EL) items can be administered to clients with expressive language
(ED) items provide alternative assessment methods for clients with expressive dysphasia

Tester's name:			Date:		
Dominant hand:	☒ Right ☐ Left	**Hand used for spoon:**	☒ Right ☐ Left		

	ITEM	ABLE (YES)	UNABLE (NO)	FURTHER PROMPTS OR ASSESSMENTS REQUIRED	HYPOTHESES, CUES AND COMMENTS
1	(EL) Identifies spoon through touch.	☐ Right ☐ Left	☒ Right ☒ Left	Put in right hand, when unable to identify-prompted to try with left.	Once he looked at and touched the object he was able to demonstrate use but not name.
2	Scans table for objects.		*	Needed verbal prompt to scan whole table.	Scanning deficit.
2	Fixes gaze on objects.	*			
2	Recognizes objects by (EL) naming or (ED) pointing.		*	Prompted to handle objects when he was unable to name.	Hesitant,unable to identify bowl until he touched it. Query object recognition and/or language deficit.
3	Puts spoon on table on right of bowl.		*	Prompted "is that your right?"	Right/left discrimination deficit.
4	(EL) Describes use of objects.	*		Verbal prompt x 1.	Hesitant – said "soup".
5	Mimes use of objects.		*	Verbal prompt x 2. Held hands to prevent touching objects.	Unable to grasp concept of mime, picked up objects. Decreased comprehension.
6	Demonstrates use of objects.	*			
7	Correctly identifies colours of all objects by (EL) naming or (ED) pointing.		*	Unable to point to colours on command "which is the red blue object?"	Colour agnosia. Unable to respond "what colour are the objects?"
8	Initiates eating on command.	*			
8	Reaches for spoon.	*			Dropped spoon first time. Decreased grasp.
8	Judges distance to spoon.	*			
8	Required prompt (handed spoon) to initiate eating.	☐ Yes ☒ n/a	☐ No ☐ n/a		

Figure 8–3. (continued)

Task 1: Eating

	ITEM	ABLE (YES)	UNABLE (NO)	FURTHER PROMPTS OR ASSESSMENTS REQUIRED	HYPOTHESES, CUES AND COMMENTS
9	Places spoon in bowl.	*			Holds spoon awkwardly, decreased grip, manipulation and fine co-ordination.
9	Judges distance from spoon to bowl.	*			
9	Puts food on spoon.	*		Prompted to stabilize the bowl with left hand.	Very slow, needed several attempts. Decreased bi-lateral integration.
10	Lifts spoon to mouth.	*			
11	Takes food into mouth.	*			
12	Correctly identifies or describes taste of food.		*	Asked to describe, then asked ... "is it pears, peaches, etc"	Taste discrimination deficit, and/or language deficit.
13	Chews food.	*			
13	Swallows food.	*			
14	Replaces spoon in bowl.	*			
15	Repeats sequence.	*			
16	Stops sequence when food is finished.	[*] Yes	[ ] No		
17	Neglects food in bowl.	[ ] Yes	[*] No		
18	Puts spoon on the left of the bowl.			Prompted "is that your left?"	Right/left discrimination deficit.
19	Puts spoon in front of the bowl.				Spatial problems. Position in space deficit.
20	Puts spoon behind the bowl.				Spatial problems. Position in space deficit.
21	Puts spoon in the bowl.				Spatial problems. Position in space deficit.

Summary: **Observations/Hypotheses**

Able to eat from bowl using spoon. Decreased scanning of visual field. Right/left discrimination and position in space deficits. Decreased manipulation and fine co-ordination on right. Decreased bilateral integration. Problems with tactile discrimination. Complex pattern of deficits – hypothesize receptive and expressive language deficits and/or visual object and colour agnosia. Able to demonstrate use of objects but not name them – query word finding deficits. Difficulty comprehending concept of "mime", "pantomime", "show how you would use without touching?" Query taste discrimination problems. Needed lots of verbal prompts.

Signature: **Date:**

Figure 8–3. (continued)

Task 2: **Washing**

Key: (EL) items can be administered to clients with expressive language
(ED) items provide alternative assessment methods for clients with expressive dysphasia

Tester's name:				Date:	
Dominant hand:	[*] Right [ ] Left		Hand used to pick up soap:	[ ] Right	[*] Left

	ITEM	ABLE (YES)	UNABLE (NO)	FURTHER PROMPTS OR ASSESSMENTS REQUIRED	HYPOTHESES, CUES AND COMMENTS
1	(EL) Identifies soap through touch.	[ ] Right [ ] Left	[*] Right [*] Left	Put soap on table – asked "point to the object you just felt?"	
2	Scans table for objects.	*			No problem with scanning this task.
2	Fixes gaze on objects.	*			
2	Recognizes objects by (EL) naming or (ED) pointing.		*	Asked "what can you see on the table?", then asked "point to the ...."	Unable to identify through naming or pointing. Visual object agnosia.
3	Puts soap on table on right of bowl.	*			Put on right correctly this task.
4	(EL) Describes use of objects.		*	Unable to describe until item 6 – demonstrate use – once he touched objects he was able.	Hesitant – touched objects. "Washing up dishes."
5	Mimes use of objects.		*	Verbal prompt x 2.	Doesn't seem to understand concept of mime.
6	Demonstrates use of objects.	*			
7	Correctly identifies colours of all objects by (EL) naming or (ED) pointing.		*	Tried naming and pointing commands.	Unable to name colours. Says he just doesn't know, says he had no problems prior to stroke.
8	Initiates washing on command.		*	Verbal prompt x 2. (See next item)	Query decreased comprehension – appeared frustrated.
8	Reaches for soap.		*	Repeated whole instruction.	
8	Judges distance to soap.		*		
8	Required prompt (handed soap) to initiate washing.	[*] Yes [ ] n/a	[ ] No [ ] n/a	Handed him the soap and re-peated instruction, first part "wash your hands."	Proceeded once given soap.

Item 8: could initiate "eat from the bowl" command, but not "wash your hands in the bowl using the soap and dry your hands on the towel" – unable to follow complex commands.

Figure 8–3. (continued)

Neuropsychological Checklist

DEFICIT	SCREENING ASSESSMENT	EATING TASK 1	WASHING TASK 2	POURING AND DRINKING TASK 3	DRESSING TASK 4
SPATIAL RELATIONS					
Figure-ground discrimination					
Position in space		*	*	*	*
Form constancy					
Spatial relations					
Depth perception				?	
Distance perception				?	
PERSEVERATION					

OCCUPATIONAL PERFORMANCE	INDEPENDENT	NEEDED VERBAL ASSISTANCE	NEEDED PHYSICAL ASSISTANCE	UNABLE TO PERFORM TASK	UNABLE TO TEST
Eating: Client's ability to eat independently from a bowl.	*				
Washing: Client's ability to wash and dry hands.			To initiate task. *		
Pouring and Drinking: Client's ability to pour from a jug and to drink from a cup.	Some spill. *				
Dressing: Client's ability to put on a front-fastening, long-sleeved garment.			Help with buttons. *		

Summary:

Language: understands simple commands, needs some repetition – problems with complex instructions, eg., mime. Two part wash and dry – responded to first part "wash" with physical cue of soap in hand. Problem with naming, especially on command – able to describe/name with a delay – several items later, when has tactile stimulus in addition to visual stimulus. Object recognition problems with one stimulus – improves with both visual and tactile stimuli. Colour agnosia. Problems with taste and temperature discrimination. Right/left discrimination and position in space deficits. Increased tone, decreased strength and manipulation on right, decreased bilateral integration. Initiation problems seem to relate to understanding complex 2/3 part instructions. Client became frustrated towards end of testing.

Signature: **Date:**

Figure 8–3. (continued)

Task 2: Washing

	ITEM	ABLE (YES)	UNABLE (NO)	FURTHER PROMPTS OR ASSESSMENTS REQUIRED	HYPOTHESES, CUES AND COMMENTS
9	Picks up soap.	*			Used left hand to pick-up soap.
10	Places hands in water.	*			Decreased function in right upper limb
10	Judges distance to bowl.	*			
11	Rubs soap between hands.		*		Decreased bilateral integration, dropped soap twice.
12	Correctly identifies or describes temperature of water.		*	1. What temperature is the water? 2. Is it cold, warm, hot?	Said he could feel the temperature, but could not describe it or respond to options
13	Puts down soap.	*			
14	Rinses hands in water.	*			
14	Continues soaping hands unnecessarily.	☐ Yes	☒ No		
15	Reaches for towel.	*			
16	Picks up towel.	*			
16	Dries hands.	*			
17	Uses correct sequence.	☒ Yes	☐ No		
18	Puts soap on the left of the bowl.		*	Prompted "is this your left?" Client looked confused "why, is it wrong?" "Try again". Moved from right to left.	Right/left discrimination deficit.
19	Puts soap in front of the bowl.		*		Problems with position in space.
20	Puts soap behind the bowl.		*		Problems with position in space.
21	Puts soap in bowl.		*	Client frustrated – didn't really try.	Problems with position in space.

Summary: **Observations/Hypotheses**

Once initiated task, was able to wash and dry hands.
Language deficits - expressive and receptive, but also appears to have object, colour and tactile recognition deficits. Unable to point to objects and colours on command which he should be able to do if it was just a word finding problem. Once he has <u>both</u> visual and tactile cues, is able to describe use and demonstrate use. This task he did not initiate on command. Continued evidence of right/left and position in space deficits, decreased bilateral integration and manipulation.

Signature: **Date:**

Figure 8–3. (continued)

Task 3: **Pouring and Drinking**

Key: (EL) items can be administered to clients with expressive language
(ED) items provide alternative assessment methods for clients with expressive dysphasia

Tester's name:			Date:	
Dominant hand:	☐ Right ☐ Left	Hand used to pour:	☐ Right ☐ Left	

	ITEM	ABLE (YES)	UNABLE (NO)	FURTHER PROMPTS OR ASSESSMENTS REQUIRED	HYPOTHESES, CUES AND COMMENTS
1	(EL) Identifies cup through touch.	☐ Right ☒ Left	☒ Right ☐ Left	Tried right first – prompted to try on left.	Identified cup with left hand, unable with right.
2	Scans table for object.	*			
2	Fixes gaze on objects.	*			
2	Recognizes object by (EL) naming or (ED) pointing.		*	Client got quite frustrated. 1. naming; 2. pointing.	Named cup as had already identified. Unable to point or name jug/mat.
3	Puts cup on table on left of jug.		*		Right/left deficit.
4	(EL) Describes use of objects.		*	"Drink" I prompted "What would you use this for?" pointed to jug.	Described use of cup, but not jug.
5	Mimes use of objects.		*		
6	Demonstrates use of objects.	*		"Oh, it's a pitcher, I'd pour a drink" prompted to demonstrate use of cup.	Once he touched jug – was able to identify it and demonstrated pouring and drinking.
7	Correctly identifies colours of all objects by (EL) naming or (ED) pointing.		*	"I just can't."	Colour agnosia.
8	Initiates pouring on command.	*		Broke command down second time "pour a drink".	Didn't respond to complex command, initiated after prompted with simple command. Decreased receptive language.
8	Reaches for jug.	*			
8	Judges distance to jug.	*			
8	Required prompt (handed jug) to initiate pouring.	☐ Yes ☒ n/a	☐ No ☐ n/a		

Figure 8–3. (continued)

Task 3: Pouring and Drinking

	ITEM	ABLE (YES)	UNABLE (NO)	FURTHER PROMPTS OR ASSESSMENTS REQUIRED	HYPOTHESES, CUES AND COMMENTS
9	Picks up jug.	*			Tried right but decreased strength, so used left hand.
10	Pours drink into cup.	*			
10	Judges distance from jug to cup.		?		Initially when starts to pour – then waivers.
11	Stops pouring before cup is full – no spill.		*	Check depth and distance perception.	Spilled a little water. Query distance/depth perception or holding cup steady.
12	Puts down jug.	*			Decreased bilateral integration.
13	Reaches for cup.	*			
14	Picks up cup.	*			
15	Lifts cup to mouth.	*			
15	Takes drink into mouth.	*			
16	Correctly identifies taste of drink.		*		Was unable to identify orange juice.
17	Swallows drink.	*			
18	Replaces cup on table.	*			
19	Uses correct sequence.	[*] Yes	[ ] No		
20	Puts cup on the right of the jug.		*		Impaired right/left discrimination.
21	Puts cup in front of the jug.		*		Impaired position in space.
22	Puts cup behind the jug.		*		Impaired position in space.

Summary: **Observations/Hypotheses**

This task identified cup with left hand. Seems to be learning test format – did he guess? He had cue of jug but he did have trouble naming this initially. Needed to hold and see jug to recognise it and demonstrate use.

Decreased strength on right, couldn't lift and pour with right so used left. Some spillage, could be because left is non-dominant and this was awkward for him. Decreased bilateral integration led to problems stabilising cup with right and co-ordinating right and left. Need to check depth perception. Consistent right/left, position in space and colour recognition deficits.

Signature: **Date:**

Figure 8–3. (continued)

Task 4: **Dressing**

Key: (EL) items can be administered to clients with expressive language
(ED) items provide alternative assessment methods for clients with expressive dysphasia

Tester's name:				Date:			
Dominant hand:	[*] Right	[ ] Left	**Hand used to pick up shirt:**		[ ] Right	[*] Left

	ITEM	ABLE (YES)	UNABLE (NO)	FURTHER PROMPTS OR ASSESSMENTS REQUIRED	HYPOTHESES, CUES AND COMMENTS
1	(EL) Identifies button through touch.	[ ] Right [ ] Left	[*] Right [*] Left		
2	Scans table for objects.	*			
2	Fixes gaze on objects.	*			
2	Recognizes objects by (EL) naming or (ED) pointing.	*		Pointed to jacket and button.	
3	Puts button on table on right of garment.		*		Right/left discrimination deficit.
3	Puts button on table on left of garment.		*		Right/left discrimination deficit.
4	(EL) Describes use of objects.	*			
5	Mimes use of objects.	*		I held onto the jacket so he couldn't touch it.	Managed to mime this time.
6	Correctly identifies colours of all objects by (EL) naming or (ED) pointing.		*	Needs further assessment and investigative questioning.	Unable to name or point. Very frustrated. Colour agnosia.
7	Initiates dressing on command.	*			
7	Reaches for garment (shirt).	*			
7	Judges distance to garment (shirt).	*			
7	Required prompt (handed garment) to initiate dressing.	[ ] Yes [*] n/a	[ ] No [ ] n/a		

Figure 8–3. (continued)

Neuropsychological Checklist

To score: Place ticks in the boxes that correspond to the deficits you feel are indicated by the client's performance and the tasks in which the indicative performance was observed. Look down the left-hand column for deficit(s) and across the columns at the top for tasks.

Client's name: Sam

Tester's name: **Date of testing:**

Diagnosis: Stroke

DEFICIT	SCREENING ASSESSMENT	EATING TASK 1	WASHING TASK 2	POURING AND DRINKING TASK 3	DRESSING TASK 4
LANGUAGE					
Comprehension		*	*	*	*
Expression	?	*	*	*	*
HEARING					
Hearing acuity					
Auditory agnosia					
COGNITION					
Orientation					
Attention					
Short-term memory					
Long-term memory					
Initiation			* Linked to receptive problems? Problem initiating following complex command.		
MOTOR					
Abnormal tone (spasticity or flaccidity)	Increased on right. *				
Bilateral integration		*	*	*	*
Fine motor coordination/dexterity on Right.		*	*	*	*
SENSATION					
Proprioception					
Tactile discrimination		*	*	*	
Taste discrimination					
Temperature discrimination					

Figure 8–3. (continued)

Neuropsychological Checklist

DEFICIT	SCREENING ASSESSMENT	EATING TASK 1	WASHING TASK 2	POURING AND DRINKING TASK 3	DRESSING TASK 4
VISION					
Visual acuity					
Visual attention					
Visual scanning		*			
Visual field loss					
Visual neglect					
AGNOSIA					
Visual spatial agnosia					
Visual object agnosia		*	*		
Colour agnosia		*	*	*	*
Tactile agnosia		*	*	*	*
APRAXIA					
Constructional apraxia					
Motor apraxia					
Ideomotor apraxia					
Ideational apraxia					
Dressing apraxia					
BODY SCHEME					
Somatognosia					
Unilateral neglect					
Anosognosia					
Right/left discrimination		*	*	*	*

Figure 8–3. (continued)

Task 4: Dressing

	ITEM	ABLE (YES)	UNABLE (NO)	FURTHER PROMPTS OR ASSESSMENTS REQUIRED	HYPOTHESES, CUES AND COMMENTS
8	Picks up garment.	*			With left hand.
9	Organizes garment (shirt) before putting on.	*			Rather hesitant.
10	Locates sleeve.	*			
11	Puts correct arm into sleeve.	*			Dresses right arm first – rather slow.
12	Puts collar behind neck.	*			
13	Puts other arm into correct sleeve.	*			
14	Fastens garment (shirt) correctly. Note type of fastening: buttons, zip, poppers, velcro.		*		Decreased find co-ordination and bilateral integration. Got quite frustrated trying. Needed physical help.

Summary: **Observations/Hypotheses**

Client getting quite frustrated with some items this task. Showed improved function in this task – hypothesis: that practice and repetition helps this client and that a teaching-learning approach might be helpful, eg., Sam was able to point to button on command, managed to mime use of jacket in this fourth task.

Continues to show a consistent right/left discrimination deficit and consistent problem with colour recognition. (Note: this client's occupation is art/animation so colour agnosia will have a significant impact for worker roles.) Says everything looks "dull".

Decreased bilateral co-ordination and fine manipulation on right. Needed physical assistance to do up buttons on jacket.

Showed better comprehension of instructions.

Client was right-handed and worker role is art so decreased prehension and manipulation on dominant side is a problem.

Signature:

Date:

Figure 8–3. (continued)

Table 8–4. Problem list

OCCUPATIONAL ROLE LIMITATIONS

Worker role	Sam was unable to work in his occupation as an animator
Partner	Sam thought that he was unable to be an equal provider in his home and an adequate sexual partner

OCCUPATIONAL PERFORMANCE TASK DYSFUNCTION

ADLs (priority area for intervention)	On the SOTOF Sam had difficulty with buttoning and fastenings, spilled liquids (e.g., when pouring a drink), and dropped objects (e.g., the soap)
IADLs	Sam was not doing any IADL tasks independently and he wanted to be involved with meal preparation (top priority for intervention), financial management, shopping, and housework
Productivity	Sam had difficulty with computer use (top priority for treatment), writing, and drawing
Leisure	Sam had difficulty with most of his leisure tasks, including reading (top priority for intervention), going to the movies, cycling, and socializing with friends

PERFORMANCE COMPONENT DEFICITS

Achromatopsia	On the SOTOF Sam was unable to name colors or point to colors on command; when questioned further he could discriminate light from dark tones; he said everything "looks kind of grey, like a black and white TV screen . . . seems fuzzy, things aren't as clear as they used to be"
Visual object agnosia	Sam could not identify all the SOTOF objects on command, either by naming or by pointing to named objects; sometimes he was able to recognize SOTOF objects when he was allowed to view and touch the objects simultaneously, and he could recognize objects by reaching for them and handling them when asked to demonstrate their use
Temperature discrimination	Sam was unable to indicate the temperature of the water in the SOTOF washing task and

(continues)

(continued)

Table 8–4. Problem list

PERFORMANCE COMPONENT DEFICITS

Temperature discrimination	was unable to indicate the temperature of the water with a Yes/No answer when asked, "Is it hot . . . cold . . . warm . . . ?"
Taste discrimination	Sam was unable to describe the taste of the food in the SOTOF eating task; he was able to discriminate sweet from salty but was unable to indicate what the fruit was with a Yes/No answer when asked, "Is it pears . . . peaches . . . strawberries?"
Expressive and receptive verbal language	Sam had some difficulty following complex commands, had some word-finding problems, and spoke slowly and hesitantly
Alexia	Sam had difficulty comprehending written language
Bilateral integration	Sam had difficulty coordinating his hands together (e.g., when trying to button his jacket)
Fine motor skills	Sam was unable to button up his jacket
Tactile discrimination	Sam was unable to identify objects with vision occluded when manipulating objects in either hand; he had some success identifying larger objects (such as the cup) with his left hand
Right/left discrimination	Sam had variable performance with the SOTOF right-left discrimination items; sometimes he put the object on correct side on command but then reversed right and left on other tasks
Position in space	Sam was unable to place objects in front, behind, in, right, and left on the on command on the SOTOF spatial items
Spatial relations	Sam had some difficulty perceiving spatial relationships between objects or between objects and himself

---

difficulty. Because the focus of this book is perceptual and cognitive deficits, Sam's psychosocial and sexual functioning will not be addressed; this chapter will focus specifically on Sam's simple perceptual problems (agnosias). Other perceptual problems, such as spatial relations syndrome, are addressed in depth in Chapter 10.

THERAPY GOALS

The therapist and Sam's long-term goals were for Sam to:

● Be independent in his personal care
● Be able to manage an equal share of IADLs, such as meal preparation, shopping, managing finances, and housework
● Be able to resume some sort of paid employment
● Be able to engage in enjoyable leisure activities with family and friends
● Be in a position in which he feels able to proceed with his plans to marry and have a family

The therapist began by setting short-term objectives related to Sam's self-care and IADL goals. She wanted to help Sam to improve his color and object recognition, taste and temperature discrimination, spatial awareness, fine motor skills, and bilateral integration in order to increase independence in self-care IADL and work.

SELECTION OF INTERVENTION STRATEGIES AND ACTIVITIES

The initial assessment process relied mostly on a top-down approach by beginning with an exploration of Sam's roles, activities, and environment before analyzing his performance to understand the impact of his performance component deficits on occupational performance. For the treatment approach, Eva decided to use a multicontext approach as described by Toglia (1989b). This approach aims to:

> . . . maximize existing visual function by providing strategies to enhance the patient's ability to assimilate visual information efficiently... [and to help] the patient to understand the underlying characteristics of the disorder... The patient's lack of understanding can produce anxiety as well as a feeling of loss of control. Treatment aims to help patients gain the ability to predict whether a situation will cause them difficulty. Once patients recognize the type of tasks that will cause difficulty, they can initiate the use of strategies that will help them overcome these limitations (p. 592).

This multicontext approach involves three intervention tools: teaching-learning, use of the environment, and body alignment (Toglia, 1989b). It combines remedial, functional, and environmental adaptation approaches:

● The remedial aspect of intervention involves the practice of weak visual perceptual skills
● The functional component of intervention is carried out at the same time and involves the practice of important functional activities

● The therapist also uses environmental adaptations to increase the efficiency of the client's visual processing (Toglia, 1989b; Neistadt, 1988)

When using this approach, the intervention and evaluation phases are not really separate and distinct but are interwoven. The therapist is continually observing and using investigative questioning to understand the client and his or her problems, priorities, feelings, and responses to the intervention strategies. Eva reports that she often begins intervention with a combined remediation and functional (or bottom-up) approach and if this appears unsuccessful switches to a compensatory/adaptation (or top-down) approach. In general, Eva states that a mix of approaches is useful with clients similar to Sam who have a complex pattern of deficits and related dysfunction. Eva adds some further insights to her approach to intervention in Box 8–5.

INVESTIGATIVE QUESTIONS RELATED TO AGNOSIAS

In Table 8–5, Eva describes the questions she asked Sam to better understand his agnosia. Eva reported drawing on the work of Humphreys and Riddoch (1987), Toglia (1989b), and Grieve (1993) to develop these questions for Sam's intervention.

BOX 8–5. THERAPIST REASONING—APPROACH TO INTERVENTION

I began Sam's intervention using a remedial approach. I selected an information processing "bottom-up" approach (as described by Abreu and Toglia, 1987). Sam had significant agnosia deficits, and I wanted to break down Sam's information processing to examine his problems in depth and explore related intervention strategies in his sensory detection, analysis, hypothesis formation, and response phases. Therefore, at the beginning of Sam's intervention program, I explored the questions outlined in the next section with Sam to:

● Gain a better understanding of the exact nature of his deficits (this is a continuation of the diagnostic reasoning process used in the SOTOF and involves cue acquisition, hypothesis formation, and hypothesis testing),

● Identify his level of insight into his deficits,

● Examine the ways in which he was already trying to overcome these deficits in his daily life, and

● Postulate, implement, and evaluate the most useful intervention strategies.

Table 8–5. Understanding the client's agnosia: Therapist questions and reasoning

QUESTION	THERAPIST REASONING
Are you able to describe to me what you can see, feel, taste?	These descriptions help me to understand what Sam was perceiving (these questions examine sensory detection). Sam revealed that his world appeared as shades of grey rather than color and that he perceived objects as "rather fuzzy and unclear."
When you are looking at an object and trying to identify what you are seeing, what are you thinking? Look at this object and tell me all your thoughts out loud as you try to identify it.	By listening to a breakdown of Sam's thought process, I could examine how Sam analyzed his visual input and raised hypotheses about what the object was.
Although you are not able to recognize objects when you see them, are you able to remember what a particular object should look like or what color an object should be?	This question is important because object recognition units are stored descriptions of known objects (Grieve, 1993). Part of object recognition depends on the client's correctly matching the visual input from the currently viewed object to his memory of known objects in order to find the name, meaning, and function of the object. The link between the client's visual and semantic systems are these object recognition units (Grieve, 1993), so I needed to know whether Sam had intact memories of what objects should look like.
Although you are not able to identify an object when you feel it with your eyes closed, are you able to identify the weight, size, and shape of the object? Can you remember objects that have the same weight, shape, and size?	I wanted to explore whether Sam could use other cues (e.g., weight) to help identify objects and work through an analysis and hypothesis-formation process.

(continues)

(continued)

Table 8–5. Understanding the client's agnosia: Therapist questions and reasoning

QUESTION	THERAPIST REASONING
When you recognize an object and can match it to a picture or memory of other similar objects in your head, can you find the name or word for the object and speak it out loud?	I wanted to examine if Sam had problems with the response phase of object recognition, if he knew what the object was, such as if he had the name "on the tip of his tongue" (i.e., had word-finding problems).
How did you know it was a cup? or Why did you think it was a spoon instead of a fork?	Toglia (1989b) suggests using questions like these after the client has given a correct or incorrect response to an object-recognition task in order to explore the client's rationale, confirm the therapist's hypothesis, and provide insight into the underlying deficit.
Can you recognize faces of people you know? Can you recognize your own face in the mirror?	I wanted to examine whether his visual object agnosia also affected his ability to recognize his friends and family.
Since your discharge, have you been managing to recognize common objects? How do you try to recognize common objects?	This question examines the ways in which Sam was already trying to overcome his visual object agnosia in his daily life.
What do you see on the page when you try to read? How do you approach a page or sentence when you try to read? Do you try breaking down the sentence and focusing on one word or letter at a time?	Sam also had some alexia; it was hard to discriminate between the problems he had experienced with dyslexia since childhood and the additional problems he was experiencing since his stroke. Because he had been treated for his dyslexia in school, I wanted to find out if he knew of successful strategies that helped him to read.

BOX 8–6. THERAPIST REASONING—TASK GRADING AND SYSTEMATIC CUEING

In addition to investigative questioning, I used task-grading and systematic cueing to establish Sam's level of visual object recognition. Grading the task demand for simple perceptual disorders can be undertaken in several ways, including:

- Changing the environmental context in which the objects are viewed from a normal context to a contrived context,
- Increasing the number of objects presented for recognition from a single object to multiple objects,
- Varying the client's level of familiarity with the objects from common self-related objects to unconventional objects, and
- Altering the spatial arrangement from a usual view with well spaced central placement to an unusual view with a scattered, crowded arrangement (Toglia, 1989b).

I would begin by changing one parameter at a time to increase task demand over treatment sessions.

I follow Toglia's (1989b) graded cueing system, which provides four levels of systematic cueing: repetition cues (which involved asking Sam to "look again"); analysis cues (which involved asking Sam to describe the attributes [e.g., size, shape, weight] of the object that was misidentified); perceptual cues (which involved directing Sam to attend to a critical feature of the object; this was accomplished by repositioning the object so that the critical feature was in the center of his vision or pointing to the feature and asking Sam to "look here"); and semantic cues (which involved providing him with a choice of several categories, such as "is it food, a tool, or clothing?") (p. 591).

In Box 8–6, Eva discusses her use of task grading and systematic cueing in addition to investigative questioning.

INTERVENTION FOR VISUAL OBJECT AGNOSIA

Grieve noted (1993) that if there is no deficit in the semantic system, objects may be matched by function and used appropriately. Sam was able to use objects appropriately when he was assessed using the SOTOF. In Box 8–7, Eva explains the reasoning behind the intervention she used with Sam to overcome his visual object agnosia.

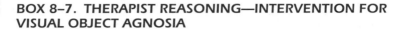

BOX 8–7. THERAPIST REASONING—INTERVENTION FOR VISUAL OBJECT AGNOSIA

I started treatment by asking Sam to match the same objects presented in the same view. I used familiar, everyday objects and placed them in a contextual setting. After Sam had mastered this, I increased the task demand to matching the same object in different views. Sam had some initial problems with **form discrimination**. I used an open box that had mirrors on the bottom and three sides to help Sam examine the object from all angles and build up memory units of what the object looked like from different angles. Then Sam graduated to matching objects that were different but had the same function, such as cups of different shapes, materials, and sizes. When Sam could do this, I set up tasks in which he had to discriminate between objects; for example, drinking versus eating objects. Sam also practiced naming the objects he was matching. Initially he could only name an object after he had picked it up, handled it, and tried to use it. Sam was prompted to use cues such as shape, size, weight, and function in his hypothesis formulation. Gradually he learned to use visual cues instead of visual and sensory cues to identify common objects. The context affected Sam's performance. For example, he found it easier to identify crockery, cutlery, and cooking utensils that were placed in the EASY STREET ENVIRONMENTS kitchen area than when the same objects were presented to him in the treatment room. After Sam mastered identifying objects in their normal context, the task demand was increased by presenting objects out of context; for example, cooking utensils in the EASY STREET ENVIRONMENTS bank environment.

INTERVENTION FOR ACHROMATOPSIA

Achromatopsia is a rare deficit, and there is very little literature concerning its intervention. Sam's intervention program was developed through trial and error. Grieve (1993) reported that color is processed separately from shape and depth and that clients can be taught to attend to shape and depth cues to help identify objects (see previous description of object recognition treatment plan). The reasoning behind Eva's approach to treating Sam for this problem is outlined in Box 8–8.

INTERVENTION FOR TACTILE AGNOSIA

In Box 8–9, Eva details her work with Sam to reduce the impact of tactile agnosia on his performance.

BOX 8–8. THERAPIST REASONING—ACHROMATOPSIA INTERVENTION

Sam could discriminate light from dark and perceive shades of gray, so I started by asking him to discriminate between light and dark shades on color cards. I gradually increased the number of color cards and asked Sam to sequence them from the lightest to the darkest color. I asked Sam if he remembered what color an object was, for example, the color of a mail box. He then looked at that object, for example, the mail box in EASY STREET ENVIRONMENTS, and attended to the shade of gray that he perceived. Then he was presented with a few color cards (one of which was red) and asked to pick out the same shade as the mail box. Sam was able to match colors quite well and sequence shades correctly. However, he was unable to name colors accurately, and he reported that he continued to perceive the world in shades of gray; therefore, compensation and adaptation methods were explored.

The main task for which Sam needed color recognition was his animation work, so it was in this area that compensation strategies needed to be devised. Sam's employer said that when he returned to work he could produce black-and-white line drawings, which would then be colored by another animator. Sam also reported that he wanted to work on mastering animation software on his computer. The software program had a color chart from which Sam would select colors for his drawings. The program allows the user to print the color chart because sometimes there is variance between the color on the screen and the color printed; Sam printed the chart on his color printer. Lisa then labeled the colors (darkest pink, purpley pink, orangey pink, pale pink, and so on). Sam had this labeled color chart pinned to a board on the wall by his computer, and he used the written color description to make his selections based on the location of that color square on the chart and the corresponding computer chart. Lisa viewed his work to ensure the colors looked coordinated on his pictures. Using his computer, Sam started working in animation part time from his home, which seemed to increase his confidence and his level of satisfaction with life.

JOURNAL WRITING AS A REFLECTIVE TOOL TO DEVELOP INSIGHT AND EVALUATE PROGRESS

Eva began each intervention session by focusing on a particular deficit area, such as color agnosia. She encouraged Sam to try to generalize what he had learned to other environments, such as his home. One of Sam's COPM goals was to improve his performance using the computer, so Eva adapted the task of keeping a written journal and asked him to keep

BOX 8–9. THERAPIST REASONING—TACTILE AGNOSIA INTERVENTION

I drew on the work of Zoltan (1996) to guide my treatment of Sam's tactile agnosia. I began by asking him to discriminate between different sizes and weights of objects, first using vision and then with vision occluded. Sam was instructed to hold two objects (one in each hand simultaneously or one after another into the same hand) and then identify which was the larger, smaller, heavier, or lighter object. Sam tried to identify through verbal description with his eyes closed. If this was difficult, I instructed him to feel an object with his eyes closed. Then I arranged the object with others on the table in front of him (starting with very different objects and then making the objects more similar in terms of shape, size, and so on). Then I asked him to open his eyes and point to the object he had just been handling. If he was unable to accomplish this through visual input alone, he handled each of the objects with his eyes open and then tried to pick out the one he had just been given to identify with his eyes shut.

Next we worked on recognizing the textures of objects. Sam started by using a texture board to match textures (e.g., sandpaper, silk, wood, metal, plastic). He was given two objects and asked to describe the textures and to identify which was the rougher, smoother, or softer object. The task demand was increased by using tasks that involved the discrimination of different everyday objects (e.g., cup, spoon, pen, soap, book). Sam began by manipulating objects while looking and then with vision occluded. If he had difficulty naming the object, he was prompted to attend to the different cues, which helped him to identify the object (i.e., to describe the weight, shape, and texture of the object). He was then coached to use this subcomponent information for hypothesis formulation to identify the object. Finally, one or two everyday objects were placed in a container that was filled with rice or beans. Sam had to use tactile discrimination to find the object or objects. Okkema (1993) also supports this approach because it makes clients more aware of their altered sensations.

a daily journal on his computer. He began with a few sentences and increased this to half a page per entry. Eva provided Sam with a printed list of short questions to guide his journal writing (this gave him a targeted reading task as well). In his journal Sam reflected on the tasks he had undertaken or attempted at home. He recorded how easy or difficult he had estimated the task would be, how easy or difficult the task actually was to perform, if he had decided to use a compensation technique or strategy to help him with the task, what strategies had worked or not worked, and what he thought might make it easier next time. The journal task gave

Sam a reason to use his computer frequently. He brought printed entries to treatment sessions. The entries provided a focus for discussion at the beginning of each session. They helped Eva understand how Sam's level of insight was improving and how he was able to gradually establish the task demand and choose whether or not he needed to implement a strategy or to request help from Lisa. The journal helped Eva to evaluate how he was generalizing his treatment sessions to his home environment and everyday context. Because progress was slow, reviewing past entries gave Sam and Lisa tangible evidence of his progress.

Lisa also kept a written journal in which she recorded Sam's performance and the level of assistance she needed to provide. She also used it to record her own coping strategies and experiences of physical and emotional burden as Sam's primary caregiver. Lisa joined a caregivers' support group and used her journal to reflect on these group sessions, record helpful advice from other caregivers, and make notes on educational group sessions provided by staff on the unit. The caregiver groups were run jointly by the occupational therapist and social worker who invited other professionals, special interest group leaders (e.g., from the Stroke Recovery Association), and experienced caregivers to present information and experiences at some group sessions.

INTERVENTION PROGRESS

The early intervention sessions involved breaking down the information process into phases and working on each part of the process. The approach also involved breaking down tasks (e.g., pouring and drinking) into subcomponents and working on each component separately (e.g., recognizing the object, judging distance to object, lifting object, coordinating cup and jug while pouring). Sam made progress while working on the separate components of visual, tactile, and color recognition. He was able to assess the demands of self-care tasks and use cues to help him with object recognition tasks. He reported improvement in his performance of self-care tasks but was daunted by the thought of attempting higher-demand tasks at home. Eva wanted to help Sam generalize his abilities from the self-care to the IADL domain and decided to implement a functional multicontext treatment approach to work on Sam's IADL goals. Eva and Sam began by working on one task at a time. After a few months Sam was ready to try stringing several tasks together. The following outline presents one of these treatment sessions with Sam.

OUTLINE OF AN INTERVENTION SESSION

After Sam had been attending outpatient occupational therapy for about 4 months, Eva developed the following short-term objectives to be achieved by Sam during a 2-hour intervention session:

Sam, given verbal prompts from the therapist and using compensatory strategies and devices, will be able to mobilize independently within the EASY STREET ENVIRONMENTS treatment area in order to (1) obtain sufficient money from the bank area for the food items he needs for lunch (he may chose to use the ATM or to interact with the therapist who will play the role of the bank clerk); (2) purchase food items he needs for lunch from the grocery store area; (3) safely prepare a light lunch and drink, which is nutritious and tasty, in the kitchen area; and (4) eat and drink without spillage. Eva describes this intervention session in Box 8–10.

PROGRESS REPORT

After 6 months of outpatient occupational therapy, Sam was ready for discharge. At this point Eva asked Sam to reevaluate his five COPM goals, and she re-administered the SOTOF, MBPC, and Burden Interview with Sam and Lisa.

CANADIAN OCCUPATIONAL PERFORMANCE MEASURE

On reviewing the COPM (Law et al., 1994), Sam's self-care scores each increased from 1/10 to 9/10 for performance and 7/10 for satisfaction. For simple meal preparation, the performance score increased from 4/10 to 8/10, and satisfaction increased from 5/10 to 7/10. In the area of work, Sam now rated his performance as 6/10, an increase of four points, and his satisfaction as 4/10, an increase of three points. His fourth goal area was reading. At discharge Sam rated this area as 5/10 for performance (which was a two-point increase) and 3/10 for satisfaction (which was a two-point increase). His last goal was computer use, and his performance rating was increased by four points to become 9/10, and his satisfaction rating increased by two to become 7/10. Sam's original overall performance score was originally 4.4; by the time of discharge from outpatient therapy, it had increased to 7.4. His original overall satisfaction score was 3.6, which increased to 5.6. Validity studies conducted on the COPM have indicated that a change of between one

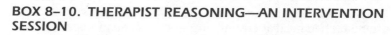

BOX 8–10. THERAPIST REASONING—AN INTERVENTION SESSION

In this session I wanted Sam to work toward independence in providing himself with a nutritious meal. This included planning what to eat, buying the ingredients, preparing the meal, and eating it. Lisa was leaving pre-prepared cold meals for Sam's lunch, and Sam had mastered reheating meals in the microwave but wanted to be able to "prepare a meal from scratch and help out with the shopping and stuff." Sam decided what to prepare on the Tuesday session so that I could purchase the necessary ingredients for the EASY STREET ENVIRONMENTS store for his Thursday appointment. To begin, he chose to make lasagna because "I used to make great lasagna for dinner parties." I asked him to estimate how difficult this meal would be to prepare. I was concerned that if he chose a task that was demanding, he might be frustrated with the results, so I wanted him to choose something that he should be able to achieve. Sam was daunted by attempting IADL tasks in his local community so I wanted the EASY STREET ENVIRONMENTS session to help build his confidence in a supportive environment. Sam agreed that lasagna might be "tricky to start with" and "involved lots of steps and ingredients." Instead, he chose to make soup from a can and a cheese, tomato, and lettuce sandwich. He prepared a written list of ingredients to work on his writing skills.

BANKING

To begin the session, I established that Sam was familiar with the different areas in the EASY STREET ENVIRONMENTS, especially the shop, bank, and kitchen areas. I told him I would stand back and observe, making comments and suggestions when he asked for them or when I thought it was appropriate to help him solve problems throughout the task. Sam stood for quite a while, so I prompted him by asking him what he needed to do first. He said he needed to get some money from the ATM machine. I asked him to judge how difficult this task would be. He thought he could manage the fine coordination required for putting his card in the machine, although it might take him "a few tries to see exactly where the hole was and line the card up just right." He thought he would be able to read the instructions because he had been using his computer everyday for the past few months and was familiar with looking at words on a screen. Furthermore, the bank only gives one short instruction at a time, which would help him. He said it would take him longer than most people to read the instructions and he might get anxious doing this out in the community if there were people in line behind him and he thought he was holding them up. Sam was aware that his function deteriorated with anxiety. He hypothesized that the movement of the money and paper slip coming out of the machine would help

(continues)

BOX 8–10. THERAPIST REASONING—AN INTERVENTION SESSION (CONT.)

cue him to their location. He thought the hardest thing would be the bilateral coordination and fine motor coordination required to put the money in his wallet. The ATM machine in the EASY STREET ENVIRONMENTS doesn't actually dispense money but it does take the client through the usual commands for obtaining money or a bank balance. As soon as Sam put his card in he realized that he had forgotten his personal identification number (PIN) (Fig. 8–4). Sam hadn't used his card since his stroke. I asked him if he knew how to find out what his PIN was, and he said it was written in a file somewhere at home. He agreed to find and memorize the number, and we decided to try the ATM again at the next session. I then asked Sam how he would get money from the bank if he forgot his PIN and he said he "would go and cash a check." We roleplayed this task, and I played the role of bank clerk (Fig. 8–5). Sam asked me how much money to get out, and I responded by drawing his attention to the shopping list and asking him to estimate the cost of the items he needed. He said that 20 dollars should cover it. Sam managed to fill out the check with difficulty. However, his writing was not very legible and he had to ask me what the date was and how to spell "twenty." At the end of the task I asked Sam to evaluate how he had done and think about what he could do to make it easier in the future. Sam said that if he had his PIN it would be easier to use the ATM than write out a check but if he had to write a check he could write it out at home, get Lisa to check it for him, and then he would only have to sign it at the bank.

SHOPPING

Next Sam went to the EASY STREET ENVIRONMENTS grocery store. He collected a basket without prompting and started to look for items along the shelves. He walked around the store for several minutes without picking up any objects. I asked him what he was thinking. He said he couldn't find what he needed, he couldn't see the colors, and the writing was hard to read. I asked him what he could try doing to help him identify objects and, after some reflection, he said he could try picking them up and looking at them from different angles (Fig. 8–6). I suggested he start by finding a loaf of bread and asked him to describe what a loaf would look and feel like. Sam said it was a "rectangular object, wrapped in a plastic bag . . . it should feel quite light and be soft and squidgy if I squeeze it." Focusing on these cues, Sam found the bread quite quickly. He was pleased with his success and systematically worked down his list, verbalizing a description of each object and picking up objects to help identify them.

Sam had some difficulty with the soup because there were several different cans in the store. He realized that he would have to read the labels to

(continues)

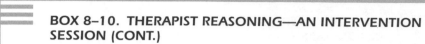

BOX 8–10. THERAPIST REASONING—AN INTERVENTION SESSION (CONT.)

find out what was in them. He was daunted by this until I pointed out that he had the words "tomato soup" already written on his shopping list and that he could match the letters on the tin to those on the list. I was surprised that Sam was having such difficulty with reading because he had been doing well with reading text on his computer when completing his journal. I asked him about this and he said that he was much more anxious about this shopping task and that when he got stressed, his "mind just went blank." He agreed that a written shopping list would be a good support for targeting the words he was searching for in the store. When Sam came to pay for his items, I roleplayed the cashier. He hesitated over which note to give me, and I asked him what he was thinking. Sam (who lives in Canada) said that he used to identify notes by their colors (blue for 5 dollar note, green for a 20, and so on) and now that he couldn't identify the color, he was confused. I asked what else he could look at, and he realized that he could focus on the numbers; he found the note easily using this cue.

MEAL PREPARATION

I was concerned that Sam was tired because he had struggled quite a bit with the shopping and banking tasks, so I asked him if he had enough energy for the kitchen task. Sam was very motivated to continue but decided just to make soup and leave the sandwich for another treatment session. He found the saucepan and can opener quite easily but had difficulty coordinating the movement for opening the can. I got him to try the electric can opener, and he found this much easier. He was able to pour the soup into the pan without spillage; he was pleased with this and said that "practicing pouring drinks had paid off!" Sam had some trouble identifying which knob turned on which ring on the cooker; he said he still got confused with front and back. We discussed strategies for making this easier at home, and he thought he would ask Lisa to stick different-shaped labels by corresponding knobs and rings because he found matching shapes quite easy. I showed him which knob to turn for the front ring he wanted to use (Fig. 8–7). Sam was nervous about pouring the soup into a bowl after it was hot, but when I reminded him how well he had done with pouring from the can, he agreed to try. A little soup spilled over the edge of the bowl onto the counter, but I reassured him that we could easily wipe this up and pointed out that 95% of the soup had ended up in the bowl. Sam carried the bowl to the table and was able to eat without spillage. At the end of the session he was tired but pleased with his accomplishment. He set two goals to do at home that weekend; first, to find his PIN number and try the ATM machine with Lisa; and second, to go shopping with Lisa and try to find a few items in the store.

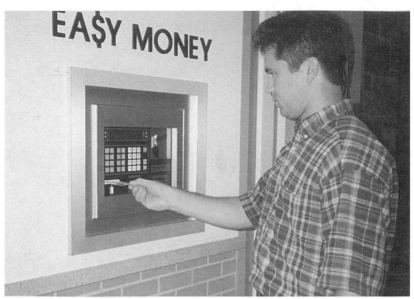

Figure 8–4. "Sam" is involved in an intervention session at the EASY STREET ENVI-RONMENTS bank. In this photograph Sam is depicted using an automated teller machine.

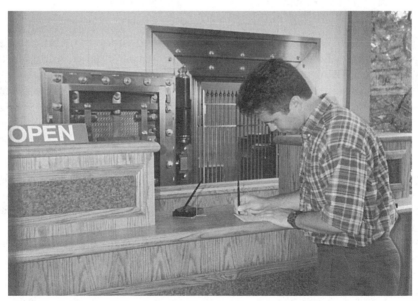

Figure 8–5. As part of the intervention session at the EASY STREET ENVIRON-MENTS bank, Sam practices writing a check.

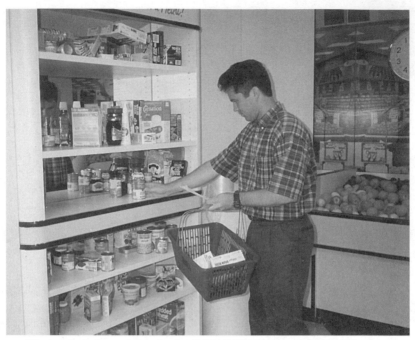

Figure 8–6. Sam shops in the EASY STREET ENVIRONMENTS store.

(or more conservatively, 1.5) and three is considered to be clinically important by the client, family, and therapist (personal communication, Dr. Mary Law, August 29, 1995). Sam's change scores were above 1.5 for both performance and satisfaction, indicating clinically relevant change for both ratings.

STRUCTURED OBSERVATIONAL TEST OF FUNCTION

Sam's overall performance on the SOTOF (Laver and Powell, 1995) at discharge indicated that he was independent on the four self-care tasks. He showed improvement in some areas of neuropsychological functioning but continued to exhibit deficits in other areas. For example, he was able to identify objects both in the tactile discrimination and visual recognition items but was unable to recognize colors (i.e., achromatopsia) and continued to exhibit color agnosia. Both expressive and receptive language had improved. Sam now initiated all tasks on command and did not require additional prompting. He had improved bilateral

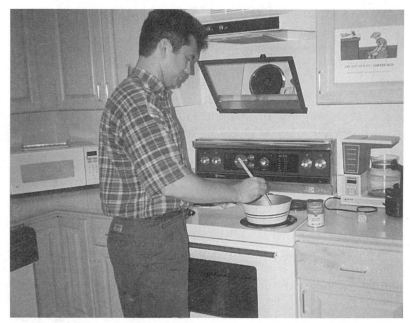

Figure 8–7. Sam cooks soup in the center's Activities of Daily Living Apartment kitchen.

coordination and fine motor skills across all four tasks and was able to button his shirt with some struggle. Reassessment indicated improved distance and depth perception in the pouring and drinking task, and Sam was able to pour a drink without spillage. Across the four tasks, he showed improved perception for position in space ("in front," "behind," and "in" items) but continued to exhibit difficulties on some right/left discrimination items. He was able to identify the temperature of the water in the washing task but still exhibited deficits with taste discrimination on the feeding and drinking tasks.

MEMORY AND BEHAVIOUR PROBLEMS CHECKLIST AND THE BURDEN INTERVIEW

Lisa's reassessment on the MBPC and the Burden Interview indicated:

● A reduction in the amount of assistance that Sam now required at home for self-care and IADL tasks,

- A reduction in problems such as "difficulty remembering things" and "not completing tasks," and
- A corresponding reduction in her experience of physical and emotional burden.

The MBPC score at beginning of the intervention program for frequency was 15/104, and at discharge it had reduced to 9/104 (for reaction, the score at admission was 10/104 and at discharge was 8/104); the initial Burden Interview score was 46/88, and at discharge it had decreased to 30/88.

CLIENT DISCHARGE FROM THERAPY AND FUTURE RECOMMENDATIONS

At discharge Sam was independent for his personal care and was beginning to take some responsibility for cleaning, meal preparation, and shopping, although Lisa reported that it was often quicker and easier to do these tasks herself. They decided that Sam would take responsibility for planning and cooking a special meal once a week on the weekend. This way he had more time to shop and cook and he thought he was making a contribution. Sam was able to travel independently in his community by train and bus, but he disliked rush hour because he was worried he might fall if he was pushed in a crowd (even though his mobility was good, he thought that his balance and righting reactions had not returned to normal). Lisa drove Sam to work each morning and he made his way home by public transport. He was able to use the ATM to withdraw money but continued to wait until there was no line because he became anxious if he thought people were waiting because he was slow.

At the time of discharge Sam was working part-time for his previous employer 2.5 days a week and was assigned the production of hand-drawn black-and-white line drawings. He was also working on other animation projects as a consultant from home by producing computer-constructed animation images for advertisements. Lisa continued to support him with the color aspect of his computer work at home. Before discharge, Sam was put in touch with other young stroke survivors at the local Stroke Recovery Association for ongoing mutual support. Lisa had made friends with two other women in her caregivers' support group, and they had started to meet twice a month outside of the group for dinner. She planned to continue these gatherings as an informal support mechanism. Sam and Lisa became actively involved in the Stroke Recovery Association's fund-raising and research activities. Eva met them again 11 months after Sam's discharge at the Stroke Recovery Association's research planning meeting; they had been married 2 months earlier and were hoping to start a family the next year.

SUMMARY

The agnosias are a complex and poorly understood set of problems. This chapter presented the reasoning behind an occupational therapist's assessment of and intervention with a client who had several forms of agnosia. Background details on agnosias were presented in terms of the kinds of agnosias that have been identified and possible lesion sites that result in these problems. The case of Sam was introduced with a description of Sam's background, his therapist, and the outpatient rehabilitation center where he was treated for 6 months. The case study provided factual details and clinical reasoning related to the therapist's data gathering (including initial interview and standardized assessment); therapy goals; rationale for the intervention approach adopted; specific treatment strategies for visual object agnosia, achromatopsia, color agnosia, and tactile agnosia; an outline of a functional treatment session; a progress report including formal reassessment; and a discharge summary.

☰ REVIEW QUESTIONS

1. Review Table 8–1 and list the brain regions where lesions would be most likely to produce agnosias.
2. For one of his final intervention sessions, Sam decided to make lasagna (a dish he enjoyed making in the past). Using the EASY STREET ENVIRONMENTS, devise an intervention session to assist Sam to purchase the necessary ingredients and prepare this dish.

● Consider where you think Sam will have problems and devise strategies to overcome these.
● Success in this activity will be important to Sam. If Sam appeared to be fatiguing halfway through the preparations, what steps could you take?

3. What is prosopagnosia? Imagine that Sam also experienced prosopagnosia. Based on the intervention ideas presented in this chapter, devise

a remedial approach to treat this problem and a compensatory approach to overcome it if remediation was unsuccessful.

≡ ACKNOWLEDGMENTS

The authors gratefully acknowledge Diane Tait, Director of Occupational Therapy at St. Peter's Hospital in Hamilton, Ontario, Canada, for providing information about the EASY STREET ENVIRONMENTS and Dr. Barbara Acheson Cooper, Associate Professor, School of Rehabilitation Science, McMaster University, Ontario, Canada, for her insights into color agnosia. We would also like to thank Bradley Jacobson, BSc(OT) candidate at McMaster University, for posing for the EASY STREET ENVIRONMENTS photographs. Finally, we extend our thanks to the client, his now-wife, and his family, who provided the inspiration for the case study described in this chapter.

9

Evaluation and Intervention with Unilateral Neglect

LOUISE CORBEN, BAppSci (Occ Ther), and
CAROLYN UNSWORTH, PhD, OTR

- Anosognosia
- Contralesional
- Extinction
- Hemianesthesia
- Hemianopia

- Hemiplegia
- Ipsilesional
- Perceptual Anchor
- Scanning
- Unilateral Neglect

On completion of this chapter, the reader will be able to:

- Define neglect
- Describe the anatomical basis for neglect
- Describe the two main theoretical approaches that have been developed to understand the unilateral neglect phenomenon
- List at least three remediation and three adaptation (compensatory) strategies that a therapist can use in an intervention program with a client who has unilateral neglect
- Plan appropriate evaluations and interventions to use with clients who have unilateral neglect
- Successfully work through the Review Questions

☰ INTRODUCTION

Unilateral neglect is one of the most puzzling cognitive disturbances. Clients who experience unilateral neglect may find that the problem resolves, that they can functionally overcome problems by using compensatory strategies, or that they may be so severely disabled by this problem that they cannot live alone. The purpose of this chapter is to examine what unilateral neglect is and to present the reasoning behind evaluating and conducting interventions with a client who is experiencing unilateral neglect after a stroke. The chapter opens with a brief review of the features of this disorder and its anatomical basis and mechanisms. The case of Alan is then presented. A review of standardized and nonstandardized assessments used with clients who experience neglect is provided, together with Alan's assessment results. Remediation, adaptation (compensation), and education intervention strategies used with Alan are examined in detail.

WHAT IS UNILATERAL NEGLECT?

Definition of Unilateral Neglect

Unilateral neglect is an extraordinary disorder of space-related behavior and spatial cognition (Bradshaw & Mattingley, 1995). Unilateral neglect is most often seen after damage to the right cerebral hemisphere (Vallar, 1993) and may occur after stroke or neoplasm affecting this region (Halligan & Marshall, 1993). A client with a unilateral neglect caused by a right lesion may neglect the left hemispace and body side. Since neglect can occur in either the right or left hemispheres, in this text we simply discuss a client who is neglecting the **contralesional** (i.e., the side of the person opposite to the side of his brain lesion), or left, side. In the acute phase the client may present with his head and gaze orientated toward the side of the lesion (i.e., **ipsilesionally**). For example, if the client has a right hemisphere stroke and consequent left-sided paralysis, he would orient himself only to the right side. Persons with neglect may appear to not perceive or to ignore auditory, visual, or tactile stimuli coming from the opposite (contralesional) side of space despite intact sensory abilities. Paradoxically, persons with neglect may appear overattentive and distracted by stimuli coming from the ipsilesional side. Unilateral neglect is particularly apparent when the client is involved in daily living tasks. The client may fail to eat food from one half of the plate or may fail to dress one half of his body. The client may be unable to successfully negotiate his way around seemingly familiar surroundings because of an inability to attend to the contralesional side. Reading, writing, and drawing present new challenges. For example, a client may be unable to read effectively because he or she omits the contralesional side of the text or individual words (Worthington, 1996). In addition, a person with neglect may begin writing in the middle of the page or omit or transpose details on the contralesional side of his drawings (Halligan, Marshall, & Wade, 1992). A classic example of a drawing of a house scene is presented in Figure 9–1A, illustrating omission of the details on the left side of the scene in Figure 9–1B.

Perhaps the most perplexing aspect of the phenomenon of neglect is the apparent lack of awareness on the part of the client regarding the loss of half of his world. It seems as though this half of his world has ceased to exist. In some cases, this may extend to the point where a client may deny any dysfunction or presence of paresis on his contralesional side. This particular problem is referred to as **anosognosia**. Anosognosia, although not necessarily always occurring in the presence of unilateral neglect, compounds efforts made by therapists in the acute stages of recovery to establish some "knowledge" of the hemiplegic side with the client (Halligan & Marshall, 1993).

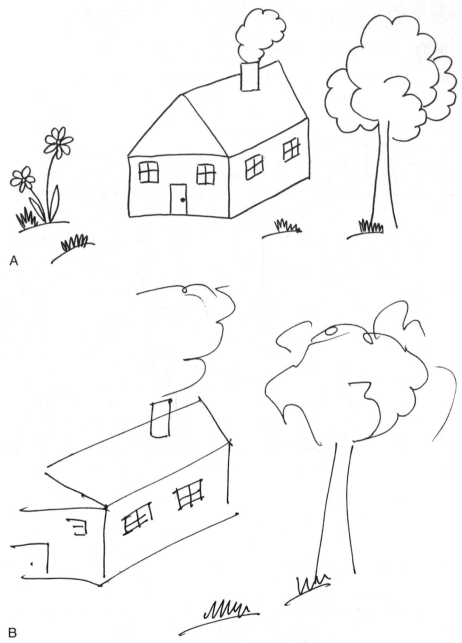

A

B

Figure 9–1. An example of drawing with a unilateral neglect—environment neglect. **(A)** The example house. **(B)** The client's attempt to copy this drawing.

The client with unilateral neglect presents as being unable to see, hear, or feel contralesional stimuli. However, this cannot be assumed unless, of course, the client has a concomitant primary sensory loss such as **hemianopia** (i.e., visual field cut that usually reduces part or all of the contralesional visual field) or **hemianesthesia**. In cases in which the client does not have a sensory loss, there is considerable speculation as to the extent the person is able to process visual, tactile, and auditory information. Studies such as those conducted by Halligan and Marshall (1988) indicate that clients with a neglect without a primary sensory loss may well process apparently "neglected" information at a subconscious level. A number of models have been proposed as to why this seemingly tacit knowledge does not generate an appropriate, conscious response. We will return to this point later when discussing the mechanism of neglect.

Unilateral neglect is not easily classified because clinical presentations may vary with each client depending on the size and location of the lesion. Therefore, the degree to which each client "neglects" varies enormously. Some clients may respond to prompting or require hands-on guidance to complete a task. Others may completely neglect the left side of their bodies or may demonstrate neglect in the form of overattending to the right side of their bodies and only a cursory attention to the left side. Whereas some clients are able to spontaneously track across to the left, others are unable to cross the midline. Consequently, clients may show significant differences in their ability to perform daily living tasks. In an attempt to encapsulate the phenomenon of neglect, a bewildering array of terminology has arisen. Terms such as *unilateral spatial neglect, hemi-inattention, hemineglect,* and *unilateral visual inattention* are all used to describe the presentation of unilateral neglect. Variations in classifications of neglect may well be due to the diversity of presentation of the disorder. For ease of discussion, this chapter continues to use the term *unilateral neglect*, particularly relating to the left body side and hemispace (i.e., as a result of right hemisphere damage).

Therapists can attempt to understand unilateral neglect by examining the functional impact for the client. This involves an examination of the difficulties clients have with activities of daily living (ADLs). Therapists also need to consider which sensory modalities are affected, including visual, tactile, and auditory. One or all of these modalities may be neglected. Neglect can also be understood in terms of the ways the client perceives the world around him and the area of space that is neglected. For example, unilateral neglect may express itself as a disorder of attention and goal-directed behavior in:

● Contralesional personal space (defined as pertaining to the body), such as shaving only the right half of the face or failing to wash the left side of the body, or

- Contralesional peripersonal space (i.e., the area of space within arm distance), such as failing to use objects on the contralesional side of the meal tray, or
- Contralesional extrapersonal space (i.e., the area of space beyond arm length), such as failing to negotiate obstacles, doorways, and so on when mobilizing (Bradshaw & Mattingley, 1995).

Unilateral neglect is also demonstrated through a client's impaired ability to attend to either the object or the environment as a whole. In other words, either half of the environment is neglected or half of objects are neglected. In the first case, the client may neglect the left side of the entire visual scene (Fig. 9–1). In the second case, a client may neglect the left side of an object, regardless of its absolute position in the visual display. For example, the client may neglect the left side of a cup even though it is on his right side. This is most apparent when a client copies a multicomponent drawing. The left side of each component of the drawing (e.g., a house, tree, flower) is omitted (Fig. 9–2). For further information, the reader is referred to an excellent case study illustrating the phenomenon of an object-centered neglect (in contrast to a spatial- or environment-centered neglect) by Driver and Halligan (1991).

The phenomenon of **extinction** must also be discussed in relation to unilateral neglect. Extinction is evident in situations in which the client can attend to isolated stimuli coming from either the contralesional or the ipsilesional side. However, when presented with double or simultaneous stimuli (i.e., stimuli from both sides), the client may respond to the ipsilesional stimuli only, thus "extinguishing" the concurrent, contralesional stimuli. Motor extinction is particularly evident in bilateral tasks (particularly if the client has good motor control of the affected side). In motor extinction, the client typically fails to use the limb normally in bilateral tasks, such as holding a cup or catching a ball. Whereas some researchers consider that extinction is a component of unilateral neglect, others believe it may be a separate and distinct disorder. It appears that extinction is more subtle and resilient than pure unilateral neglect. In some cases, neglect may be seen as resolving into an extinction phenomenon (Robertson & Eglin, 1993).

It is important to note that despite the apparent disparity of presentations, all clients with unilateral neglect tend to have a common underlying dysfunction. This may be seen in terms of a lateralized attentional disorder (Bradshaw & Mattingley, 1995) as evidenced by their diminished or reduced response (hypoattention) to contralesional stimuli and an over-response (hyperattention) to ipsilesional stimuli. Alternatively, it may also be seen as a lateralized disorder of spatial representation (Bisiach & Luzzatti, 1978).

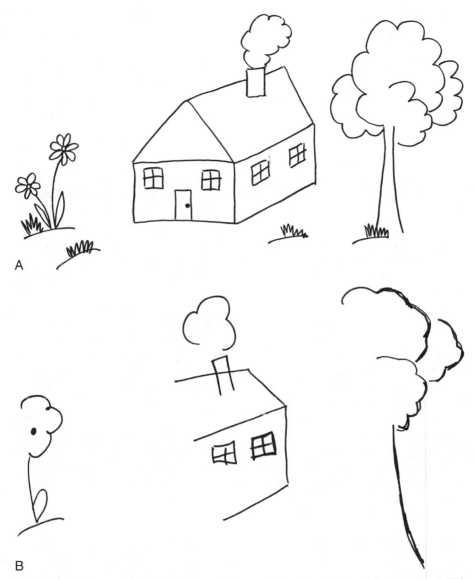

Figure 9–2. An example of drawing with a unilateral neglect—object neglect. **(A)** The example house. **(B)** The client's attempt to copy this drawing.

Anatomical Basis and Mechanisms
of Unilateral Neglect

Unilateral neglect may occur after lesions in either the left or the right cerebral hemispheres. However, as discussed previously, this disorder is more frequently seen and more severe after a lesion in the right hemisphere (Vallar, 1993). Lesions may occur at either a cortical or subcortical level and be either anterior or posterior. It has been suggested that lesions involving the inferior-posterior regions of the right parietal lobe are significant determinants of neglect (Vallar, 1993). Lesions to subcortical structures, such as the thalamus, basal ganglia, and internal capsule, have also been associated with the presentation of unilateral neglect. Correlational studies between the clinical and anatomical presentation of neglect indicate that unilateral neglect may be produced by a disruption of the complex neural networks that underlie spatial cognition (Demeurisse et al., 1997). A breakdown in the neural circuitry linking anterior and posterior areas (often through subcortical structures) may account for the apparent diversity of the neglect syndrome and qualitatively different manifestations of neglect.

Unilateral neglect is often a confusing disorder, and considerable research attention has been directed in this field to attempt to understand why it occurs. There are two major theoretical models that seek to explain its mechanisms. The first model is based on the notion of neglect's occurring as a result of a disrupted attentional system, and the second model of neglect is based on the representation of space (i.e., neglect's occurring from a deficit in the ability to form a complete spatial representation). These models are by no means mutually exclusive, and they can both be considered as providing a sound rationale for the underlying mechanisms of neglect. The central theme in the first model is asymmetry of attention, particularly in the dominance of the right hemisphere, in mediating attention (Heilman & Van den Abell, 1980). Damage to the attentional circuits in the right hemisphere results in failure to attend to (i.e., to notice) or intend to (i.e., to move toward or act on) stimuli in the contralesional hemispace, resulting in a unilateral neglect.

Kinsbourne (1993) also proposed an attentional model for neglect. However, this model is quite different from the one proposed by Heilman and Van den Abell (1980). Kinsbourne's model adopts a similar notion to that of hypertonicity, suggesting that neglect is the result of an imbalance between the inhibitory effect of opponent processors. The undamaged hemisphere is disinhibited and largely in control, causing hyperattention to the unaffected side. Neglect is therefore said to occur as a result of dysfunction in the ability to focus, sustain, detach, and divide attention. Posner and Peterson (1990) approach the attentional model from a different perspective. They adopted a "top-down" approach (different from the top-down treatment approach described in Chapter 1) that attempts to understand neglect within the context of the overall human attentional system. The basis of this approach is the ability to disengage, shift, and engage attention. Clients with neglect typically demonstrate difficulty disengaging from stimuli to shift and engage with the new stimuli. This causes two problems: (1) initial, automatic attention to ipsilesional stimuli and (2) impairment in the ability to shift attention to the contralesional side. The attentional model of neglect has spawned many fascinating studies, the description of which is beyond this chapter. For a detailed explanation, the reader is referred to Mesulam (1981), Gainotti (1994), and Rizzolatti and Berti (1993).

As mentioned, the second model of neglect is based on the representation of space. Bisiach and Luzzatti (1978) argue that neglect originates from a deficit in the ability to form a complete spatial representation. Space is representationally organized across the two cerebral hemispheres. Damage in one area is presumed to produce a damaged representation in the contralesional side of space. Rizzolatti and Berti (1993) attempt to combine these two models (both the attentional and representational models) in their premotor theory of neglect. The basis of this theory is that spatial attention is dependent on several independent neural circuits. Attention toward, and therefore perception of, stimuli is enhanced as a direct result of activation of motor circuits, as occurs when a person moves. Therefore, activating motor circuits of the ipsilesional hemisphere (through voluntary movements of the left upper or lower limbs) may facilitate associated sensory circuits. Such movement may in turn lead to improvements in the processing of stimuli from the contralesional (left) side. In other words, the premotor theory of neglect suggests that by working with the client to increase movement on his contralesional side (e.g., the client's left arm), that attention to the left hemispace is heightened, thus increasing the possibility of perceiving stimuli on this side. Evidence to support this approach was gained through a study by Robertson et al. (1994) in which six clients with left unilateral neglect were asked to walk through a doorway. Each of their walking trajectories (or pathways) was measured, and it was found that all trajectories were significantly deviated to the right of center. Clients were then asked to clench and unclench their left hands before and during walking through the doorway. The researchers found that this procedure significantly assisted clients in centering their walking trajectories. These two models that seek to explain neglect are by no means mutually exclusive. Taken in part or together, both can provide sound rationale for therapeutic intervention in cases of neglect. For further information relating to research on unilateral neglect in occupational therapy, the reader is referred to Van Deusen (1988, 1993).

≡ CASE STUDY: ALAN

BACKGROUND

This section provides background information on the case study client presented to illustrate the therapist's reasoning behind conducting evaluations and interventions.

THE ACUTE CARE SETTING

Alan was admitted to a 738-bed acute care hospital in a suburb close to his home. The hospital has an emergency department, and clients with stroke and head injury are often admitted through this department. Clients generally stay in the acute care setting for 5 to 7 days before being discharged to either a rehabilitation facility (if required), home, or to alternative accommodation, such as an assisted-living retirement village or nursing home.

INTRODUCTION TO THE OCCUPATIONAL THERAPIST AND THERAPY MODEL

Sarah is a 37-year-old senior occupational therapist with 14 years' experience in her field. Initially Sarah worked in a slow-stream rehabilitation hospital for clients with acute brain injury. After that she worked in a day center/short-term stay facility for clients with multiple sclerosis. Sarah currently works on the neurological and neurosurgery wards of an acute care hospital; she has had this job for 5 years. Although she enjoys this work, she states that she is frustrated by how little time she spends with her clients before they are discharged. Sarah says that ideally she would like to return to work in a rehabilitation hospital. She is currently doing some research in the assessment of unilateral neglect.

   Sarah states that she uses a variety of models to guide her work with clients in this field. However, on further discussion it seems that Sarah prefers to use the Retraining Approach (Averbuch & Katz, 1992) and the Rehabilitation Frame of Reference (Trombly, 1995a) to guide her practice. She states that she always begins therapy with a "bottom-up" approach and addresses underlying skill deficits primarily because she works with clients in an acute phase, in which there is greater potential for recovery of basic skills. Sarah believes that on a client's transfer to rehabilitation, the therapist may then choose to work on a "top-down," or adaptive, approach. In such cases, the therapist may introduce adaptive (or compensatory) strategies when the client is not making progress in therapy and discharge is imminent. She bases her interventions with clients who experience unilateral neglect on the attentional theory of neglect. The remaining section of this chapter outlines the story of Sarah and Alan in occupational therapy.

INTRODUCTION TO ALAN

Alan is a 62-year-old man who has a history of hypertension and stress and anxiety. He was admitted to the emergency department at the hospital with a sudden onset of left face, arm, and leg weakness. A computerized tomography (CT) scan on admission revealed an old right parietal infarct (i.e., stroke) with a possible extension or new infarct in the same area. A CT scan on the tenth day after admission revealed a right parietal infarct. On admission, Alan experienced a mild hemiplegia of the left upper and lower limbs and was able to transfer from his bed to a chair with assistance from one person. At this stage, he was not able to walk. He experienced reduced functional control of his left upper limb because of reduced coordination and a decrease in fine motor skills.

INITIAL INTERVIEW: PROCEDURAL AND INTERACTIVE REASONING

Initially Sarah interviews her clients to better understand who they are and to begin to gather information about their functional abilities. Box 9–1 and Box 9–2 provide descriptions of her first session with Alan.

BOX 9–1. THERAPIST REASONING—INITIAL SESSION

One of my interests is unilateral neglect. When I see a client for the first time after a right hemisphere stroke, I am alert to the possible presence of a neglect. Generally I follow the procedure as outlined in Box 9–2 to determine if the client is experiencing this problem. On the first day after his stroke, I went to see Alan. He was resting in bed when I saw him for this initial assessment. I introduced myself to Alan and explained how I would see him for occupational therapy and what this would involve. As I approached him I had already begun my assessment. I noted that he had turned his head toward the right side and seemed to be lying asymmetrically in the

(continues)

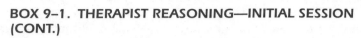

BOX 9–1. THERAPIST REASONING—INITIAL SESSION (CONT.)

bed (i.e., he was lying across the bed rather than in the middle). I pointed this out to him and invited him to assist in straightening himself. Despite having adequate motor skill to do so, he seemed unable to work out how to correct this asymmetry. I had initially approached Alan from his left side but since he seemed unable to maintain his attention to this side, I relocated to the other side of the bed. All this information seemed to suggest to me that Alan might be experiencing unilateral neglect.

Alan seemed drowsy but was able to rouse sufficiently to answer my questions appropriately. I found he was better able to talk to me when I was on his right side. First, I wanted to get an idea of Alan's orientation. This tells me whether he has been following what has happened to him. I found that he was able to indicate that he knew where he was and why he was in the hospital. Next I wanted to find out more about Alan's lifestyle before his hospital admission. This achieves two things: first, I begin to form a picture in my mind about who this client is and what is important to him; second, asking the client about his lifestyle provides me with information about how much he remembers of his life and whether he is a good historian. This is important because if the client cannot provide details on his lifestyle, then I need to get this information from a family member or friend.

Alan told me that he lived with his wife and one of his four adult children. He told me that the family owned a bakery, which he ran in conjunction with his wife and one of his sons. I asked Alan how he liked this work, and he told me how he found work really stressful at the moment and that his financial situation was of concern. I asked him about his ability to manage activities of daily living (ADLs). He told me that he had been independent in all personal ADLs and that his wife had assisted in domestic tasks. Alan reported that he drove a manual-transmission car before his stroke. When I prompted him to talk about his home, Alan told me that he lived in a two-story house. The house is accessed by about five steps at the front and a couple of steps at the back entrance.

Throughout the interview Alan seemed to have a rather flat affect. This, coupled with his past history of work-related anxiety and stress, made me wonder if he was also depressed. I decided to investigate this more in the future. By this stage, Alan seemed to be tiring and was having considerable difficulty maintaining his attention answering questions. I decided to change focus to his physical abilities and give him a rest from answering questions.

BOX 9–2. CONFIRMATION THAT A CLIENT HAS A NEGLECT

1. Referral received for a new client with stroke.

2. I consider the site of the lesion as described in the computed tomography scan or documented in the referral. If certain areas of the brain are lesioned, particularly the right parietal lobe, then I may suspect the presence of unilateral neglect.

3. Next I'll go see the client. I observe his posture and spatial orientation while conducting the initial assessment. In particular, I look at things like how the client responds to where I am (spatial relationships), his or her ability to attend to my questions, and so on. If it appears that the client is neglectful of one side, then I'll conduct a visual confrontation test (described further on in the chapter).

4. After this, I'll observe the client doing an ADL, such as dressing or grooming.

5. At this stage I'm pretty confident about whether he has a neglect or not. If I think he does, I'll do a formal screening assessment to confirm my clinical judgment.

PHYSICAL AND SENSORY EVALUATION

After questioning Alan about his lifestyle, Sarah conducted a brief evaluation of his upper limb function, which revealed normal control of his right arm. His left arm demonstrated full passive and active range of motion; however, strength was reduced. He also demonstrated reduced coordination in fine motor skills and altered sensation. Sarah noted that when she suspects a neglect may be present, it is very important to determine whether or not the client has any visual deficits, particularly because a neglect can mask a visual problem and it is not uncommon for clients to experience both a unilateral neglect and a visual impairment after stroke. A visual confrontation test (Pedretti, 1985; Gainotti, D'Erme, and Bartolomeo, 1991) (Fig. 9–3) and extinction test (as developed by Robertson and cited in Rafal, 1994) (Fig. 9–4) are generally used to determine whether or not a client has a unilateral neglect, homonymous hemianopia (i.e., a defect of either the left or the right half of the visual field), or both. The therapist assessed Alan's visual fields with the visual confrontation test, which indicated that Alan had a left homonymous hemianopia. Table 9–1 outlines some of the clinical differences between unilateral neglect and homonymous hemianopia.

Visual confrontation test (examining for neglect and homonymous hemianopia). The visual confrontation test is a nonstandardized assessment of a person's ability to "see" and "attend" to stimuli in both left and right visual fields. Versions of the assessment have appeared in Pedretti (1985), Zoltan (1996), Gainotti, D'Erme, and Bartolomeo (1991), and Walsh (1994). This assessment can be completed with each eye separately by using an eye patch (Zoltan, 1996).

Description:

In this assessment, the therapist and client sit opposite each other (about 1 yard apart). The client is asked to look directly at the therapist's nose at all times. The therapist holds up both hands about 12 inches from the client at the periphery of his visual field. The therapist points his or her first finger toward the ceiling. Then the therapist brings in a finger on one side and then brings in the other finger on the other side in an arc shape and asks the client to report when he or she can see the finger. The client can indicate when he or she saw a finger either verbally or by pointing. The therapist should do around 3 trials: one at eye level, one in a plane above the client's head, and one in a plane below the client's head.

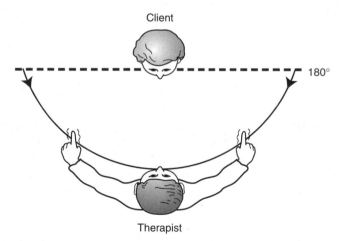

Figure 9–3. Instructions and diagram on how to complete a visual confrontation test.

Extinction test (isolating to determine if extinction of contralesional visual stimuli is present).

The "double simultaneous extinction test" is a nonstandardized assessment of a person's ability to attend to stimuli in both the left and right visual fields at the same time. Similar to the visual confrontation test, versions of this assessment have appeared in Rafal (1994), Gainotti, D'Erme, and Bartolomeo (1991), Zoltan (1996), and Walsh (1994). Advocates of this assessment warn not to assess the client in an area of known visual loss (for example, homonymous hemianopia).

Description:

In this assessment, the therapist and client sit opposite each other. The client is asked to look directly at the therapist's nose at all times. The therapist holds up both hands about 12 inches from the client. The therapist points his or her index fingers of both hands toward the ceiling. Then the therapist wiggles either the index finger on the right, left, or both hands. The client can indicate which finger is wiggling, either verbally or by pointing. The therapist should do around 18 trials in the three levels (midline, upper, and lower quadrants), randomly applying single or double stimulation. Clients are considered to show extinction when at least 3 out of 9 double stimuli are extinguished (Gainotti, D'Erme, & Bartolomeo, 1991).

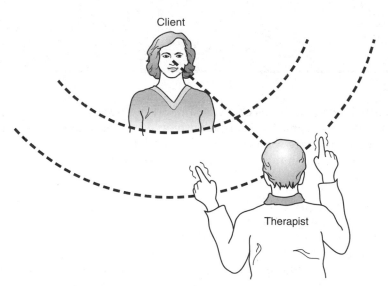

Figure 9–4. Instructions and diagram on how to complete an extinction test.

Table 9–1. Distinguishing between a unilateral neglect and homonymous hemianopia

HOMONYMOUS HEMIANOPIA	UNILATERAL NEGLECT
Sensory base	Attentional or representational base
If client turns his head, information can be seen	If client turns his head, he will still have difficulty attending to information
Client demonstrates insight into visual loss	Client demonstrates little insight into the deficit
Simultaneous extinction not present	Simultaneous extinction may be present
During ADLs, a consistent loss is noted	During ADLs, an inconsistent performance is noted (i.e., responds appropriately to some visual input from the left side)
No evidence of visual processing	May demonstrate some evidence of visual processing
In clinical tests such as star cancellation and line crossing, clients demonstrate evidence of attempts to compensate for their visual loss by scanning. This often results in correct cancellation of targets or line bisection	Evidence of neglect apparent in clinical tests such as star cancellation, line bisection, and line crossing through failure to accurately cancel all targets (particularly those on the contralesional side), and a tendency to bisect lines toward the ipsilesional side (Bradshaw & Mattingly, 1995)

At this stage in his recovery, Alan had not been out of bed, so Sarah concluded the initial evaluation with an explanation about the next occupational therapy session, which would be in the form of a functional ADLs session including showering and dressing.

PERSONAL ACTIVITIES OF DAILY LIVING EVALUATION AND RETRAINING

Sarah saw Alan the day after his initial evaluation to assess his personal ADLs (PADLs). Box 9–3 details Sarah's description of this evaluation session with Alan.

Table 9–2 describes what Sarah did during the showering and dressing assessment and the areas with which Alan had problems. The information in the second column of Table 9–2 discusses Alan's difficulty in

BOX 9–3. THERAPIST REASONING—PADL ASSESSMENT

The next day I saw Alan to assess his PADLs and commence retraining. This involved taking him through the tasks of transferring him out of bed into a shower/commode chair for showering, washing, and drying; grooming (cleaning teeth, shaving, combing hair); and dressing himself. Alan was resting in bed when I arrived to assist with his shower. He was able to transfer himself from lying to sitting on the edge of the bed with supervision only. Alan said he wanted to transfer himself onto the portable shower chair without any help. I explained to him how the stroke affected his mobility. However, he shrugged this off, attributing any weakness to his extended time in bed. I noted that he was possibly denying his problems and suspected that he might have a mild form of anosognosia as well as the neglect. I encouraged him to accept my assistance because I thought he would not safely transfer alone.

completing tasks related to the left side of his body and an overattentiveness to his right side. These observations of Alan during his ADL assessment seem to demonstrate evidence of a unilateral neglect.

Although Sarah chose to use a showering and dressing assessment, a therapist may observe a new client during a number of ADLs to look for signs of neglect and other cognitive and perceptual problems. For example, Table 9–3 provides an overview of some of the observations a therapist may make when a client with neglect is involved in a variety of ADLs. It is important to note that observations listed in Table 9–3 may vary in quality for different clients. As discussed earlier, neglect varies enormously in terms of severity and therefore in the ways it manifests itself. For example, if we take the first ADL observation of the client dressing, the quality of the performance could range as follows:

1. Client neglects to dress left side of body
2. Client dresses ipsilesional (right) side of body and some parts of the contralesional (left) side
3. Client dresses body, but clothing looks untidy on the contralesional (left) side because the shirt is not tucked in, the trousers are all twisted, and the bottom of the trouser leg is tucked into the sock

However, each of these performances may suggest the presence of a unilateral neglect.

As outlined in Box 9–2, after Sarah has observed a client completing ADLs, she often selects and administers one or more standardized

Table 9–2. Showering and dressing assessment tasks and problems experienced by Alan, as reported by the occupational therapist

THERAPIST ACTIONS AND REQUESTS	THERAPIST OBSERVATIONS AND REASONING
I wheeled Alan into the shower area and instructed him to start undressing in preparation for his shower.	Alan removed his hospital gown from his right arm (with a shrugging action of his right arm) and after a prompt from me, removed the gown from his left arm. His inability to spontaneously remove the gown from his left side gave me further reason to suspect a neglect.
I adjusted the water and gave Alan the soap and washcloth.	Alan was able to use his left arm to wash himself; however, he continually dropped the soap or washcloth from this hand. He seemed unaware of this and continued the task until I intervened. I pointed out to him that he had dropped the soap. He began washing his body on the right side and did a thorough job (he seemed to be overattentive to washing on this side). Although he did wash his left side, it was only a minor flick with the washcloth. Again, his overattention to the right side and lack of attention to the left further supported my observation that Alan was experiencing a neglect.
When he finished washing his body, I suggested he turn off the taps.	Alan did this; however, he neglected to turn off the hot water tap on the left side of the pair of faucets.
Alan reached spontaneously for the towel, which was hanging on his right side.	Drying his body produced a similar attentiveness to drying the right side of his body and a cursory wipe to the left leg.
Given that Alan was still in acute care, he was only required to don underclothes and a hospital gown.	Alan had trouble managing his underpants, and I had to assist him in placing his left leg into the correct leg hole. Similarly, he seemed determined to place his right arm in both sleeve holes of the hospital gown. He could not seem to recognize that there was a problem with this.
When he was dressed, I encouraged Alan to attend to his personal grooming tasks.	At first, Alan cleaned his dentures. I noted that he frequently dropped the dentures when he held them in his left hand. He seemed

(continues)

(continued)

Table 9–2. Showering and dressing assessment tasks and problems experienced by Alan, as reported by the occupational therapist	
THERAPIST ACTIONS AND REQUESTS	**THERAPIST OBSERVATIONS AND REASONING**
	unaware that at times the brush was actually connecting with his hand more than with the dentures. Again, Alan did not turn off the hot water tap after brushing his dentures. Alan was unable to replace the dentures in his mouth because he did not allow for the left side of the denture to negotiate the left side of his open mouth. Alan also had difficulty shaving. After shaving the right side of his face, he did shave the left side. However the end result was quite rough and haphazard compared with the right side of his face.
By this stage Alan was tired and anxious to return to bed.	During the transfer back into bed, Alan required more assistance than the initial transfer out of bed, possibly because of his fatigue. He required considerable reinforcement to systematically weight-bear on both legs while standing (tending to favor weight through his right leg).

assessments to confirm her judgments about the nature of the client's problems. (It is important to note that some therapists may prefer to administer standardized assessments *before* observing ADLs to provide direction for their functional assessments.) The next section of this chapter outlines Sarah's reasoning behind the assessments she used with Alan.

SELECTION OF STANDARDIZED ASSESSMENTS

If the therapist suspects that the client has unilateral neglect, visual and somatosensory assessments should be performed in an effort to decide whether deficits in the primary sensory areas are contributing

Table 9–3. Behaviors possibly observed in clients with unilateral spatial or body neglect

MOBILITY

The client . . .

- does not symmetrically weight-bear while standing.
- demonstrates difficulty initiating movement through the left side. For example, the client has greater difficulty transferring to the left rather than the right side.
- bumps into people or objects when walking or wheeling self around.
- does not spontaneously move the affected side of his body even when movement is present during transferring or walking.
- may demonstrate reduced left arm swing when mobilizing.
- does not check the placement of his limbs before transferring.
- has difficulty taking left hand turns.

ADLS

The client . . .

- fails to dress the affected side of his body, or the activity is not completed on the left side (e.g., tucking in shirt on left side).
- does not groom one half of the face.
- ignores food on one side of plate or does not empty food completely out of left side of mouth when eating.
- may complain that he was not given something that was on his affected side (e.g., toiletries beside the wash basin).
- may complete the activity in half of the space available (e.g., may place cookies on only half of the cookie sheet).
- demonstrates difficulty locating objects on shelves or in cupboards.

GENERAL

The client . . .

- demonstrates reduced ability to attend to the task at hand and is highly distracted by tasks, events, and conversation on the ipsilesional side.
- requires prompting to attend to tasks, events, and conversation on the contralesional side.
- fatigues easily.
- fails to respond to people approaching from contralesional side.

(continues)

(continued)

Table 9–3. Behaviors possibly observed in clients with unilateral spatial or body neglect

---

GENERAL

- has poor eye contact with people placed on contralesional side and difficulty establishing and sustaining interaction with people on this side.
- constantly turns head to ipsilesional side and appears to pay excess attention to this side.
- fails to care for the affected side of his body (e.g., may leave arm dangling in wheelchair spokes or lie on arm while in bed). Signs of injury may be visible (e.g., a bruised hand).
- denies affected half of body as being paralyzed or impaired in any way or belonging to self (anosognosia) or fails to recognize body parts or the relationship between body parts (somatoagnosia).
- drops items from affected hand and does not appear to notice (e.g., soap or an eating utensil).
- does not scan environment effectively for hazards (e.g., open overhead cupboards).

---

to the client's poor functional performance. It is particularly important to determine whether or not the client is experiencing homonymous hemianopia, neglect, or both (this assessment and results for Alan were described previously).

There are few standardized assessments of unilateral neglect; however, many cognitive and perceptual assessment batteries contain items to screen for this problem. One assessment that is often used is the Behavioural Inattention Test (BIT) (Wilson, Cockburn, & Halligan, 1987a). In the case study described in this chapter, Sarah chose to conduct some parts of the BIT to confirm that Alan was experiencing a neglect. Although it is generally recommended that therapists use an assessment in its entirety (to preserve standardization), each component of the BIT has been standardized and can therefore be administered alone. Sarah chose to use the following subtests from the BIT (Wilson, Cockburn, & Halligan, 1987a): (1) star cancellation, (2) line crossing, and (3) line bisection. Her reasoning for selecting these three subtests is outlined in Box 9–4.

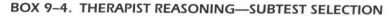

BOX 9–4. THERAPIST REASONING—SUBTEST SELECTION

Although I would like to use all of the BIT, I just find that I don't have time to do it. I find that the most useful parts of this assessment to test for unilateral neglect are the line crossing, line bisection, and star cancellation subtests, so I chose to use these with Alan. These subtests usually confirm quickly and accurately whether or not a client is experiencing a degree of unilateral neglect.

ALAN'S ASSESSMENT RESULTS

Alan's assessments from the BIT line-bisection, line-crossing, and star-cancellation subtests are provided in Figures 9–5, 9–6, and 9–7, respectively. Sarah's observations about Alan's results are presented in Box 9–5.

PRIORITIZED PROBLEM LIST

The findings from Sarah's formal and informal evaluations led to the construction of the following problems list for Alan and Sarah to work on:

1. Reduced attention to the left side of personal, peripersonal, and extrapersonal space (indicating presence of unilateral neglect)
2. Reduced ability to attend to tasks without fatiguing
3. Reduced function and strength of left upper and lower limbs
4. Sensory changes in left upper limb
5. Left homonymous hemianopia
6. Depression, or flat affect

These problems have led to a reduced independence in Alan's current ability to care for himself in the acute care setting and point to future difficulties in engaging in work and leisure activities.

MEDICAL COMPLICATIONS AND A CHANGE IN THERAPY FOCUS

Shortly after Sarah had set these goals to work on with Alan, he experienced a medical complication. For some months before his stroke, Alan had been experiencing chest pain. While resting in his room, he had an episode of severe chest pain, and a mild heart attack was suspected. Al-

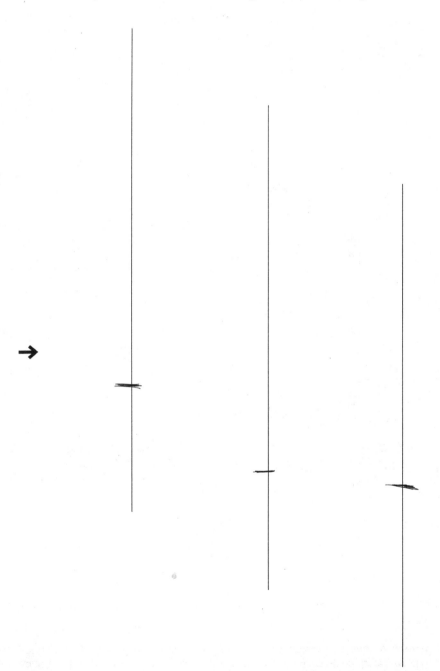

Figure 9–5. Alan's result on the line bisection subtest from the BIT (Wilson, Cockburn, & Halligan, 1987a). (Reprinted with permission from Thames Valley Test Company, Bury St. Edmunds, England.)

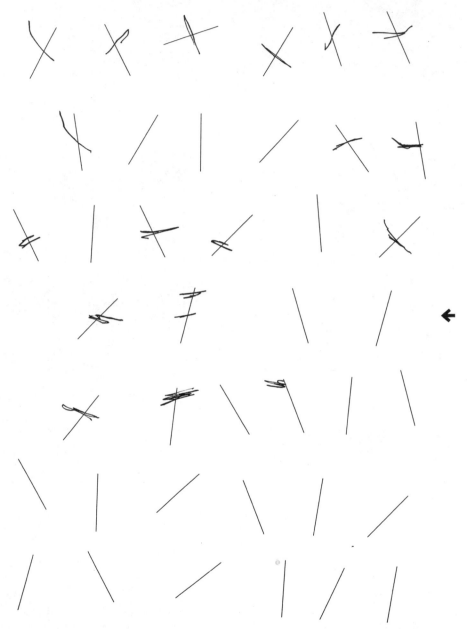

Figure 9–6. Alan's result on the line crossing subtest from the BIT (Wilson, Cockburn, & Halligan, 1987a). (Reprinted with permission from Thames Valley Test Company, Bury St. Edmunds, England.)

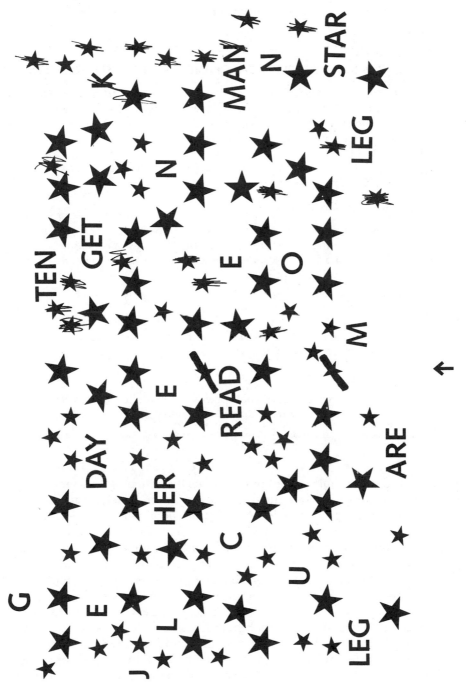

Figure 9–7. Alan's result on the star cancellation subtest from the BIT (Wilson, Cockburn, & Halligan, 1987a). (Reprinted with permission from Thames Valley Test Company, Bury St. Edmunds, England.)

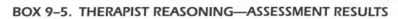

BOX 9–5. THERAPIST REASONING—ASSESSMENT RESULTS

I think it's pretty clear from these three components of the BIT that Alan has a unilateral neglect. It is also interesting to note how he has perseverated in marking the stars and several of the lines on the line-crossing subtest. This overattention to stimuli on the ipsilesional (right) side is quite typical of patients with unilateral neglect. I compared Alan's scores for each of the subtests with the norms provided in the BIT manual (Wilson, Cockburn, & Halligan, 1987a).

1. STAR CANCELLATION

Although there are 54 small stars on the page to be crossed (27 right and 27 left—the two in the center are not scored), Alan was only able to score 18. You can also see how he cancelled one large star and two letters. The acceptable range is 52 to 54.

2. LINE CROSSING

The manual indicates that the maximum score for this test is 36 lines crossed (18 right and 18 left—the four central lines are not scored). Alan scored 16; the acceptable range is 35 to 36.

3. LINE BISECTION

The BIT manual suggests that the acceptable range is 8 to 9 points and the cut-off score for neglect is 7. Alan scored only one point.

though Alan was able to continue with his therapy program, he required further medical tests, treatment, and observation in regard to his heart condition. It was predicted that Alan would remain in the acute care facility for 2 more weeks. At this point, Sarah decided that she would begin a rehabilitation program with Alan that would continue after he was transferred to the nearby rehabilitation facility. Initially Sarah was planning to work with Alan from a more bottom-up perspective to identify his problems and work on remediation-type strategies. Sarah believes this approach works well in acute care and that she is able to provide the occupational therapist at the rehabilitation center with a useful acute care discharge summary. However, given his extended stay, Sarah decided to revise her focus and to include top-down functional and adaptive (or compensatory) activities as part of the total therapy program. Sarah envisioned this program continuing in the rehabilitation facility, which is affiliated with the acute care center.

GOAL SETTING WITH ALAN

The therapist's long-term goal was for Alan to return home; to manage his PADLs; walk safely; and perform simple instrumental daily living activities (IADLs), such as meal preparation, making phone calls, and simple home maintenance. In order to achieve this, Sarah wanted to facilitate improvement in Alan's attention (to be able to maintain attention, disengage from a right-sided stimulus, shift attention, and engage with a left-sided stimulus) and for Alan to develop an awareness of the existence of the left side of personal, peripersonal, and extrapersonal space (Box 9–6). The following short-term objective was devised to be attained in one intervention session. This objective is written in the "who, given what, does what, how well, by when" format discussed in Chapter 3.

> **Who:** Alan
> **Given what:** Given opportunities to attend to objects in his left hemispace, verbal prompts from the therapist, the use of his left hand during the activity (to activate motor circuits), and compensatory devices such as a chopping board with stabilizers
> **Does what:** Will be able to safely prepare a simple lunch consisting of a sandwich and hot drink
> **How well:** That is both nutritious and tasty
> **By when:** During the course of a 1-hour therapy session

BOX 9–6. THERAPIST REASONING—GOAL SETTING

I think Alan needs to be able to perceive and act on information from both the left and right sides equally. Only then can he possibly achieve a degree of independence in PADLs and mobility. The majority of Alan's PADLs and mobility dysfunction is symptomatic of his underlying lateralized spatial and attentional disorder. Intervention needs to be addressed by treating both the underlying dysfunction and then when as much success has been achieved as possible with this remediation approach, to intervene at a symptom level. By this I mean we will introduce some adaptive strategies to overcome difficulties in ADLs. Before Alan can begin to benefit from any intervention strategy he has to have the capacity to attend to the intervention process. He has to have sufficient spatially representative knowledge of his own body and the space around him. I think that achievement of both these goals must be uppermost in the mind of the therapist.

INTERVENTION

PATTERNS OF RECOVERY

Studies based on the rehabilitation of unilateral neglect have established that over time, some clients may show improvement in their ability to redirect attention to the contralesional side (Weinberg et al., 1977). In addition, clients with chronic neglect can learn task-specific compensatory **scanning** responses. Although the client may learn to redirect attention to the contralesional side in automatic, learned, familiar tasks, the underlying asymmetry is often revealed when the client is presented with a novel or complicated task (Lennon, 1994; Robertson, 1994). The severity of neglect may resolve over time; however, the phenomenon of extinction may be more subtle and resilient to intervention (Robertson & Eglin, 1993). For example, a client with neglect may learn to attend to both sides of the plate when eating a meal, with no apparent rivalry between left and right sides. However, if the same client is asked to cross a busy road with traffic approaching from both sides, the ipsilesional bias in attention may reemerge with potentially catastrophic results because the client may only attend to traffic on the right side.

SELECTING INTERVENTION STRATEGIES

Remediation, adaptive (or compensatory), and education strategies all form the basis of intervention with clients who have neglect. Each of these approaches was used with Alan and is discussed Box 9–7. Sarah talks about how she selects intervention approaches to use with clients who have neglect.

BOX 9–7. THERAPIST REASONING—SELECTING INTERVENTION STRATEGIES

When considering the selection of intervention strategies I need to decide if I'll follow a remediation (or restitution) approach or an adaptive (or compensatory) approach. I generally find a mix of both approaches to be useful, particularly because I constantly review and check the client's progress and alter intervention as appropriate. For example, if a client clearly is unable to feed himself without external structure, then it is appropriate to instigate compensatory tools such as highlights (colors) on the left side of his plate. Educating the client and his family about neglect is really important. Often caregivers get very frustrated with their relative's inability to correctly complete a task when it appears to them that he should be able to do it.

Remediation

Table 9–4 provides an outline of strategies and interventions that may be considered appropriate when pursuing the remediation of function approach with clients who have unilateral neglect. In Table 9–4 , a *strategy* may be defined as an approach to assist the client to engage in the activity. On the other hand, an *intervention* may be defined as the activities and approaches used to implement the strategy during interven-

Table 9–4. Intervention strategies and intervention ideas for clients with neglect

STRATEGY	INTERVENTION
Use generalized attentional training (i.e., training client to gain voluntary control over previously automatic functions to be able to attend (engage), shift attention (disengage), and reengage attention).	Work within attentional limits. Be mindful that these clients will fatigue and be easily distracted by items and events on the right side. Initially modify the environment to decrease the distractions, then gradually increase the complexity of the task. Use functional activity whenever possible (i.e., shaving, dressing, reading recipe, scanning a cupboard). Encourage visual tracking across midline and to the left. If attention wanes, use verbal prompts to redirect attention to the task at hand.
Use perceptual "anchoring" (i.e., place and find left arm at edge of an activity client is involved in) (Robertson, North, & Geggie, 1992).	Use PADL tasks such as shaving and bathing. Teach client to start activity with perceptual anchor and then go onto left side of body. Place left arm next to food while eating.
Use contralesional limb movement to increase attention to the left. (Note: using both right and left limbs together may reduce the positive effect of increased attention to the left. Bilateral activities may inhibit the latent function of the damaged hemisphere.) (Robertson, North, & Geggie, 1992; Robertson & North, 1993)	Contralesional limb movements before or during a task. Encourage movement in the left hemispace. Use what little movement is available in the hemiplegic limb.

tion. The remediation approach with clients who have neglect has been widely reported by Robertson and North (1993); Robertson, North, and Geggie (1992); and Robertson et al. (1995) and is based on the theoretical work of Posner and Peterson (1990). The fundamental premise of this approach is that by improving sustained attention, there may also be an associated reduction in unilateral neglect (Robertson et al., 1995). Treatment aims at improving a client's ability to self-alert and sustain attention. Remediation includes the technique discussed earlier in which increasing activation of motor circuits on the contralesional side is believed to produce increased attention to this side. Although it is understood that unilateral neglect is often accompanied by a dense left hemiplegia, even the use of gross motor skills, such as shoulder elevation, is of potential benefit.

Adaptation (or Compensation)

As described in Chapter 1, adaptive approaches involve teaching the client strategies to overcome the effects of his or her disability and adjustments to the environment so that the client can be as independent as possible. A range of adaptive strategies may be taught to the client with neglect; these include:

- Placing a red ribbon on the left margin of reading material to ensure the client always starts the line from the marker
- Directing as much information to the client as possible from the right side
- Using techniques to "pattern" attention to the left; this involves teaching the client to begin scanning to the left side by first locating the left arm at the left side of the task, thus using the arm as a **perceptual anchor** (Robertson, North, & Geggie, 1992)

Adaptive strategies often revolve around ensuring that the home environment is safe for those who may have a chronic neglect. For example, an occupational therapist may conduct a home visit and recommend some or all of the following changes:

- Use a temperature guard on hot water taps (if hot tap is on left side)
- Use appliances that automatically switch off (e.g., iron, kettle)
- Use fire screens or guards for fireplace
- Rearrange cupboards, drawers, and wardrobes to promote ease of locating items
- Remove loose rugs and ornaments that are easily knocked over
- Remove hanging baskets of flowers or foliage at the entrance to a house; also be alert to overhead cupboards

- Use a spike board in the kitchen to stabilize food for chopping, which minimizes the need for a client to use his or her left hand
- Rearrange furniture to promote left turns in the house, particularly if the bathroom involves a left turn to enter it

Education

An important factor in determining recovery from neglect is the client's level of insight or awareness into the deficit (Mattingley, 1995); therefore, education is an essential part of any occupational therapy intervention. Clients with unilateral neglect, as well as their families, usually require considerable education and reassurance about the nature of the client's difficulties, the reason for the problems observed, the ways the problems may respond to treatment, and the possible long-term outcomes. Education must also be provided about safety in the home and in the community, making left turns, and protecting the body from injury on the left side, particularly the hand. In particular, it must be made clear to both the client with persistent neglect and his caregivers that the client is not safe to drive a car, motorbike, or bicycle. In cases in which the client has little or no insight into his problems, education and counseling may be more effectively given to the caring relatives instead of the client alone.

OUTLINE OF AN INTERVENTION SESSION

Box 9–8 outlines an intervention session that Sarah undertook with Alan. In this session, Sarah uses both remediation and compensatory strategies to assist Alan in completing the task of making a sandwich and a hot drink. The behavioral objective for this session was outlined earlier in the section on goal setting.

BOX 9–8. THERAPIST REASONING—OUTLINE OF INTERVENTION SESSION

In this session I wanted Alan to work toward independent preparation of a simple meal. When he returns home, I know his wife will be at work during the day, so he needs to be safe and independent in preparing himself a light lunch. Alan and I had spent some time yesterday deciding what to make. I encouraged him to make a simple choice, bearing in mind his reduced attention and increased fatigue level. He chose to make a tomato, cheese, and lettuce sandwich and a cup of coffee. We prepared a list of in-
(continues)

BOX 9–8. THERAPIST REASONING—OUTLINE OF INTERVENTION SESSION (CONT.)

gredients together and I purchased these in readiness for today's session. Before the session I made sure that we would have the occupational therapy kitchen to ourselves. I thought it was important to reduce the distractions as much as possible so that Alan could focus on the task.

To begin the session, I made sure Alan was familiar with the layout of the kitchen and reminded him of the location of food and utensils. Then I explained to Alan that I would observe and intervene when I thought appropriate. I asked Alan to go ahead and make his sandwich and asked what he would do first. Alan replied that he would need to collect all the ingredients from the refrigerator, and he began this task. Alan had considerable difficulty locating some items, especially those on the left side of the refrigerator. After an unsuccessful search for the sandwich ingredients, I encouraged him to use his left hand to locate the ingredients (thus activating motor pathways in order to facilitate increased attention to this side). I find that this remediation approach often works well. He was able to locate most of the items; however, he needed a verbal prompt to locate the cheese and butter on the shelf of the refrigerator door (on his left). He placed all these ingredients on the table in the center of the kitchen. Next he scanned the cupboards and drawers for the necessary utensils. I adopted similar strategies as described above to assist him to locate a cutting board, knife, and plate.

Alan began to make the sandwich by removing the bread from the package. He had some difficulty with this task because his left hand continually let go of one side of the package, making it difficult to remove the bread. After three or four unsuccessful attempts, he clearly did not know what was stopping him. At this point, I prompted him to "look what your hand is doing," and told him, "You may need to change your grip." In this way, I am constantly educating the client about how to successfully complete the activity. Alan carefully observed his left hand and with ongoing verbal prompts was able to successfully obtain two slices of bread. He buttered each slice of bread. I encouraged him to hold the bread steady on the cutting board with his left hand, making sure that he scanned over to his left hand before he began buttering. Therefore, Alan used his left hand as a perceptual anchor. Alan then prepared the sandwich ingredients (tomato, cucumber, lettuce) by washing them first at the sink. He failed to notice that he did not turn the left tap off and required a verbal prompt to do this.

While he was cutting the tomatoes, I observed how closely Alan placed his stabilizing left hand to the cutting edge of the knife, and I was concerned about his cutting his left hand. I pointed out this safety issue and suggested he distance his fingers from the knife. At first he was able to do this, but then again his fingers crept back toward the cutting edge of the

(continues)

BOX 9–8. THERAPIST REASONING—OUTLINE OF INTERVENTION SESSION (CONT.)

knife. I intervened again, instructing him to attend to the position of his left hand. Alan appeared to be tiring at this stage, and I was not surprised given the amount of scanning and attending he had done over the course of the session. At this point to ensure his safety, I provided a vegetable cutting board with prongs to stabilize the vegetables. I used this as a compensatory mechanism to remove the necessity of having his left arm actively involved in the task (and to reduce the danger of his cutting himself). Instead, I encouraged Alan to use his left arm as a perceptual anchor by placing it alongside the left side of the board and scanning to it before cutting each item.

After preparing the sandwich ingredients, Alan placed them on the buttered bread with his left hand (thus encouraging a symmetrical placement and stimulating attention to this side). Alan completed preparation of the sandwich by cutting it in half diagonally. I encouraged him to visually locate both corners of the bread before he made the cut. At this stage Alan was to prepare a hot drink; however, he was obviously fatiguing and his attention was waning. I reinforced the success of all that he had completed during the session and suggested we prepare the drink at a later time.

CLIENT DISCHARGE FROM THERAPY

Alan's medical condition stabilized, and he was discharged to the rehabilitation facility after 17 days in acute care. Mattingley and Fleming (1994) refer to the discussions that surround a client's medical condition and the reports filed in a client's medical record as "chart talk." The discharge report presented in Figure 9–8 was filed by Sarah on Alan's discharge from the acute care facility and is written in chart-talk style.

SUMMARY

This chapter has explored the phenomenon of unilateral neglect: its definition, the kinds of brain damage that may produce this disorder, and the theories that have evolved to assist us in understanding the disorder. The case study of Alan was presented to illustrate the reasoning used by a therapist when assessing and treating a client with neglect. Remediation, compensation, and education intervention strategies used by occupational

OCCUPATIONAL THERAPY REPORT
DISCHARGE/TRANSFER REPORT

To: O.T. Rehabilitation Program - Re: Alan, 62 y.o.

Date of admission: 14/02/xx

Date of discharge: 28/02/xx

PREVIOUS MEDICAL HISTORY: Hypertension, stress, anxiety

SOCIAL HISTORY: Married - has four children, one of which lives with him. Owns family business - bakery. (Alan works with his wife and one of his sons in the business.)

HISTORY OF PRESENTING COMPLAINT: Admitted to the emergency room with a sudden onset of left face, arm and leg weakness. CT scan on admission revealed an old right parietal infarct with a possible extension or new infarct in the same area. CT scan on day 10 confirmed new right parietal infarct.

PREVIOUS LEVEL OF FUNCTION:

Mobility: Independent

Personal ADLs: Independent

Domestic ADLs: Independent

Community ADLs: Independent

Cognition: Independent

CURRENT LEVEL OF FUNCTION:

Balance: Sitting: ✓ (static/dynamic) Standing: Reduced dynamic balance

Transfers: Requires supervision only

Bed mobility: Independent

Mobility: Ambulates ~ 30 meters with standby assistance

Figure 9–8. Alan's discharge summary.

Patient's Last Name:_____ UR No:_____

UPPER LIMB DOMINANCE: right/left   **PRESENCE OF SHOULDER PAIN:**   Yes/No

AFFECTED LIMB: right/left   **TONE:** Increased tone in a flexo-pattern in L UE._____

PROM: Full PROM both upper extremities (UEs)   **Sensation:** N.A.D._____

AROM: Full AROM both UEs . Reduced strength distally in left UE._____

CO-ORDINATION: R arm L arm - reduced (overshoots target)._____

FINE MOTOR SKILLS: R arm L arm - reduced._____

COGNITION:

Orientation: ✓_____

Attention: Reduced. Fatigues easily, distractable._____

STM/LTM: Reduced STM.

Perception: Left unilateral neglect of personal, peripersonal and extrapersonal space._____

Behaviour: Appropriate in therapy sessions. Flat affect._____

Insight: ✓_____

Planning/Problem Solving: ✓_____

Motor Planning/Presence of Dyspraxia: Not observed._____

Communication: Mild dysarthia apparent._____

ADLs	Depend-ent	With Assist	With Aid	With Sup'vision	Independ/ Age Approp	
Eating			✓			
Dressing		✓				
Showering		✓				
Toileting		✓				
Grooming		✓				
Continence:						
Bladder				✓		
Bowel				✓		
Barthel	(Modified)		62/100			

HOME LAYOUT: - Two-storey house

Access - Front: 5 steps (no rail)_____   Rear: 3 steps (no rail)_____

Bathroom: Separate shower stall_____   Toilet: Separate_____

Seating: Lounge and kitchen type chairs_____   Other: _____

EQUIPMENT PROVIDED: None provided as yet.

CONTINUING AIMS/RECOMMENDATIONS:

Alan continues to display a L sided neglect and reduced function of his UE and L/LE. He would benefit from _____
ongoing inpatient rehabilitation to maximise his independence in (P) ADL and mobility._____

Thank you for continuing this person's management.

Please do not hesitate to contact me if you require any further details. **Occupational Therapist**

Figure 9–8. Continued

therapists when working with clients who experience unilateral neglect were discussed.

≡ REVIEW QUESTIONS

1. Damage to which brain areas are thought to produce a unilateral neglect? On what side of the brain (left or right) is damage more likely to produce unilateral neglect?
2. When you suspect that your client has unilateral neglect, what other disorder do you want to assess for to rule out as a possible explanation for the observations you have made? Why? What assessment could you perform?
3. Describe three remediation and three compensatory strategies therapists can use when treating a client with neglect.
4. Plan a 1-hour intervention session in which Alan will prepare a hot drink for lunch. First write a behavioral objective. Then describe the (a) steps involved in making coffee with milk and sugar, (b) problems Alan may have, and (c) treatment strategies you will use with Alan to overcome these problems.

≡ ACKNOWLEDGMENTS

We would like to thank Sally Stevens and Kate Rickard, occupational therapists at Hampton Rehabilitation Hospital, Melbourne, Australia, for providing the case notes that assisted with developing the case study of "Alan."

10

Evaluation and Intervention with Complex Perceptual Impairment

GUDRÚN ÁRNADÓTTIR, MA, BOT

- Anosognosia
- Apraxia
- Body Scheme
- Constructional Abilities
- Depth Perception
- Figure/Ground Discrimination
- Finger Agnosia

- Form Discrimination
- Right/Left Discrimination
- Somatoagnosia
- Spatial Relations
- Topographical Orientation
- Unilateral Neglect (Spatial and Body)
- Visuospatial Disorders

On completion of this chapter, the reader will be able to:

- Define complex perception including visuospatial disorders and body scheme disorders
- Describe the anatomical basis for visuospatial disorders and body scheme disorders
- Describe at least three standardized assessments to screen for the disorders
- Describe at least three treatment techniques that a therapist can use to treat a client who has complex perceptual disorders
- Successfully work through the Review Questions

≡ INTRODUCTION

The purpose of this chapter is to present the reasoning behind assessment and intervention with client who experienced a cerebrovascular accident (CVA) resulting in impairments, some of which can be classified as complex perceptual disorders. In the literature, there are various classifications of impairments that can be related to complex perceptual disorders, and the conceptual definitions of these differ. The classification used in this textbook assigns disorders of visuospatial and body scheme components to complex perceptual disorders. The chapter further provides definitions of complex perceptual disorders and the neuroanatomical basis for them.

Occupational performance is the ability of an individual to accomplish tasks required by his or her role within a given context. *Performance components* are functional elements necessary for task performance. *Impairments* are dysfunction of performance components. In order to discuss dysfunction of performance components such as various visuospatial impairments, the necessary components for task performance are reviewed and related to central nervous system (CNS) function. The case of Mr. H, who sustained a right CVA, is presented together with the reasoning behind his occupational therapy intervention. The theoretical approach taken in working with Mr. H is outlined. The approach used for assessing Mr. H and gathering information for problem resolution is based on the factor-relating theory behind the A-ONE (Activities of Daily Living Neurobehavioral Evaluation) (Árnadóttir, 1990). The theory provides guidance regarding the ways neurobehavior relates to activities of daily living (ADLs) and can easily be matched with options for intervention, depending on the therapist's beliefs. The instrument used to evaluate Mr. H, the A-ONE, is described. The A-ONE simultaneously evaluates ADL performance and neurobehavioral impairments that interfere with independent task performance. Based on assessment results, choices for intervention and reasoning for these are outlined. Finally, an example of an intervention session and discharge recommendations for this client are provided.

WHAT ARE COMPLEX PERCEPTUAL DISORDERS?

Complex perceptual functions take place in the tertiary functional area of the cortex located in the inferior part of the parietal lobe. This area combines and integrates sensory information from more than one of the three posterior lobes (i.e., parietal, occipital, and temporal) into complex functions. Because the function of this area is complex, it can be difficult to analyze in terms of input, output, and intrinsic organization. It includes processing of visuospatial information, body scheme, and complex forms of gnosis, which in cases of dysfunction can lead to **anosognosia** and **somatoagnosia** (both of which can also be viewed in relation to body scheme disorders) as well as praxis. This chapter focuses on visuospatial functioning and body scheme. *Visuospatial abilities* are the abilities to relate objects to each other or to the self. This includes the following components: spatial perceptions, object relationships (sometimes combined and referred to as **spatial relations**), **constructional abilities**, **figure/ground discrimination**, **form discrimination**, **depth perception**, unilateral spatial attention, and **topographical orientation**.

Body scheme abilities are perceptions of body position, including and involving the relationship of body parts to each other. **Body scheme** is dependent on information from somesthetic sources, attention, memory, visual information, and language. It is necessary to have comprehension and be able to use words such as "left" and "right," as well as words referring to the naming of the different fingers. Visuospatial information is needed for relating body parts to each other as well as limiting the boundaries between different body parts and different persons. It is also needed for relating body parts and positions to the external space (Árnadóttir, 1998; Zoltan, 1996). Chapter 7 presents more detailed information on praxis and **apraxia**, and Chapter 8 presents further information on the simple, or "pure," forms of gnosis and agnosia (i.e., those related to secondary association areas of the cerebral cortex).

Visuospatial disorders, also referred to as *spatial-relations disorders*, have been conceptually defined as difficulties relating objects to each other or to the self. This may include difficulties with figure/ground discrimination, depth and distance perception, perception of form discrimination, perception of position in space, or constructional deficits (Árnadóttir, 1998). Benton and Tranel (1993) differentiate between visuoperceptual, visuospatial, and visuoconstructive dysfunctions. Table 10–1 provides conceptual definitions and anatomical location for performance components dysfunction, or impairments related to the complex perceptual disorders.

Body scheme disorders have been conceptually defined as perceptual deficits regarding one's own postural model. Body scheme disorders are defined as "defective perception of body position, including and involving the relation of body parts to each other" (Árnadóttir, 1998, p. 308). Body scheme disorders are usually related to dysfunction in the inferior parietal lobe and include anosognosia, finger agnosia, difficulties with **right/left discrimination** of body sides, unilateral body neglect, and somatoagnosia (Árnadóttir, 1998).

Occupational therapists are concerned with the task performance of their clients. The foundation of task performance is based on the function of the CNS. Different tasks require different types of performance components. The *Uniform Terminology for Occupational Therapy*, third edition (AOTA 1994a, 1994b), classifies occupational performance into three groups: performance components, performance areas, and performance contexts. The group of performance components can be further subdivided into three groups: (1) sensorimotor components, (2) cognitive integration and cognitive components, and (3) psychosocial skills and psychological components. According to Árnadóttir (1990, 1998) the "performance components are based on neurological function, which takes place at different levels of the central nervous system" (p. 293). Therefore, the different performance components can be related to functional areas of the brain responsible for different neurological-processing functions. Furthermore, "during activity performance different types of processing mechanisms may also be taking place simultaneously" (p. 293). Neuronal processing within the brain varies in complexity (see Árnadóttir, 1990, for more detailed information on the functional organization of the cerebral cortex). Although certain functions can be assigned

Table 10–1. Conceptual definitions of complex perceptual impairments and their anatomical locations

IMPAIRMENT	DEFINITION	ANATOMICAL LOCATION
VISUOPERCEPTUAL		
Figure ground disorders (visual analysis and synthesis)	Trouble differentiating the foreground from the background. The foreground is a part of the field of perception that is the center of attention (Zoltan, 1996)	Parieto-occipital lesions of the right hemisphere and less frequently the left hemisphere (Benton & Tranel, 1993)
Form discrimination	Inability to distinguish between different types of forms (Zoltan, 1996)	Different cortical regions (Zoltan, 1996)
VISUOSPATIAL		
Defective judgment of depth and distance	Misjudges depth and distances (Zoltan, 1996)	Posterior right hemisphere lesions; superior visual association cortices; bilateral or right-sided lesions (Benton & Tranel, 1993)
Spatial relations disorders	Difficulties in relating objects to each other or to the self (Árnadóttir, 1990; Zoltan, 1996)	Inferior parietal lobe lesions or parieto-occipital-temporal lesions, usually of the right side (Árnadóttir, 1990; Luria, 1973)
Topographical disorientation	Difficulty finding one's way in space as a result of amnestic or agnostic problems; it manifests in problems with finding one's way in familiar surroundings or in learning new routes (Árnadóttir, 1990)	Inferior parietal lobule or occipital association cortex; occipito-temporal cortex, particularly on the right side; bilateral parietal lesions are also possible as well as occasional left-sided parietal lesions (Benton & Tranel, 1993; Walsh, 1994)

(continues)

Table 10–1. Conceptual definitions of complex perceptual impairments and their anatomical locations

IMPAIRMENT	DEFINITION	ANATOMICAL LOCATION
VISUOSPATIAL		
Unilateral spatial neglect	Inattention to or neglect of stimuli presented in the extrapersonal space of the side contralateral to a cerebral lesion as a result of visual perceptual deficits or impaired attention (Heilman et al., 1993) (see Chapter 10 for more detailed discussion of neglect)	Inferior parietal lobule, right cingulate gyrus, and prefrontal cortex, reticular formation, specific sensory thalamic nuclei, and posterior internal capsule
BODY SCHEME		
Somatoagnosia	A disorder of body scheme; diminished awareness of body structure and the failure to recognize one's body parts and their relationship to each other (Zoltan, 1996); clients with this disorder also have difficulties relating their bodies to objects in the external environment (Árnadóttir, 1990)	Right inferior parietal lobe; left-sided lesions have also been reported (Árnadóttir, 1990)
Defective right/left discrimination	A lack of ability to discriminate between right and left body sides or to apply the concepts of left and right to the external environment; the impairment is composed of several factors, including a verbal component, nonverbal component of tactile	Right-sided lesions, usually inferior parietal lobe; could also be left temporal or parietal lobe dysfunction (Árnadóttir, 1990, 1998; Benton & Sivan, 1993)

(continues)

Table 10–1. Conceptual definitions of complex perceptual impairments and their anatomical locations

IMPAIRMENT	DEFINITION	ANATOMICAL LOCATION
BODY SCHEME	sensory discrimination and stimuli location as well as spatial relations and visuo-spatial components (Árnadóttir, 1990, 1998; Benton & Sivan, 1993)	Left- or right-sided lesions depending on dysfunctional components, particularly parieto-temporal occipital junction (Árnadóttir, 1990; Benton & Sivan, 1993)
Finger agnosia	Impaired ability to identify the fingers of one's own hand or those of another person. The impairment affects both the ability to name the fingers and knowledge of which one was touched; it is a collective term for diverse types of defective performances in finger identification, depending on type of stimuli (verbal, visual, tactile) as well as the type of response (Zoltan, 1996; Benton & Sivan, 1993)	
Unilateral body neglect	Failure to report, respond, or orient to a unilateral stimulus presented to the body side contralateral to a cerebral lesion; it can be a result of either defective sensory processing or attention deficit, resulting in ignorance or impaired use of the extremities; it usually occurs toward the left body	Inferior parietal lobule, right cingulate gyrus, and prefrontal cortex, reticular formation, specific sensory thalamic nuclei, and posterior internal capsule (Árnadóttir, 1990, 1998; Heilman et al., 1993; Heilman & Van Den Abell, 1980)

(continues)

(continued)

Table 10–1. Conceptual definitions of complex perceptual impairments and their anatomical locations

IMPAIRMENT	DEFINITION	ANATOMICAL LOCATION
BODY SCHEME		
Anosognosia	side (Árnadóttir, 1990, 1998; Heilman et al., 1993; Heilman & Van Den Abell, 1980) A person's denial of a paretic extremity as his or hers accompanied by lack of insight with regard to the paralysis; the person may refer to paralyzed extremities as objects or may perceive the extremities out of proportion to other body parts (Árnadóttir, 1990, 1998)	Right inferior parietal lobule; specifically sensory thalamic nuclei, reticular formation, basal ganglia; prefrontal and premotor frontal lobe (Starkstein & Robinson, 1994)

to specific lobes, several CNS areas frequently contribute to the processing of particular performance components. Several different processing models indicating processing sites of different functions within the cortex have been constructed (Árnadóttir, 1990, 1998). An example of these models is the processing of visuospatial information.

Visuospatial Processing

Visuospatial processing, the processing of visual stimuli and spatial information within the CNS, depends on visual information and involves many different cerebral areas. These include the primary visual cortex, the visual association cortex, the frontal eye fields, the dorsolateral prefrontal cortex, and the limbic cortex. Visual information from the left visual hemi-field travels through the visual pathway to the right primary visual cortex in the occipital lobe and visa versa. From the primary visual cortex on either side of the calcarine fissure, information travels to the visual association cortex in each hemisphere. Whereas the secondary association cortex is within the occipital lobe on either side of the primary visual cortex, the tertiary cortex is mainly situated in the inferior parietal lobe, which combines and processes information from all three posterior lobes (i.e., somesthetic information from the parietal lobe, auditory information from the temporal lobe, and visual information from the occipital lobe). Information is integrated with previous information in the visual association areas, and visual memory traces are formed.

Two major intercortical visual pathways have been proposed for processing different aspects of visual stimuli. One pathway runs from the primary visual cortex to the inferior temporal lobe and is sometimes called the *inferior occipitotemporal pathway*; it is involved in object recognition, including perception of form, color, and size. The other pathway runs from the primary visual area to the posterior parietal lobe; this pathway has been termed the *occipital parietal pathway* and is involved in attention to stimulus components, perception of movement, and appreciation of spatial relationships (e.g., object location in space and object relation to other objects and to one's own body). The two pathways are connected at different levels, providing a basis for almost endless analysis of vision (Árnadóttir, 1990; Benton & Tranel, 1993; Kandel, 1985; Warren, 1994).

The frontal eye fields in the premotor cortex are involved in directing the eyes toward a stimulus, and the limbic and prefrontal cortical areas are important in attending to visual information. There are two routes for visual information and visual attention to reach the cortex. One is from the reticular activating system (RAS) through the lateral geniculate body in the thalamus to the primary visual cortex and then to the visual association cortex. The other route is from the RAS through the limbic system, which activates the entire cortex and prepares it for stimulus arrival. This route further activates the prefrontal cortex, which is important in determining, for example, whether to attend to information arriving in the visual cortex or not. Thus, the limbic system influence is important in determining the significance of the stimulus and the needs of the individual, which play a role in goal-directed behavior. The limbic system provides emotional meaning to visual information and thereby influences motivation (Árnadóttir, 1990, 1998; Heilman & Van Den Abell, 1980; Heilman, Watson, & Valenstein, 1993; Warren, 1994). One set of these attention pathways (including both the route through the specific thalamic nuclei to the sensory cortex and the route going through the limbic system to the cortex) reaches each hemisphere; the pathway reaching the right hemisphere is dominant. If there is a lesion in the left hemisphere, the right hemisphere, which attends to bilateral visual information, can still attend to information arriving from the right visual field. The left hemisphere, on the other hand, only attends to information coming from the right visual field and therefore cannot compensate for dysfunction of the right hemisphere in attending to stimuli from the left (Árnadóttir, 1990; Heilman & Van Den Abell, 1980). Figure 10–1 depicts the visuospatial processing pathway. In the figure, information enters the primary visual cortex and is further processed by the association cortex. There are two intercortical visual pathways, the inferior occipitotemporal pathway and occipital parietal pathway. These pathways process different aspects of visual stimuli. The frontal eye fields are important in directing the eyes toward a stimulus and the cingulate gyrus and the prefrontal cortex play roles in visual attention.

In addition to visuospatial processing, the visual system assists the somesthetic system in formation of the visuokinesthetic motor engrams, which are memory molecules for movement. Therefore, the visual system also affects motor learning and praxis, and visual feedback also affects motor control. Furthermore, there are spatial components to movement (Árnadóttir, 1990; Heilman & Gonzalez-Rothi, 1993; Warren, 1994).

Warren (1994) refers to two approaches for viewing the visual system. The first approach refers to the ability to see objects and includes components such as visual acuity, visual fields, and oculomotor control. The second approach, which is often adopted by occupational therapists, includes visual closure, figure/ground discrimination, form constancy, spatial relations, and position in space. Warren further discusses a hierarchy of visual skills in which visual cognition is dependent on underlying skills, such as visual acuity, visual fields, visual attention, pattern recognition, and memory.

Benton and Tranel (1993), on the other hand, recognize that there has always been controversy regarding the nature of agnostic disorders, including

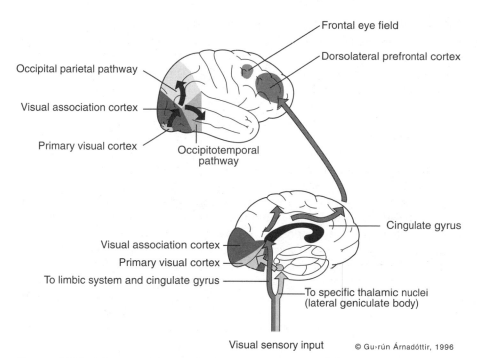

Frontal eye field

Dorsolateral prefrontal cortex

Occipital parietal pathway

Visual association cortex

Primary visual cortex

Occipitotemporal
pathway

Cingulate gyrus

Visual association cortex

Primary visual cortex

To limbic system and cingulate gyrus

To specific thalamic nuclei
(lateral geniculate body)

Visual sensory input   © Gu·rún Árnadóttir, 1996

Figure 10–1. Visuospatial processing pathway. (From Árnadóttir, A-ONE course notes, 1996, with permission from author.)

visual-processing disorders. They propose that some definitions in the literature claim that there is adequate sensation but that perceptual-integrative (i.e., apperceptive agnosia) or associative processes (i.e., associative agnosia) are impaired. Other definitions claim that the disorders occur as a result of sensory defects and incomplete information on which to base perceptual recognition. According to these authors, there are problems with both classifications because there is no way to clearly distinguish between perception (i.e., higher-order processing) and recognition (i.e., basic deficits pertaining to form, color, and texture).

Processing During Task Performance and Possible Lesion Sites

The pathway involved in the processing of visuospatial information (as described previously) is only one type of performance component that can be related to neurobehavior. Performance of different tasks or activities requires several different performance components. The type of component and the degree of involvement depend on the particular task to be performed. As mentioned previously, activities of several processing mechanisms may be simultaneously involved for performance of function. This has been demonstrated by Árnadóttir (1990, 1998) through her analysis of an activity such as the dressing task of putting on a shirt (Fig. 10–2). In the figure, different types of sensory information regarding the task reach the cortex by different routes, resulting in simultaneous processing of different information. Sensory information arrives in primary sensory areas for the different sensations and is subsequently processed further by the appropriate association areas. Sensory information is integrated with previous experiences. Attention is necessary and memories are brought into play, along with ideation, resulting in the subject getting the idea that he is to put on the shirt. Responses include thoughts related to how the shirt should turn, emotional responses, motivation processes, and motor planning as well as motor execution, in which the man grabs the shirt and puts it on. A series of feedback movement interactions and readjustments follow in combination with manipulation of the shirt. These are based on continuous sensory information from the activity. An example of this would be the spatial perceptual and visual analysis regarding which parts of the garment are the sleeves, what is the top and the bottom of the shirt, and what is the inside and outside of the garment. The task performance that is the result of this kind of processing can reveal substantial information regarding function and subsequently dysfunction of the cerebral cortex. See Árnadóttir (1990) for details on the different processing models.

According to Figure 10–2, the CNS works in a holistic way—a number of parallel-processing mechanisms may contribute to the same function. Therefore, it is not possible to consider one performance component without paying attention to how it is influenced by and influences other components. The concept of spatial relations, for example, is formed by visual, tactile, auditory, and even vestibular information but requires the attention mechanism, memory functions, and often motor output for manipulation of objects to gather further information.

A lesion affecting the visuospatial processing pathway (e.g., in the inferior part of the parietal lobe in the right hemisphere) may result in dysfunction of spatial relations and subsequent problems in, for example, aligning buttons; figuring out which side of the shirt is the front and which is the back and which armhole is for the right arm and which one for the left; or difficulties perceiving whether the arm went through the armhole or the neck hole.

The processing model outlined in Figure 10–2 indicates that a lesion in several cortical areas may affect visuospatial processing, although the most common lesion site is the inferior parietal lobe of the right hemisphere. However, it should be kept in mind that this area processes information

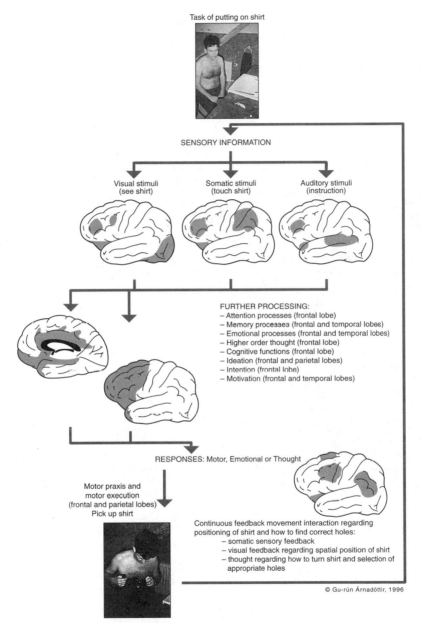

Task of putting on shirt

SENSORY INFORMATION

Visual stimuli
(see shirt)

Somatic stimuli
(touch shirt)

Auditory stimuli
(instruction)

FURTHER PROCESSING:
– Attention processes (frontal lobe)
– Memory processes (frontal and temporal lobes)
– Emotional processes (frontal and temporal lobes)
– Higher order thought (frontal lobe)
– Cognitive functions (frontal lobe)
– Ideation (frontal and parietal lobes)
– Intention (frontal lobe)
– Motivation (frontal and temporal lobes)

RESPONSES: Motor, Emotional or Thought

Motor praxis and
motor execution
(frontal and parietal lobes)
Pick up shirt

Continuous feedback movement interaction regarding
positioning of shirt and how to find correct holes:
– somatic sensory feedback
– visual feedback regarding spatial position of shirt
– thought regarding how to turn shirt and selection of
appropriate holes

© Gu·rún Árnadóttir, 1996

Figure 10–2. Processing during performance of the task of putting on a shirt. (From Árnadóttir, A-ONE course notes, 1996, with permission from author.)

from the occipital lobes as well as the parietal and temporal lobes and thus is dependent on the processing taking place in these areas. It is also dependent on frontal lobe functions, such as the frontal eye fields, attention processes, and, in some instances, memory and cognitive processes. Table 10–2 provides the terminology used in this chapter to refer to components

Table 10–2. Complex perception: Components and impairments matched with items on the A-ONE

COMPONENTS	IMPAIRMENTS	ITEM NAMES ON THE A-ONE
PRAXIS		
Ideational praxis: concept formation	Ideational apraxia	Ideational apraxia
Ideomotor praxis: planning, programming, sequencing and timing of movement	Ideomotor apraxia	Motor apraxia
Motor components		
Somatosensory components		
Memory components (visuokinesthetic motor engrams)		
Spatial components of movement		
Visuospatial components	Constructional deficits	
BODY SCHEME		
Somesthetic components	Finger agnosia	
Attention components	Impaired right/left discrimination	Impaired right/left discrimination
Memory components	Unilateral body neglect	Unilateral body neglect
Visuospatial components (relating body parts to each other and the external space)	Anosognosia	Anosognosia
	Somatoagnosia	Somatoagnosia
Language (related to body parts and the concepts of right and left)		

(continues)

(continued)

Table 10–2. Complex perception: Components and impairments matched with items on the A-ONE

COMPONENTS	IMPAIRMENTS	ITEM NAMES ON THE A-ONE
SPATIAL RELATIONS		
Spatial relations (including spatial perceptions and object relationships)	Spatial relations impairment, including difficulties with:	Spatial relations impairment including visual spatial agnosia
Figure/ground discrimination	● Figure ground discrimination	
Depth and distance perception	● Depth and distance discrimination	
Form discrimination	● Form discrimination	
Perception of position in space	● Perception of position in space	
Constructional abilities	● Constructional deficits	
Visual attention	● Unilateral spatial neglect	Unilateral spatial neglect
Topographical orientation	● Topographical disorientation	Topographical disorientation

of complex perception and impairments and corresponding items assessed using the A-ONE (Árnadóttir, 1990).

Evaluation of Visuospatial Disorders

The traditional way of evaluating visuospatial disorders is by using the deficit-specific approach, also referred to as the *bottom-up approach*. Many of these assessments have been borrowed by occupational therapists from the disciplines of neurology or neuropsychology (Árnadóttir, 1990). Similarly, items on many deficit-specific tests developed by occupational therapists have been borrowed from the same sources. Recently, many authors within occupational therapy have emphasized the importance of focusing on task performance or occupational functioning when assessing clients rather than their impairments. They have also emphasized the importance of developing standardized tests that relate occupational performance to components of task performance (Árnadóttir, 1990, 1998; Christiansen, 1993; Fisher & Short de Graf, 1993; Holm & Rogers, 1989; Mathiowetz, 1993; Trombly, 1993). Table 10–3 provides examples of deficit-specific tests and assessments of occupational functioning used by occupational therapists to evaluate complex perceptual disorders.

Rehabilitation interventions for complex perceptual disorders reported in the literature (Brockmann Rubio, 1998; Neistadt, 1990, 1994c; Toglia; 1991; Zoltan, 1996) include both bottom-up approaches (also called *remedial* or *restorative approaches*), which focus on the impairments, and top-down approaches (also referred to as *adaptive approaches*), which focus on environmental adaptation to improve task performance. Restorative approaches require learning capacity and are generally more time consuming than adaptive approaches (Brockmann Rubio, 1998). This needs to be kept in mind because cuts in funding for rehabilitation are common, resulting in shorter hospital stays. Toglia (1991) describes transfer of learning as a phenomenon that ranges through four levels, from near transfer (i.e., transfer over to very similar tasks, in which only one or two surface characteristics have been changed) to very far transfer (i.e., spontaneous application of the things that have been learned in remedial treatment over to everyday functioning, or generalization). The intermediate level and the far level of transfer refer to increasing numbers of surface characteristics that are changed. Research with brain-injured individuals indicates that this population may only be able to transfer from perceptual retraining to very similar tasks in 5 to 6 weeks of intervention (Neistadt, 1994c). Whereas the adaptive approaches place little (near or intermediate transfer) or no requirement on transfer of learning, remedial approaches have traditionally assumed that transfer of training from tabletop activities or sensorimotor exercises to functional performance does take place. However, this is only true for individuals who have insight into their own capacities, and lack of insight or awareness is a frequent problem for individuals with cortical dysfunction (Toglia, 1992b; Neistadt, 1994c). This ability to transfer learning should be considered when choosing intervention methods. Abreu et al. (1994) have described a "new functional approach" in cognitive rehabilitation. This is a factor-relating theory (as is the A-ONE theory, mentioned earlier) that recognizes a relationship between bottom-up and top-down levels of occupational performance. This approach uses the tasks that are most appropriate to the individual according to set goals. The tasks are presented so that cognitive performance components are "appropriately engaged and challenged." As Brockmann Rubio (1998) pointed out, although the intervention may be focused on performance components, the intervention modality is always daily occupation. According to Abreu et al. (1994), this

Table 10–3. Examples of evaluations used to detect complex perceptual impairments

ASSESSMENT	SOURCE	TYPE
VISUOPERCEPTUAL IMPAIRMENTS		
FIGURE/GROUND		
Overlapping figures subtest of the LOTCA	Katz et al., 1989	Bottom-up approach, deficit-specific testing
Sensory integration and praxis tests: Figure/Ground Visual Perception Test	Ayres, 1989; Zoltan, 1996	Bottom-up approach, deficit-specific testing
The embedded-figure test	Spreen & Benton, 1969; Spreen & Strauss, 1991	Bottom-up approach, deficit-specific testing
Hooper visual organization test	Hooper, 1983	Bottom-up approach, deficit-specific testing
VISUOSPATIAL IMPAIRMENTS		
SPATIAL RELATIONS		
Sensory integration and praxis tests: space visualization	Ayres, 1989; Zoltan, 1996	Bottom-up approach, deficit-specific testing
A-ONE	Árnadóttir, 1990	Top-down approach
TOPOGRAPHICAL DISORIENTATION		
Functional test: find his or her way to the ward or dining room	Zoltan, 1996	Top-down approach
A-ONE	Árnadóttir, 1990	Top-down approach
UNILATERAL NEGLECT		
BIT	Wilson et al., 1987a	Bottom-up approach, deficit-specific test
Functional tests of reading and writing		Top-down approach
A-ONE	Árnadóttir, 1990	Top-down approach

(continues)

(continued)

Table 10–3. Examples of evaluations used to detect complex perceptual impairments

ASSESSMENT	SOURCE	TYPE
VISUOCONSTRUCTIVE IMPAIRMENTS		
Graphic design	Zoltan et al., 1983	Bottom-up approach, deficit-specific test
Block design	Zoltan et al., 1983	Bottom-up approach, deficit-specific test
BODY SCHEME AND BODY IMAGE IMPAIRMENTS		
Right/left orientation	Benton et al., 1983	Bottom-up approach, deficit-specific test
Unilateral body neglect: draw a man	Zoltan, 1996	Bottom-up approach, deficit-specific test
The Rabideau kitchen evaluation-revised: an assessment of meal preparation skill	Neistadt, 1992b	Top-down approach
A-ONE	Árnadóttir, 1990	Top-down approach

For evaluation of visual skills as opposed to visual perception, see Aloisio, 1998; Warren, 1996, 1993a, 1993b, 1994.
A-ONE = Árnadóttir Occupational Therapy Activities of Daily Living Neurobehavioral Evaluation; BIT = Behavioral Inattention Test; LOTCA = Lowenstein Occupational Therapy

approach rejects the treatment dichotomy between remedial/restorative and adaptive approaches that suggests a causal unidirectional relationship between the two. The outcome of this new approach is defined as *effective adaptation*, emphasizing that adaptation is the outcome of treatment and not a treatment format. It should be noted that neurobehavioral impairments do usually not appear in isolation. For many diagnostic categories, impairments are grouped together. In terms of intervention, the therapist needs to take all impairments into consideration because focusing on only one particular impairment may not lead to an improved outcome.

CASE STUDY: MR. H

BACKGROUND

INTRODUCTION TO THE CLIENT, MR. H

Mr. H is a 71-year-old man. He was admitted to a 60-bed rehabilitation unit with outpatient facilities after a short stay in an acute hospital ward after experiencing a CVA. He was referred to occupational therapy on admission to the rehabilitation unit for an ADL evaluation as well as a cognitive and perceptual evaluation.

INTRODUCTION TO THE OCCUPATIONAL THERAPIST, CAROL

Carol, the occupational therapist assigned to treat Mr. H, works in a hospital that has an acute care facility with a rehabilitation unit attached to it. The rehabilitation unit has both in- and outpatient services. Carol works in the rehabilitation unit with a mixed caseload of mainly neurological and orthopedic clients. Clients are referred to the rehabilitation unit as soon as their medical condition has stabilized, and their length of stay varies from 1 week to several months, depending on the severity of disability and availability of placement resources. However, there is a pressure for early and even premature discharge because of financial restrictions in the health sector. Carol has 6 years of clinical experience, during which time she has undertaken several continuing education courses, including the 1-week-long certification course required for reliable administration and scoring of the A-ONE (Árnadóttir, 1990).

INFORMATION GATHERING

REVIEW OF MEDICAL RECORDS

Before meeting Mr. H, Carol reviewed his medical records. According to the records, Mr. H is retired, and 1 week earlier, he fell down when walking as a result of a right-side cerebral infarct. The infarct led to decreased strength in his left body side. Clumsy movements were also manifest as well as subtle facial paresis on the left side, dysarthria (which resolved after a few days), and a left visual field defect. Eye movements during neurological evaluation were reported to be normal. Somatic sensory testing, including tactile, proprioceptive, and pain sensation, was also reported to be normal. Mr. H was reported to be oriented regarding time and place. Some **unilateral neglect** of the left body side was noted.

The medical history indicated that Mr. H had experienced a minor stroke 7 years earlier, resulting in reduced strength in his right arm and difficulties with writing. These symptoms persisted for a few days and then resolved. The history also revealed a transient ischemic attack (TIA) 2 years earlier, which caused some "confusion" and dysarthria lasting for only a few hours. There was further a history of one isolated incidence of atrial fibrillation and diabetes mellitus that was controlled through diet and medication. The current computed tomography scan revealed three older infarcts located at the anterior horns of both lateral ventricles and a new one in the right parieto-occipital area.

SELECTION OF A THEORETICAL BASIS FOR THERAPY

After reviewing the medical record, Carol was able to combine the obtained information with the expectations she had about the case based on her previous experience of working with clients who have had CVAs. Thus, she was able to generate narrative hypotheses (Dutton, 1995) that she could use to construct a prospective story for intervention before selecting the appropriate evaluation tools. The hypotheses included her client's potential assets and deficits, including:

- The right body side seems to be unaffected, and the left body side has decreased strength but not paralysis; therefore, some bilateral manipulation might be possible.
- Mr. H is retired, so he does not need to support a family or go back to a previous job; this removes financial pressures. However, there may be other tasks that he needs to be able to master, such as household or leisure activities.
- Mr. H has apparently normal language functions, and sensory input would aid in task performance.
- Signs of neurobehavioral impairments, such as unilateral neglect, point to the possibility of other impairments that need to be evaluated.
- Neurobehavioral impairments may affect ADL performance in household or leisure activities

Based on these hypotheses, Carol decided to use the theoretical base behind the A-ONE (Árnadóttir, 1990) for working with Mr. H because it provides guidance regarding the ways neurobehavior relates to ADLs and can be matched easily with intervention possibilities, depending on the therapist's beliefs. The A-ONE theory is a factor-relating theory according to the conceptual framework described by Dickoff et al. (1968)

because it relates factors from neurobehavioral performance components to ADL task performance without implying causality. Neurobehavior is concerned with the ways environmental stimuli and different performance components are processed within the CNS through different mechanisms to affect behavioral and emotional responses (Llorens, 1986). Thus, neurobehavior is the basis for task performance.

According to Árnadóttir (1990, 1998), when using the A-ONE theory, the behaviors that are required for task performance are subsequently related to neuronal processing at the CNS level in the theory. Furthermore, ". . . performance of daily activities requires adequate functioning of specific parts of the nervous system. Consequently, impairment of certain components of the CNS may result in dysfunction of specific aspects of ADL" (1990, p. 289). An example of a relational statement from the theory is that a massive posterior inferior parietal lobe lesion in the left hemisphere may cause bilateral motor apraxia. This neurobehavioral impairment may make manipulation of objects difficult during functional activities such as combing hair, brushing teeth, or holding a spoon when eating because of "clumsy" movements. In contrast, a posterior inferior parietal lobe lesion in the right hemisphere may cause spatial-relations impairment. This neurobehavioral impairment may make figure/ground discrimination difficult as well as perception of depth but does result in motor apraxia. As a result, a person may reach out too far for a cup or may be unable to find the correct armhole when putting on a shirt. Thus, neurological impairments that can be observed through a client's engagement in ADLs may indicate the location and extent of neurological damage. Therefore, the integrity of CNS activity can be evaluated by applying the A-ONE theory. Any behavioral response observed during evaluation is classified according to the operational definitions of the theory by applying activity analysis, which reveals dysfunction in performance components. The relational statements of this factor-relating theory indicate how neurobehavior and neurobehavioral impairments are related to ADLs and task performance.

Carol therefore chose to use the A-ONE instrument, which is classified as a top-down assessment (Duchek & Abreu, 1997), to assess functional independence in ADLs and subsequently aid in detecting neurobehavioral dysfunction or impaired neurological performance components that interfere with independent task performance. When using this approach, Carol applies interactive and procedural (or diagnostic) reasoning to gather cues that she interprets to make occupational therapy hypotheses (Rogers & Holm, 1989, 1991, 1997). These hypotheses are subsequently used to form the occupational therapy diagnosis. In other words, Carol analyzes the nature or the cause of a functional problem that requires occupational therapy intervention, and her analysis is made from the view of occupa-

tion. Using knowledge of the occupational therapy diagnosis and procedural reasoning, she is able to select interventions to work with the client
to attempt to resolve his or her problems.

INITIAL INTERVIEW

After reading the medical records, Carol met briefly with Mr. H to schedule time for an assessment. Carol walked into the dining room, where she
found Mr. H sitting by himself finishing breakfast. The following dialogue ensued:

>Therapist: Good morning, Mr. H.
>
>Mr. H: Good morning.
>
>Therapist: My name is Carol, and I am an occupational therapist. How are you today?
>
>Mr. H: I am fine.
>
>Therapist: How long have you been here at the Rehabilitation Center?
>
>Mr. H: I arrived the day before yesterday.
>
>Therapist: Did you come directly from home?
>
>Mr. H: No, I came from the City Hospital.
>
>Therapist: How long were you there for?
>
>Mr. H: About a week. *(Mr. H answered promptly, and these answers were correct.)*
>
>Therapist: What happened to you?
>
>Mr. H: I had a stroke.
>
>Therapist: How did that affect you?
>
>Mr. H: Well, the left arm went out of control.
>
>Therapist: What do you mean by "went out of control?"
>
>Mr. H: Well, I could not raise it up like this. *(Abducts his fully extended left arm to 180°. He notices that he still holds a piece of bread in his left hand, which had been positioned in his lap under the tabletop. Removes the bread from his hand and raises his hand again. Carol notices that although he answers all the questions, he always looks straight ahead and does not attend to her visually [she is sitting on his left side].)*
>
>Therapist: Are you right-handed?
>
>Mr. H: I have always been able to use both hands equally.
>
>Therapist: Which hand do you write with?
>
>Mr. H: I write with the right hand.
>
>Therapist *(stands up)*: Grab both my hands and squeeze them; let's see how strong you are.
>
>Mr. H: Oh, I am afraid I will hurt you. *(He smiles.)*
>
>Therapist: Don't worry, just squeeze. *(He does so.)* Well, there is a little less strength in your left hand.
>
>Mr. H: Yes, but it has become much better. I used to forget it, for example, under tabletops, like this. *(He shows how the hand got stuck under the table.)*

Therapist: How does the stroke affect your activity performance? Anything you have problems with?

Mr. H: No, not in particular, except the hand has been difficult.

(Carol decides that although Mr. H identifies the hemiparesis as a result of the stroke, there are other impairments that he does not seem to have insight into. For example, he only refers to the unilateral body inattention when confronted with it and does not mention other problems. Furthermore, he may be unrealistic regarding his task performance.)

Therapist: Do you have a family?

Mr. H: Yes, I have a wife.

Therapist: Any children?

Mr. H: Yes, we have five children.

Therapist: Are they living with you?

Mr. H: No. They are all grown up.

Therapist: In what kind of housing do you live?

Mr. H: We live on the second floor of a condominium.

Therapist: Have you been home since you had the stroke?

Mr. H: No, I have not.

Therapist: How old are you now?

Mr. H: I am 71.

Therapist: Are you still working?

Mr. H: No, I am retired.

Therapist: When did you retire?

Mr. H: When I turned 70.

Therapist: Where did you work?

Mr. H: At an oil company.

Therapist: How do you spend your days now?

Mr. H: Oh, they pass somehow.

Therapist: Any particular interests or projects that you are working on?

Mr. H: No.

Therapist: Is there anything you like doing in particular?

Mr. H: Well, I like my Mercedes, keeping it in shape and driving it around.

Therapist: How about your wife; does she work?

Mr. H: No, she is at home too.

Therapist: How old is she?

Mr. H: She is 3 years younger than I am.

Therapist: Have you been getting assistance with getting up in the morning after your stroke?

Mr. H: Yes.

Therapist: Well, tomorrow morning I will come at eight o'clock and see how you are doing with the dressing and grooming activities before breakfast. Then I can maybe set up a treatment program for you to help you become more independent. Is that alright?

Mr. H: Yes, that's fine.

(The physical therapy assistant arrives and says it is time to come down for therapy. Mr. H gets up and starts walking. His eyes catch an object on one of

the tables as he walks through the dining room, with his left side lagging a little bit behind. He grabs the object.)
    Therapist: **What are you doing with that?**
    Mr. H: **I don't know.**
    (He puts the object down and follows the assistant out of the room. Carol thinks of field dependency together with other attention deficits as she leaves the room.)

During this interaction, Carol gained information regarding how Mr. H felt about the CVA and his activity performance. She also gathered information about Mr. H's current strengths, possible problems, and his home and family context to guide her in the areas she needed to assess and the ways she would direct intervention. During the interview she attempted to assess nonverbal cues regarding his impairments, such as unilateral neglect of body and visual field as well as field dependency, possible lack of insight into his problems, and gait dysfunction.

SUMMARY OF INITIAL FINDINGS

Mr. H's medical record information indicated reduced strength in the left body side, clumsy movements, subtle dysarthria, a visual field defect, and some unilateral neglect of the left body side. Observation during the brief initial interview confirmed the slightly reduced strength in his left body side as well as unilateral body neglect but also suggested the presence of other impairments, such as unilateral spatial neglect (i.e., visual modality), further attention deficits (including field dependency), the possibility of perseveration, and a lack of insight into his problems. Thus, some of Carol's narrative hypotheses were already confirmed. However, she reasoned that formal assessment would be needed to gather further information regarding activity performance and the ways it is affected by the mentioned impairments and possible presence of other impairments. Carol reasoned that an interview with Mrs. H might be useful to gather more information about Mr. H's interests, habits, and the situation at home.

EVALUATION

AREAS REQUIRING FURTHER EVALUATION

Box 10–1 details Carol's thoughts based on the previous information gathering related to which areas she will need to assess further.

BOX 10–1. THERAPIST REASONING—FURTHER EVALUATION

I need to investigate Mr. H's independence in ADLs and whether dysfunction of neurobehavioral components interfered with task performance in this area. I also decided to gather information in relation to Mr. H's leisure activities because he was retired and would need some occupations to balance his life. I was also interested in whether his reading and writing skills had been affected by the stroke because reading is a common leisure task that is also necessary in order to follow what is going on in the community. Writing, on the other hand, may be necessary in dealing with financial tasks and, if affected, would require assistance from his wife. In addition, his driving skills need to be considered because this is a leisure activity and neurobehavioral impairments might make him an unsafe driver. Ability to maneuver on stairs has to be evaluated in relation to Mr. H's environmental context because his apartment is located on the second floor. This ability would be important if he is to be able to leave his apartment independently. Furthermore, simple household and kitchen activities could be assessed later on because he is retired and it might be important that he share some of the workload at home with his wife. His ability to manage medication also needs to be investigated. Additionally, information needs to be gathered regarding Mr. H's past and present interests and possibilities of using those occupations in the future or making necessary changes to them.

Table 10–4 lists Mr. H's problem areas based on the initial data gathering and the methods for follow-up assessment.

SELECTION OF A STANDARDIZED ASSESSMENT

Box 10–2 outlines the reasons Carol chose to use the A-ONE (Árnadóttir, 1990).

ASSESSMENT RESULTS: A-ONE FUNCTIONAL INDEPENDENCE SCALE

The A-ONE (Árnadóttir, 1990) is described in detail in Chapter 3. Appendix 10–1 displays Mr. H's results on the A-ONE, including the Functional Independence Scale. Mr. H used his glasses during all the testing situations. In summary, Mr. H needed physical assistance for all the dressing items (e.g., putting on shirt, trousers, and socks and manipulating fastenings) except for putting on shoes, for which he

Table 10–4. Problem areas based on initial data gathering, and methods for further evaluation

PROBLEM AREAS TO INVESTIGATE FURTHER	EVALUATION CHOSEN FOR FURTHER INVESTIGATION
Based on:	
• Data gathering	
• Cues from initial interview with Mr. H	
• Medical records	
PATHOLOGY	
R-CVA	
History CVA	
Diabetes Mellitus	
Atrial fibrillation	Diet is under control by wife
PERFORMANCE AREAS AND TASKS	
ADLs	A-ONE
Leisure and interests	Interview wife (and Mr. H when possible)
Reading	Clinical observation
Writing	Clinical observation
Driving	Consider performance in ADLs first to determine whether clinical observation is relevant
Maneuvering stairs	Clinical observation
Kitchen/household	Clinical observation
Medication management	Cognitive test item Lone Sörensen
PERFORMANCE COMPONENTS DYSFUNCTION	
COMPLEX PERCEPTUAL DISORDERS:	
Body scheme:	
Unilateral body neglect (left)	A-ONE
Right–left discrimination	A-ONE
COMPLEX PERCEPTUAL DISORDERS:	
Visuospatial impairments:	
Spatial relations impairment	A-ONE

(continues)

(continued)

Table 10–4. Problem areas based on initial data gathering, and methods for further evaluation	
PROBLEM AREAS TO INVESTIGATE FURTHER	**EVALUATION CHOSEN FOR FURTHER INVESTIGATION**
Right–left discrimination	A-ONE
Unilateral visual neglect (left)	A-ONE
OTHER IMPAIRMENTS:	
Strength and motoric left side	A-ONE or muscle testing
Coordination	Box and block, Purdue peg board
Apraxia	A-ONE
Visual field defect	Clinically confirmed
Lack of insight	A-ONE
Field dependency	A-ONE
Other neurobehavioral impairments	A-ONE
PERFORMANCE CONTEXT DYSFUNCTION	
Stairs to apartment	Clinical observation Home visit
Distance to stores	Consider wife's driving

needed verbal assistance. He exhibited severe spatial-relations problems that affected his ability to figure out the back versus the front of clothes, inside versus outside, and right versus left side. He placed both legs through the same leg hole and his arm through the neck opening. He was unable to recognize his errors, and his responses when corrected indicated lack of judgment. He also needed physical assistance to deal with unilateral body neglect because he did not manage to dress his left body side properly (i.e., pull down the shirt on that side) and he had to be reminded to use his left hand to assist in bilateral activities. He also presented with premotor perseveration, which means that he persisted with movements such as pulling on a sock even though the activity had been completed. He also pulled the sleeve all the way over his elbow on one side. Organization and sequencing of activity steps was also impaired. For example, he put his shoes on before his trousers. Attention

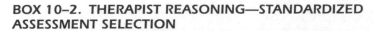

BOX 10–2. THERAPIST REASONING—STANDARDIZED ASSESSMENT SELECTION

I chose to use the A-ONE for primary data gathering because it is a standardized evaluation that provides information both on performance task dysfunction in the different ADL domains and the dysfunctional neurobehavioral components that might affect ADL performance. Based on the information gathered through administration of the A-ONE and clinical observations during task performance, deficit-specific tests could be selected if needed to evaluate dysfunction of performance components (e.g., muscle strength and tone, coordination, motor apraxia, spatial relations, neglect, and memory). Use of deficit-specific tests as a follow up of the functional evaluation has been suggested in instances in which difficulties in defining deficits are experienced, when new clinicians need to refine their observation skills (Okkema, 1993; Phillips & Walters, 1996), and when an aid in quantification of the deficit's severity is needed (Phillips & Wolters, 1996). I decided to use an informal evaluation to gather more information in the area of leisure and to add an interview with Mrs. H rather than assess Mr. H further in this area. I decided this because Mr. H seemed rather inflexible in his thinking and it was hard to get information from him other than "yes" or "no" answers to specific questions. In the initial interview, it was hard to tell from his affect what he liked and disliked and if he cared at all, and I thought Mrs. H would be better able to comment on things her husband enjoyed.

problems such as field dependency, in which he grabbed objects that did not belong to the present task or activity sequence, also interfered with performance. Bilateral motor apraxia was particularly apparent when manipulating fastenings. Refer back to Table 10–2 to relate names of items on the A-ONE to the terminology of impairments used in this chapter.

In the grooming and hygiene domain, Mr. H was independent with combing his hair, brushing his teeth, shaving, and using the toilet. He needed verbal assistance to wash the upper part of his body (i.e., face, chest, hands, and arms) because of lack of organization and sequencing and unilateral body neglect (e.g., he failed to wash and rinse his left hand). He was not able to include all activity steps, such as using soap and rinsing off the soap, without step-by-step verbal reminders. He was not consistent in placing objects out of the way after use, so they piled up in the sink. He needed physical assistance with bathing. Motor apraxia was noted in both hands during object manipulation when brushing his teeth and combing his hair but did not interfere with independent activity performance in this domain. Carol questioned this impairment because it was not consistent with the recent diagnosis of right hemisphere dysfunction. According to the processing model for praxis, whereas bilateral motor apraxia occurs with lesions in the left hemisphere, where the visuokinesthetic motor engrams or memory molecules for praxis are stored, unilateral motor apraxia of the left body side occurs in cases of a lesion in the anterior fibers of the corpus callosum or the premotor cortex in the right hemisphere, which is responsible for planning and programming of movements of the left body side (Árnadóttir, 1990, 1998; Heilman & Gonzalez Rothi, 1993). Table 10–5 provides examples of the ways critical cues were used to form hypotheses regarding impairments and occupational diagnosis. Another impairment that was noted but did not require assistance was unilateral spatial neglect—Mr. H did not pay attention to the towel's falling into the sink and onto the floor. He also gathered all items into the right visual field. Spatial relation impairments manifested as difficulty in turning his dentures the correct way and manipulating water taps. Prefrontal perseveration was evident in activity performances such as combing his hair and washing his face. Field dependency interfered with sequencing of activity steps. He grabbed things that he did not use as he saw them. For example, he grabbed the comb every time he saw it and combed his hair on three different occasions. He also grabbed the denture brush, which he had previously used for brushing his teeth, and used it as a nail brush.

Mr. H was independent with the transfers and mobility tasks on the A-ONE, except he needed assistance with bathtub transfers. He was able to walk up the stairs and use the elevator. There was some lagging of his left side (i.e., lack of strength), and he did not always account properly for distances when sitting down (suggesting spatial-relations impairment). He did get to know his way around his own room, dining room, or therapy settings in the rehabilitation center in relatively short time, but topographical disorientation was suspected in larger settings and outdoors.

In the feeding domain, Mr. H was able to eat and drink independently but needed assistance with cutting and buttering because of spatial-relations impairment, motor apraxia, and unilateral body neglect of the left hand. The spatial-relations impairment and motor apraxia required bilateral hand use for the knife, and this was not effective because of his unilateral neglect. He did not always notice objects in his left visual field but was usually able to compensate for this. For example, he did not notice his own knife in his left visual field but compensated by taking another knife that was located by the next patient's plate in his own right

Table 10–5. Problem identification: Examples of observations and explanatory hypotheses

HYPOTHESIS #1: SPATIAL RELATIONS IMPAIRMENT

CRITICAL CUES OBSERVED DURING A-ONE (AND INTERVIEW)	CUE INTERPRETATION AND HYPOTHESIS FORMATION USING A-ONE TERMINOLOGY
Problems finding correct holes on shirt, arm through neckhole	Spatial relations impairment Attention deficit
Placed both legs into the left leghole	Spatial relations impairment Unilateral spatial neglect
Jacket turned wrong front to back	Spatial relations impairment Attention deficit
Placed left arm through right sleeve	Spatial relations impairment
Took right shoe on left foot	Spatial relations impairment Field dependency
Folded Velcro fastening on right shoe back on top of D-ring rather than threading the Velcro through the D-ring	Spatial relations impairment (depth distance, figure ground discrimination) Organization and sequencing (did he leave out one step?) Ideational apraxia (did he know what to do?) Attentional deficit (did he notice the problem?)
Misjudged distances when holding jacket for zipping	Spatial relations impairment (object held too far away) Bilateral motor apraxia (clumsy movements)
Misjudged distances when stabilizing during feeding tasks	Spatial relation impairment Unilateral visual neglect
Misjudged distances when sitting down	Spatial relations impairment Unilateral visual neglect Hemianopsia
Problems orienting dentures correctly in space when placing them into mouth	Spatial relations impairment

CONCLUSION: SPATIAL RELATIONS IMPAIRMENT DUE TO RIGHT HEMISPHERE DYSFUNCTION

Cue interpretation involves consideration of the operational definitions in the A-ONE and information from the A-ONE theory regarding processing sites

(continues)

(continued)

Table 10–5. Problem identification: Examples of observations and explanatory hypotheses

---

for different functions within the cortex. Most of the critical cues listed can be interpreted as spatial relations impairment and attention deficits. The presence of other impairments suggested, such as unilateral spatial neglect and bilateral motor apraxia, are supported by other cues later on as well. Ideational apraxia is ruled out because it appeared to Carol that Mr. H did know that the Velcro had to go through the D-ring, but initially he did not attend to the fact that this was not happening and then he had problems visualizing the distance; therefore, it took many trials for him to get the Velcro through the loop and not on top of it.

HYPOTHESIS #2: UNILATERAL SPATIAL NEGLECT

EXAMPLES OF CRITICAL CUES OBSERVED DURING THE A-ONE (AND INTERVIEW) (SEE A-ONE EVALUATION FORMS IN EXHIBIT 1 FOR FURTHER CUES RELATED TO THIS IMPAIRMENT IN OTHER ADL DOMAINS)	CUE INTERPRETATION AND HYPOTHESIS FORMATION USING A-ONE TERMINOLOGY
Did not notice towel falling into sink, where water was running, on the left side	Unilateral spatial neglect Hemianopsia
All equipment was placed out of the way on the right side.	Unilateral spatial neglect Hemianopsia

CONCLUSION: HEMIANOPSIA AND UNILATERAL SPATIAL NEGLECT DUE TO RIGHT HEMISPHERE DYSFUNCTION

HYPOTHESIS #3: UNILATERAL BODY NEGLECT

EXAMPLES OF CRITICAL CUES OBSERVED DURING THE A-ONE (AND INTERVIEW): DRESSING DOMAIN (SEE EXHIBIT 1 FOR CRITICAL CUES OBSERVED IN OTHER DOMAINS)	CUE INTERPRETATION AND HYPOTHESIS FORMATION USING A-ONE TERMINOLOGY
Did not take shirt off left hand when undressing	Unilateral body neglect Impaired sensation

---

(continues)

(continued)

Table 10–5. Problem identification: Examples of observations and explanatory hypotheses

HYPOTHESIS #3: UNILATERAL BODY NEGLECT

EXAMPLES OF CRITICAL CUES OBSERVED DURING THE A-ONE (AND INTERVIEW): DRESSING DOMAIN (SEE EXHIBIT 1 FOR CRITICAL CUES OBSERVED IN OTHER DOMAINS)	CUE INTERPRETATION AND HYPOTHESIS FORMATION USING A-ONE TERMINOLOGY
Did not pull shirt down properly on left side	Unilateral body neglect Unilateral spatial neglect Impaired sensation
Shirt got stuck on left shoulder	Unilateral body neglect

CONCLUSION: UNILATERAL BODY NEGLECT DUE TO RIGHT HEMISPHERE DYSFUNCTION

Impaired sensation was ruled out by using the pervasive scale of the A-ONE. Unilateral spatial neglect was supported further by cues previously identified.

HYPOTHESIS #4: FIELD DEPENDENCY AND PREFRONTAL PERSEVERATION

CRITICAL CUES OBSERVED DURING THE A-ONE (AND INTERVIEW)	CUE INTERPRETATION AND HYPOTHESIS FORMATION USING A-ONE TERMINOLOGY
Used denture brush to brush hands when sees it during middle of the task of washing hands	Field dependency Prefrontal perseveration Ideational apraxia Lack of judgment
Grabbed comb each time he sees it and combs the hair	Field dependency Prefrontal perseveration
Grabbed shoe when he sees it and puts it on before trousers	Field dependency Organization and sequencing impairment
Grabbed food on table before sitting down to eat	Field dependency

(continues)

(continued)

Table 10–5. Problem identification: Examples of observations and explanatory hypotheses

---

HYPOTHESIS #4: FIELD DEPENDENCY AND PREFRONTAL PERSEVERATION (Continued)

CRITICAL CUES OBSERVED DURING THE A-ONE (AND INTERVIEW)	CUE INTERPRETATION AND HYPOTHESIS FORMATION USING A-ONE TERMINOLOGY
Grabbed objects on tables when passing by without purpose	Field dependency
Claimed it did not matter if clothes turned inside out or incorrectly front to back	Lack of judgment
Did not use feedback from own errors when provided by therapist	Lack of judgment
Claimed he is able to drive	Lack of insight

CONCLUSION: FIELD DEPENDENCY, PREFRONTAL PERSEVERATION, LACK OF JUDGMENT, AND LACK OF INSIGHT DUE TO RIGHT HEMISPHERE DYSFUNCTION

This conclusion was drawn given that several cues support each of the hypothetized impairments. Ideational apraxia was ruled out because Mr. H knew how to use the denture brush correctly, but his judgment should have stopped him from using it for two unrelated tasks.

HYPOTHESIS #5: BILATERAL MOTOR APRAXIA

CRITICAL CUES OBSERVED DURING THE A-ONE (AND INTERVIEW) (SEE EXHIBIT 1 FOR CRITICAL CUES IN OTHER DOMAINS OF THE A-ONE)	CUE INTERPRETATION AND HYPOTHESIS FORMATION USING A-ONE TERMINOLOGY
Clumsy movements bilaterally when manipulating fastenings	Bilateral motor apraxia Sensory deficits (ruled out) Lack of strength (very slight in left hand only)

CONCLUSION: BILATERAL MOTOR APRAXIA DUE TO PREVIOUS LEFT HEMISPHERE DYSFUNCTION

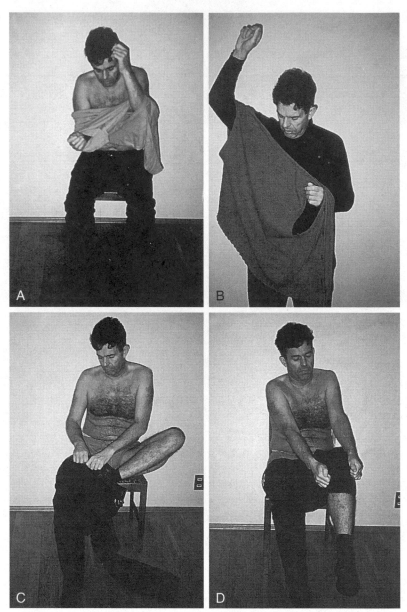

Figure 10–3. Neurobehavioral impairments manifested during the dressing domain of the A-ONE. **(A)** Spatial relations impairment manifested as the man puts the arm through the neck hole instead of the armhole. **(B)** Spatial relations impairment manifested as the man puts the right arm through the left sleeve and vice versa, resulting in the vest turning wrong from front to back. **(C)** Spatial relations impairment resulting in both legs being placed in the same leg hole. **(D)** Premotor perseveration, where the man repeats the movements of pulling up the leg hole after it has cleared the foot.

visual field. Figures 10–3, 10–4, 10–5, and 10–6 provide samples of neurobehavioral impairments interfering with Mr. H's task performance in dressing, grooming and hygiene, and feeding domains on the A-ONE. No problems were noted with comprehension and speech, and the dysarthria noted earlier seemed to have resolved. In summary, Mr. H's performance on the independence scale of the A-ONE indicated that he needed physical assistance, particularly during dressing, and verbal assistance for grooming and hygiene tasks as well as feeding. He was independent in transfers and mobility tasks, and no communication problems were detected.

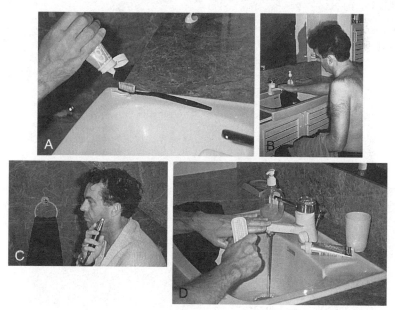

Figure 10–4. Neurobehavioral impairments manifested during the grooming and hygiene domain of the A-ONE. **(A)** Spatial relations impairment manifested in that the man misjudges distances when placing toothpaste on toothbrush. **(B)** Unilateral body neglect manifested in that the left arm has not been properly undressed before the washing task. **(C)** Motor apraxia resulting in problems with adjustment of hand movements during manipulation of the razor. The razor is turning sideways when touching the face. **(D)** Field dependency manifested in the man grabbing a denture brush when he sees it during a washing task and incorporating it into the washing activity. Further, he does not pay attention that the towel on the left side is getting wet due to visual inattention. All objects he has used are gathered in the right visual field, also suggesting unilateral spatial neglect.

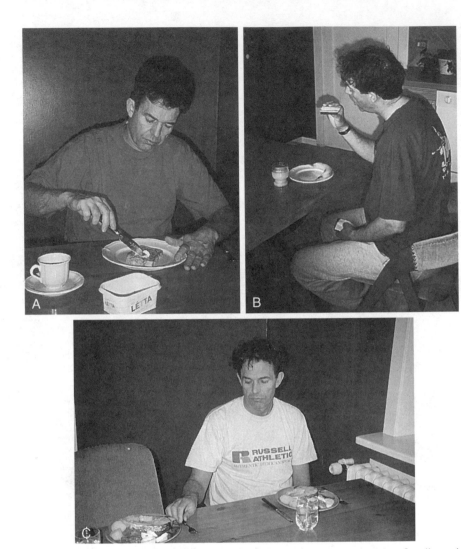

Figure 10–5. Neurobehavioral impairments manifested during the feeding do-main of the A-ONE. **(A)** Spatial relations impairment manifested in misjudgment of distances when stabilizing the bread in order to spread the butter. **(B)** Unilateral body neglect manifests as the man does not attend to the bread in the hand that has slid under the table top, and grabs another piece of bread and continues eat-ing with the right hand. **(C)** Unilateral spatial neglect, where the man does not note his own knife in the left visual field but compensates by grabbing silverware from the next person's plate.

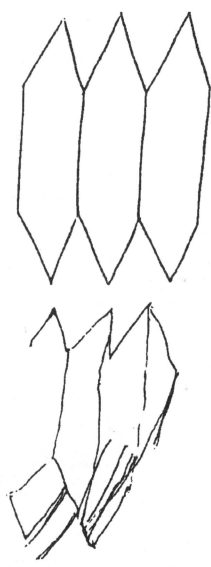

Figure 10–6. Spatial relations impairment on a two-dimensional construction task. The person has a problem aligning the lines according to the stimulus figure. A unilateral spatial neglect of the left visual field is also evident.

ASSESSMENT RESULTS: A-ONE NEUROBEHAVIORAL SPECIFIC IMPAIRMENT SUBSCALE

Mr. H had complex perceptual disorders, including spatial-relations impairments, unilateral spatial neglect, and unilateral body neglect, which interfered considerably with dressing, grooming and hygiene performance, and feeding performance. Premotor and prefrontal perseveration, bilateral motor apraxia, field dependency, and organization and sequencing problems regarding activity steps were also noted. A slight lack of strength in the left body side was also noted.

ASSESSMENT RESULTS: A-ONE NEUROBEHAVIORAL PERVASIVE IMPAIRMENT SUBSCALE

Problems with right/left discrimination manifested during dressing and upon confrontation (i.e., asking Mr. H to indicate right and left). Concrete thoughts manifested as difficulties with simple calculations, for example, related to the time of Mr. H's retirement. Lack of insight into his own condition was apparent because Mr. H was not able to identify any impairments as a result of the stroke, except for his physical weakness. However, he mentioned at other times during the evaluation that he often forgot his left hand when, for example, he was confronted with not having removed his shirt from his hand during washing activities. Mr. H did indicate that he could be discharged shortly and become an outpatient because he could "drive in every day" despite his severe spatial-relations impairments, which would certainly interfere with his driving performance. Lack of judgment manifested in comments such as, "It does not matter if the clothes turn inside-out," when that performance was pointed out to him. He did not use feedback from his errors even though they were indicated to him. He used his own denture brush to scrub his hands as if it were a nailbrush (indicating field dependency), without paying attention to the error and without judging that although the brush could be used for either task, the same brush should not be used on both occasions. Some short-term memory problems were also noted and at times instructions had to be frequently repeated. Lack of attention probably affected his short-term memory as well. Specific visual stimuli that were not relevant for a particular activity frequently distracted him. He picked up irrelevant items and at one point incorporated an item into performance of a previous activity, indicating prefrontal perseveration and field dependency.

Mr. H was able to recognize objects placed in either hand through tactile senses with his vision occluded and maintain different positions of his left arm with somesthetic sensory feedback alone. Depression was not noted at this stage. Apathy may have been questioned because extra responses were limited; however, he did grin at times, for example, regarding not squeezing the therapist's hand too hard and regarding incorrectly turning his jacket back to front. He was fully oriented to time and place (he was only two dates off the correct date, which is within normal limits). His long-term memory seemed intact because he was able to give reliable information regarding his background.

Based on the cues gathered through administering and interpreting the A-ONE, Carol formed several hypotheses (see Table 10–5) regarding the occupational diagnosis of Mr. H, as outlined in Box 10–3.

BOX 10–3. THERAPIST REASONING—HYPOTHESIS FORMATION

When determining which impairments interfered with performance of ADLs, I used the operational definitions of concepts from the A-ONE as guidelines to match with the critical cues observed during the different ADL tasks. I then used procedural, or diagnostic, reasoning to interpret the cues and differentiate between impairments. As an example, when Mr. H folded the Velcro fastening back on top of the D-ring rather than threading it through the ring, I considered the operational definitions for spatial relations, such as, "Is unable to find armholes, leg holes, or bottom of shirt; pulls sleeve in wrong direction; overestimates or underestimates distances when reaching out for objects" (Árnadóttir, 1998, p. 301), and for ideational apraxia, such as, "Does not know what to do with toothbrush, toothpaste, or shaving cream; uses tools inappropriately (e.g., smears the toothpaste on face); sequences activity steps incorrectly so that there are errors in end results of tasks (e.g., puts socks on top of shoes) (Árnadóttir, 1998, p. 302). It became evident that a lot of other cues supported the hypothesis of spatial relations impairment but only one cue supported possibility of ideational apraxia. Furthermore, Mr. H did indicate that he knew what to do, so the problem was not lack of knowledge but rather that he did not judge correctly the distance of how far he had to take the Velcro for it to go through the D-ring. Similarly, when Mr. H used the denture brush to scrub his hands, it was obvious that the brush caught his visual attention.

He became distracted from washing by the stimulus of the brush, grabbed it, and incorporated it into the previous task, a sample of field dependency including both components of dysfunctional attention and prefrontal perseveration (i.e., perseveration of activity steps, not movement). It was not an incorrect idea to scrub the hands with a brush that looked like a nail brush, but

(continues)

> ### BOX 10–3. THERAPIST REASONING—HYPOTHESIS FORMATION (CONT.)
>
> Mr. H's judgment should have stopped him from using the same brush for both tasks. The conceptual definition of lack of judgment from the A-ONE is the "inability to make realistic decisions based on environmental information; unable to make use of feedback from own errors" (p. 304). An example of operational definitions of the same concept would be: "Does not turn off water taps after washing; does not put breaks on wheelchair and makes unsafe transfers; goes to dining room without dressing or combing hair; does not care if clothes are turned inside out or back to front, even when those facts have been pointed out" (Árnadóttir, 1998, p. 304). Thus an ideational apraxia was also ruled out as an impairment in this case. I used the same kind of reasoning, simultaneously using the operational definitions from the A-ONE to determine all other impairments interfering with his ADLs, as indicated by some samples in Table 10–5 and the assessment forms in Appendix 10–1.
>
> According to the information presented in Table 10–5, many of the critical cues listed were interpreted as spatial relations impairment and unilateral spatial neglect. Many critical cues observed by using the A-ONE further support the presence of unilateral body neglect and impaired right/left discrimination. All of these impairments can be related to right hemisphere dysfunction by using the A-ONE and its theoretical background according to Árnadóttir (1990). Other cues observed and interpreted as field dependency, prefrontal perseveration, lack of judgment, and lack of insight can also be related to right hemisphere dysfunction, where the memory molecules for movement of either body side are stored. The left hemisphere dysfunction and motor apraxia would therefore be related to an older infarct, a hypothesis validated by the medical records and computed tomography scan results. In addition, Mrs. H claimed that the clumsiness had started after an earlier CVA; this should be considered in therapy. Possible interpretation of cues, including sensory disturbances, were ruled out by other observations in the A-ONE and so was ideational apraxia because the observed cues could be explained better by other impairments than by lack of knowledge. The resulting occupational diagnosis (using procedural or diagnostic reasoning, identifying cues, and forming hypotheses about the nature of the deficit) included several impairments that interfere with task performance as a result of right CVA and motor apraxia resulting from an earlier left CVA. The information presented in Table 10–5 from the problem-sensing and definition stage was used to form an occupational therapy diagnosis. This diagnosis was then used in the problem-resolution stage of the occupational therapy process, because it provided a basis from which appropriate interventions could be implemented.

FURTHER EVALUATION RESULTS

Reading, Writing, and Construction

Mr. H was able to read aloud but sometimes left out words on the left margin of the page and then had to go back and read the sentence again to obtain the meaning or guess the meaning. He used glasses for reading. He was able to write automatic information, such as his own name and address, without errors, but he had a tendency to start closer to the middle of the page rather than at the left margin. He was able to write a sentence about the weather. Some perseveration and spatial-relations problems were noted in writing forms. He had difficulty copying drawings because of spatial-relations impairment. Furthermore, he demonstrated poor performance on constructional tests, such as block constructions, because spatial-relations impairment was present.

Muscle Strength

Mr. H had slightly reduced strength on his left side, although he was able to withstand some resistance to all movements. Full range of motion was noted.

Coordination

Coordination requires good praxis and accurate judgment of visuospatial relationships for estimation of distances and reach. The results from the Purdue Peg Board Test (Tiffin, 1968) and the Box and Block Test (Cromwell, 1976; Mathiowetz et al., 1985) indicated that Mr. H's coordination was considerably impaired bilaterally. Performance was worse on the left side.

Cognitive Test Lone Sörensen (Sörensen, 1978)

Perceptual and cognitive items from this assessment (e.g., copying drawings and block constructions) indicated visuospatial impairments in two and three dimensions and unilateral spatial neglect (visual modality). Problem-solving items indicated that Mr. H was experiencing concrete thoughts. For example, he was able to figure out medication for 1 day on the medication item of the test but was not able to carry the information over to subsequent days.

RESULTS FROM INTERVIEW WITH WIFE

Carol asked Mrs. H about her husband's habits during an interview because this information had not been obtained through administering the A-ONE to Mr. H. Mrs. H confirmed that Mr. H used soap during washing (validating organization and sequencing problems identified by the A-ONE), and she identified his brush as the denture brush and not a nailbrush (supporting field dependency and prefrontal perseveration identified by the A-ONE). She revealed that Mr. H did not have many interests. After his retirement he had sat around, watched some TV, and done a little reading. Otherwise he liked driving, was very proud of his car, and never got tired of keeping it in good shape. They had occasionally gone on walks in their neighborhood. In the past they had been more active and had enjoyed going out dancing. Mrs. H was also retired and did most of the chores around the house. Mr. H had been active in shopping because his wife did not drive, although she did hold a driving license. After being made aware that Mr. H's impairments would severely interfere with his driving performance, Mrs. H indicated that she was willing to take a couple of driving instruction lessons to see if she could manage the driving. She seemed to be very positive in general, realistic about the situation, and willing to do everything in her power to help her husband to function better.

FORMULATION OF PRIORITIZED PROBLEM LIST

Carol constructed a prioritized problem list for the dysfunctions identified in performance tasks of different areas and performance components based on information obtained during assessment with Mr. H and the interviews with his wife and him (Table 10–6). Although Mr. H was not able to list goals himself due to lack of insight and apparent indifference about what was going on, Carol ensured that Mr. and Mrs. H agreed to the functional goals on the list and their importance.

GOALS AND INTERVENTION STRATEGIES

Carol used conditional reasoning (Mattingly & Fleming, 1994; Fleming, 1991) to incorporate information obtained from interviews with Mr. and Mrs. H regarding their previous lifestyle and habits to imagine what effect the stroke would have on their future lives, including activity performance, roles, and the context in which they lived. Based on this rea-

Table 10–6. Prioritized problem list: Short-term goals to be reached after 3 weeks of intervention

PERFORMANCE AREA AND TASKS	
DYSFUNCTION	**INTERVENTION**
Priority #1: Short-term goal: ADL area For Mr. H to improve all dressing tasks to independent level with intermittent verbal cues and supervision: • Grooming, especially washing • Feeding: assistance with cutting only • Transfers: assistance with bathing only • Medication management	Functional approach with repetition of tasks within daily context Use adaptation for garments in order to provide cues to look for to overcome spatial relations problems Compensate for impairments such as visual neglect and other attention problems Videotaped feedback to gain insight into problems Involve wife when needed before discharge
Priority #2: Short-term goal: ADL area Solution for problems with driving task	Impairments are too severe for safe driving; have wife take over the role of driving
Priority #3: Short-term goal: leisure area For Mr. H to be able to read newspapers and TV subtitles	Functional approach with compensation techniques, such as, "Look to the left"
Priority #4: Short- and long-term goal: work area For Mr. H to be able to participate in at least four kitchen or household tasks with verbal cues	Functional approach: practice simple meal preparation and household tasks that he could share with wife
Priority #5: Long-term goal: leisure and work area For Mr. H to be able to identify at least two possible interest pursuits before discharge	Check social resources (i.e., dancing, sheltered work) before discharge; check if he could take responsibility for cleaning the car and waxing it in order to maintain this role; check possibilities for walks with wife in neighborhood

(continues)

(continued)

Table 10–6. Prioritized problem list: Short-term goals to be reached after 3 weeks of intervention

---

PERFORMANCE COMPONENTS: INTERVENTION RELATES TO BOTH SHORT- AND LONG-TERM GOALS ADDRESSED THROUGH FUNCTIONAL ACTIVITIES

DYSFUNCTION	INTERVENTION
Priority #1: Attention problems:	Domain-specific functional approach with repeated practice in ADL tasks and compensation using diminishing cues to overcome impairments
• Unilateral body neglect or inattention	
• Unilateral spatial neglect (visual modality) or inattention	Lateralized task approach (Heilman & Watson, 1978; Keh-chung, 1996); activate right hemisphere with music and visuospatial input; avoid activating left hemisphere by unnecessary verbal comments during activity performance; use movement and music therapy group
• Field dependency or visual distraction	
• Impaired attention	
For Mr. H to be able to use three or four intermittent verbal cues during each of the dressing tasks	
Priority #2: Cognitive disturbances (higher-order cognition)	Videotaped feedback of performance errors (Söderback et al., 1992)
• Lack of judgment	Step-by-step feedback during actual performance
• Lack of insight	
• Concrete thoughts	
For Mr. H to be able to recognize at least two visuospatial and spatial in-attention errors by observing own dressing performance on a videotape	
Priority #3: Spatial relations impairment	Functional approach: use of ADLs and other tasks important for maximum independence, such as washing and waxing the car and household activities
• Spatial relations impairment	
• Topographical disorientation	
• Right–left discrimination problems	
For Mr. H to be able to perform dressing tasks with only verbal cues	
Priority #4: Strength and apraxia	Functional approach: use real activities that require strength and proprio-ceptive feedback, such as cleaning the car and waxing the car or wood-
• Bilateral motor apraxia	
• Slightly reduced strength on left side	

(continues)

(continued)

Table 10–6. Prioritized problem list: Short-term goals to be reached after 3 weeks of intervention

---

PERFORMANCE COMPONENTS: INTERVENTION RELATES TO BOTH SHORT- AND LONG-TERM GOALS ADDRESSED THROUGH FUNCTIONAL ACTIVITIES

DYSFUNCTION	INTERVENTION
• Measurable improvement on the Purdue peg board test and the Box-and-Block test	work if appropriate; keep in mind that the motor apraxia is not recent and may therefore have a different prognosis when compared with other impairments
Priority #5: Perseveration • Premotor perseveration • Prefrontal perseveration For Mr. H to be able to perform dressing tasks with only verbal cues	Feedback related to errors during ADLs
Priority #6: Organization and sequencing • Related to other impairments For Mr. H to be able to perform dressing tasks with only verbal cues	Functional approach and feedback during ADLs, such as organizing ADL tasks, cleaning the car, and light kitchen tasks
Priority #7: Short-term memory impairment possibly related to attention problems For Mr. H to be able to perform all grooming and hygiene tasks without verbal reminders	Same as for attention problems and use compensation approaches, such as writing things down where necessary.

STRENGTHS TO CONSIDER

Oriented toward time and place
Good long-term memory
Language functions intact; could be used for verbal cueing during activities
Avoid unnecessary verbal comments during task performance because of attention deficits
Good use of all four extremities and ambulant; however, this will lead to an early discharge
Relatively intact tactile and proprioceptive sensation
Supportive wife

(continues)

(continued)

Table 10–6. Prioritized problem list: Short-term goals to be reached after 3 weeks of intervention
The main emphasis of intervention is on the use of functional tasks that are important for Mr. H's occupational performance. Simultaneously, attention is given to dysfunctional performance components that interfere with independent task performance and an effort is made to diminish these by using compensation techniques and error detection to increase insight. Leisure tasks that motivate Mr. H are used to simultaneously address dysfunctional performance components.

soning, she set short- and long-term goals for intervention in agreement with Mr. and Mrs. H. The short-term goals included training of ADLs so that Mr. H would be able to dress, groom and wash, get into the bathtub, and use a knife to cut and butter, all with minimum assistance from his wife.

Carol decided to use the "new functional approach" described by Abreu et al. (1994) and practice the tasks listed as goals during intervention sessions. The "new functional approach" is a factor-relating theory that emphasizes that task performance simultaneously engages different performance components and that effective adaptation always takes place in environmental context. It rejects the treatment dichotomy between bottom-up and top-down approaches that imply unidirectional relationship between the two. It also rejects the view of selection of adaptation treatment approaches versus restorative approaches based on the perceived transfer potential. Assessment includes both micro and macro levels, establishment of observed relationships between the two, and environmental context. The intervention modality is daily occupation, taking aim at the most relevant occupational tasks possible based on the client's needs and goals. Therapists' skills are used to present the tasks in such a manner that impaired cognitive performance components are appropriately challenged. Therefore, this approach requires the therapist to be sensitive to the task itself as well as to the environmental context where the activity takes place. It incorporates use of activity analysis and adaptation as well as graded assistance and progressively more relevant occupational environments. During these ADL tasks, Carol used principles that have previously been classified as functional compensation, such as encouraging Mr. H by using verbal cues to look to the left and scan both visual fields to overcome the visual neglect. Carol also used principles previously classified as functional adaptation, in which clothes were, for example, labeled with prominent colors to emphasize the back and front to diminish the effects of the spatial-relations impairment. These two aspects of the functional approach have been classified as top-down approaches. The remedial treatment (also referred to as *deficit-specific*) approaches, classified as bottom-up approaches, are addressed simultaneously in the treatment sessions through activities because according to the "new functional approach," cognitive performance components should be appropriately engaged and challenged during task performance. Different kinds of feedback would be combined with the activity sessions in an attempt to influence Mr. H's insight into errors in task performance and to provide his wife with relevant information about his performance. The feedback about errors in performance would be provided immediately to Mr. H by using verbal cueing as well as by viewing videotapes of his performance later on (Söderback et al., 1992). Therefore, Mr. H would identify errors during observation of a videotape or be assisted in identifying them with comments on how to overcome them.

Other intervention approaches (sometimes classified as remedial approaches), such as the lateralized task approach (Heilman & Watson, 1978; Keh-chung, 1996), can be used simultaneously in treatment to further influence some of the neurobehavioral impairments that interfere with function. In the lateralized task approach, stimuli that activate an affected right hemisphere, such as visuospatial stimuli, are provided. Stimuli that activate the intact left hemisphere, such as verbal stimuli, are avoided. The lateralized task approach ensures that stimuli that activate the affected right hemisphere, such as visuospatial stimuli, are provided during activity performance. Stimulation of the unaffected left hemisphere, such as verbal stimuli, is avoided because it is believed to make the unilateral neglect worse. Carol chose to use this treatment method by including Mr. H in an established movement and music therapy group with four to six other clients. The lateralized task approach is used in the group sessions because vestibular (i.e., movement) and nonverbal auditory stimuli (i.e., music) activate the right hemisphere and are thought to affect cortical tone, mood, emotion, and attention. In addition, contralateral tactile and proprioceptive stimuli would also be provided through this activity. Attention is crucial for many cerebral functions; therefore, the emphasis would be placed on improving attention before focusing on other problems such as visuospatial problems. Box 10–4 explores the reasoning behind the selection of a therapeutic approach.

Another short-term goal (of lower priority) was to assist Mr. H in developing his leisure activities, such as improving his reading skills by

BOX 10–4. THERAPIST REASONING BEHIND SELECTION OF A THERAPEUTIC APPROACH

I chose to use activities that are a part of Mr. H's daily routine and that he has difficulty with for intervention. I am in favor of using occupational performance as an intervention medium in occupational therapy. Furthermore, the intervention time in this case will be short, and I question the transfer of learning potential that Mr. H has, given his lack of insight to his problems. I made this decision keeping in mind that studies have shown (e.g., see Neistadt, 1994c) that clients with brain dysfunction are only capable of near transfer in relatively short training periods. Since lack of insight and lack of judgment are identified as problem areas, I thought that intervention needed to address the issue of awareness and client education through feedback regarding task performance during actual occupational performance or by using videotapes (in which Mr. H is assisted in detecting the errors), particularly in ADLs, for effective use of compensation. The approach I have chosen to use in general in my practice (outlined previously), linked with the A-ONE theory and assessment results, seems to have a lot in common with the new functional approach described by Abreu et al. (1994). The new functional approach is a factor-relating approach similar to the A-ONE theory, and it simultaneously considers occupational performance and performance components necessary for task performance. In the new functional approach, the intervention modality is daily occupation, although treatment may include tasks that emphasize training in certain components. The movement-and-music group includes stimulation of attention components (music to the right hemisphere) and movement (vestibular stimulation affecting the right parietal lobe), thus also affecting the performance component dysfunction of unilateral spatial neglect in locating the ball. This activity addresses dysfunctional visuospatial components, such as spatial relations impairment, in judging the direction of the ball in the air or from the floor if it falls down. It also addresses body scheme components, such as unilateral neglect of the left body side when reaching for the ball and incorporating verbal instructions about looking to right or left. All these components are incorporated into this task, which also doubles as a leisure activity motivating Mr. H (as he identified) because he used to enjoy music and related activities, such as dancing. Although the new functional approach seems to have many similarities to the quadraphonic approach described by Abreu (1994), I feel more comfortable with the new functional approach since (1) I am not considering all four microperspectives described in the quadraphonic approach, (2) I am not using different reductionist tests for those components, and (3) I am not reducing tasks to specific exercise drills for certain components.

The approach I am using is also different from the Dynamic Interaction Approach described by Toglia (1993b) (also described in Chapter 3), which

(continues)

BOX 10–4. THERAPIST REASONING BEHIND SELECTION OF A THERAPEUTIC APPROACH (CONT.)

relies on a specific assessment that requires a high level of training in the approach that I do not have and standardized deficit specific tests. I do not find it necessary to use deficit-specific tests if I can detect impairments by using the A-ONE (which is standardized). I feel really comfortable with the A-ONE as an occupational therapist. I prefer to use it rather than using deficit-specific tests or test items that are more or less borrowed from other disciplines (e.g., neuropsychology or neurology) and in some cases even duplicate the testing performed by members of these disciplines. In the Dynamic Interaction Approach, metacognitive training is important. This training relies on insight, which is limited in Mr. H's case. I cannot rely on too much transfer of training during the short intervention time. Furthermore, the Dynamic Interaction Approach uses reductionist drills for intervention (although the items chosen can have meaning in daily activities, such as sorting cutlery, they are still reductionist), and I prefer to use intervention time to practice occupational performance in real-life situations.

using a functional approach and cueing regarding scanning of the left visual field to aid in reading newspapers and TV subtitles. The ability to perform simple kitchen and household tasks was also addressed by using a functional approach so Mr. H could eliminate inactivity by sharing the responsibility of these tasks with his wife.

Carol considered it an important long-term goal to gather more information regarding Mr. H's opportunities to engage himself in leisure activities. Household chores would be related to this goal as well as the ability to take walks with his wife and possibly join an activity center for the elderly in which movement groups, dancing, or other social engagements are offered. Carol also thought of checking on the possibility of Mr. H's attending an activity center where he could engage in some part-time work if boredom or inactivity became a problem at home. Mr. H was independent in ambulating; therefore, Carol did not expect that he would need more than 2 or 3 weeks in the rehabilitation center to reach these goals. Working with his wife and possibly involving social services at the time of discharge would therefore be crucial in achieving the long-term goals. In terms of driving, Carol did not expect that Mr. H would be able to drive safely in the near future and possibly ever. A short-term goal was set to evaluate his wife's driving skills and whether she would feel comfortable in taking over the role of driving (i.e., using a functional adaptation approach). Mr. H could then accompany her on the shopping trips and possibly be partially responsible for keeping the car in shape because the car seemed to be his primary interest. His ability to structure the task of washing the car should therefore be examined during an intervention session. In this session, verbal cues (i.e., functional compensation) could be provided to minimize, for example, the effects of spatial-relations problems and unilateral spatial neglect as well as unilateral body neglect in the initial session and an attempt made to withdraw those upon repetition of the task (domain-specific functional approach). Simultaneously this task would provide tactile, proprioceptive, and vestibular stimuli (in addition to visual and auditory stimuli) from a remedial point of view, and these would affect muscle strength, balance, and possibly praxis. Table 10–6 presents a prioritized problem list, including goals and a brief description of the intervention plan that Carol chose to achieve these goals.

INTERVENTION

OUTLINE OF A THERAPY SESSION

During his 3-week stay in rehabilitation, Mr. H had ADL training every morning and an afternoon session focusing on specific intervention activities. After the first week, he joined a movement and music group three times a week in the afternoon, one afternoon session a week for household activities, and another one for working on the car. Two extra sessions a week were kept open for various activities, such as going over videotapes of Mr. H's performance during different tasks (detecting errors resulting from dysfunction of visuospatial and other components) in order to provide feedback.

Movement and Music Group

A brief description is provided of a movement and music intervention session that Mr. H attended during his stay at the rehabilitation facility. It must be kept in mind, however, that this is just an example and does not reflect the full treatment he received. Carol and Mr. H decided that he should attend the group three times a week for 45 minutes each time. As mentioned previously, the group could be used to incorporate principles from the lateralized task approach to activate the right hemisphere and thereby enhance cortical tone and attention, which is crucial for other cerebral functions such as visuospatial functions. A movement and music group can also be used to train visuospatial functioning and to give feedback regarding errors, for example, in judging distances. There were four to six individuals in the group during each session. An example of an activity used in the group was to line up group members in an irregular circle and pass a light beach ball around the group. The ball was passed around by the participants' hitting it in the desired direction from one person to another while music was played. If a person missed the ball, that person had to bend down and pick it up to pass it on. The person holding the ball when the music stopped playing received a point score. The points were added up at the end of the session, and the person with the lowest score in the end would be the winner of the session. Missed catches were also recorded. In the latter part of the session, the ball would be passed on randomly from alternating directions. Therefore, the session provided visuospatial information regarding the location of the ball and people and required scanning of both visual fields for successful performance. Auditory input was provided through music, thus activating processing of the right hemisphere and subsequently affecting emotion and attention mechanisms. Vestibular information, which also affects these mechanisms, was provided through moving the head in space, looking in different directions, and bending down for the ball when it fell. This information was also important for balance and together with sensorimotor feedback, had the potential to affect muscle strength, balance, and praxis (praxis has spatial components, as mentioned previously).

Box 10–5 outlines Carol's thoughts on Mr. H joining this group, and Carol's reflection on the outcome of the therapy session is provided in Box 10–6.

DISCONTINUATION OF INTERVENTION AND FUTURE RECOMMENDATIONS

Upon discharge, 3 weeks after admission to the rehabilitation center, Carol reflected on whether Mr. H's treatment had been successful or not. She considered the impact of the intervention program on Mr. and Mrs. H's future using conditional reasoning (Mattingly & Fleming, 1994). In order to do this she considered the progress made toward the predetermined goals, Mr. H's change in attitude toward his condition, and the effect these would have on his life.

ACTIVITIES OF DAILY LIVING PERFORMANCE

Mr. H had improved in ADL performance so that he only needed occasional verbal cues. His wife was able to provide these cues when necessary. Mrs. H felt comfortable in taking over the driving task, and

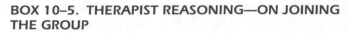

BOX 10–5. THERAPIST REASONING—ON JOINING THE GROUP

On this particular day, Mr. H was the only new member of the group. He was willing to participate in the session but did not look enthusiastic. I introduced Mr. H and then gave the group verbal instructions about how the ball should be passed around. I placed Mr. H so that the ball would arrive in his left visual field during the first part of the session. The first time the ball came to him, he noticed it too late, and it fell on the floor. I commented, "You have to be prepared to look for the ball on the left side, Mr. H. Now bend down for it and pass it on to Mrs. G." Mr. H bent down slowly and reached for the ball but had problems grabbing onto it with his right hand alone (showing unilateral body neglect). I told him, "You need to grasp the ball with both hands to be able to lift it." Mr. H then reached out with his left hand as well, grabbed the ball, raised himself up, and passed the ball to Mrs. G. The next time the ball came around to him, I alerted him to it and shouted, "Look to the left, Mr. H; the ball is coming to you." Mr. H Looked to the left in time and attempted to push the ball to Mrs. G with his right hand but did not reach out far enough (showing complex perceptual disorder of visuospatial origin), so the ball fell on the floor again. He picked it up with some instructions from me and passed it to Mrs. G. The music stopped, and Mrs. G got a point marked down on the blackboard. Another tune started, and while I was preparing for the ball to be passed around again, Mr. H uttered, "I know this music; we used to have it at home." I gave Mr. H verbal cues several times during the session when the ball approached him. Then I intermittently withdrew the cues to see if his performance would change. He was occasionally able to locate the ball by himself, reach far enough out for it, and pass it on (using complex perception such as visual attention and visuospatial processing), but at other times the ball fell to the floor. As the session went on, Mr. H felt more at ease. Now he smiled when he dropped the ball and when the music stopped and he happened to be holding the ball, thus receiving penalty points. At one point when he dropped the ball and had difficulties grabbing it again with his right hand alone (showing unilateral body neglect), I confronted him and asked what was wrong. "I need to use both hands," he said, and reached out with his left hand as well. After the session he commented that it had been fun and told me that he would be willing to participate again.

BOX 10–6. THERAPIST REASONING—INTERVENTION SESSION OUTCOME

In considering the outcome of the intervention session with Mr. H, I concluded that it had been a good practice for balance and making judgments regarding visuospatial abilities, including distance (i.e., locating and hitting of the ball). I noted that as the session went on, Mr. H was able to make use of the cues to look to the left and incorporate both hands even though the cues were intermittent and slowly reduced. However, when a group member started talking about something irrelevant, Mr. H's unilateral neglect became more apparent. I also noted a change in mood during the session—Mr. H was more cheerful toward the end of the group. It seemed that the group awakened his motivation. Mr. H's performance during the session strengthened my conclusion to avoid unnecessary verbal information and only use cues necessary for successful performance of particular tasks. I decided that immediate discussion after a group session regarding the incidences when Mr. H dropped the ball and the reasons for it (i.e., complex perceptual disorders such as spatial relations impairment and unilateral visual or body neglect) could be used to improve his insight into problems, for example, his driving ability, and the consequences these errors might have for him and others during driving. Furthermore, I thought that the social aspects of the group might make Mr. H more positive to seek company or activity centers outside his home in the future, and that might prove to be an important aspect in avoiding inactivity and depression.

Mr. H accepted this role change. The intervention sessions that aimed at making him aware of his limitations and considering the impact of his spatial relation impairments on task performance, such as driving, were successful.

Mr. H needed encouragement and verbal cues to structure a plan of action for various tasks as well as organization and sequencing hints to complete activity steps. He also needed occasional verbal cues to use his left hand in performance of bilateral activities, scanning the left visual field, and using spatial-relational information. After these verbal reminders, he could continue working, making use of the cues for some time. His wife was able to provide the cues needed for the task of keeping the car clean, and he could participate in kitchen tasks with her but could not perform them independently. Mrs. H was willing to allow Mr. H to share the homemaker role with her and understood that it was important to keep her husband motivated and active.

LEISURE ACTIVITIES

There was an activity center located a 15 minutes' walk from Mr. and Mrs. H's home. It was arranged that they would walk there twice a week for an afternoon program on a trial basis.

ENVIRONMENTAL CONTEXT

Although Mr. H did not claim to have encountered any environmental barriers at home during weekend visits, Carol conducted a home visit to see if any recommendations could be made regarding home adaptations. She recommended that improved lighting could diminish the effects of the visuospatial problems, and she rearranged loose electric and phone cords on the floor and loose carpets to minimize possible falls.

Although Carol envisioned that Mr. H would be able to perform his ADL routines with supervision and verbal cues from his wife and to participate in household chores and shopping, she was apprehensive regarding the possibility that he might become inactive and possibly depressed. Therefore, Carol decided to visit Mr. and Mrs. H in their home 1 month after discharge to assess his adjustment to his new conditions at home and to determine if social activation needed to be increased.

SUMMARY

This chapter reviewed complex perceptual functions, including visuospatial components and body scheme components, which are necessary for performing different tasks in a variety of ADLs. The chapter provided conceptual definitions for these dysfunctions. A case study of an individual who had sustained a right CVA resulting in several complex perceptual problems was presented. The factor-relating theory behind the A-ONE (Árnadóttir, 1990) was applied as the theoretical base for the occupational therapy process. Subsequently the A-ONE instrument was used to simultaneously evaluate task performance dysfunction and dysfunction of performance components that interfered with task performance. The results from the evaluation were reviewed and examples of the ways different impairments can affect task performance during ADLs were provided. Throughout the chapter interactive and procedural reasoning strategies were used during the data-gathering phase of the occupational therapy process to investigate and define the problem. Procedural reasoning was used to form a series of hypotheses to establish an occupational diagnosis in order to reflect the nature of phenomena requiring occupational therapy intervention. In addition, conditional reasoning was applied to form goals for intervention and select appropriate intervention methods. The "new functional approach" was selected to guide intervention because it involves the use of functional tasks (as determined by the goals) within their context and simultaneously engages and challenges performance components. The chosen interventions were provided with the goal of diminishing the effects of dysfunctional components on task performance, allowing for more adaptive behavioral responses. Principles from "remedial approaches," including the lateralized task approach and the use of verbal feedback regarding performance, were adopted. An intervention sample from a movement and music group was provided. Finally, procedural and conditional reasoning were used to determine the effectiveness of the overall intervention and to evaluate whether the intervention had prepared Mr. H for his new life after his stroke.

≡ REVIEW QUESTIONS

1. What suggestions do you have for gathering information and conducting an assessment if Carol had not been certified to use the A-ONE?
2. How would you change the focus of information gathering, goal formation, goal priority, and therapeutic intervention if Mr. H was:

● Still working at the office of the oil company, or
● Living alone?

3. Can you think of a situation involving a client who had problems with dressing in which you would need to differentiate between:

● Ideational apraxia and spatial-relations impairment, and
● Ideomotor apraxia and spatial-relations impairment?

How would you make a hypotheses in relation to observed critical cues for the two items above, and how would you interpret these (see Table 10–5)?

≡ ACKNOWLEDGMENTS

I would like to thank Atli Vagnsson for his assistance and support in compiling the material for this chapter and Mr. H for his contribution to the content of the chapter.

APPENDIX 10-1

Árnadóttir OT-ADL Neurobehavioral Evaluation (A-ONE) forms and results from the case of Mr. H. (With permission from author.)

Árnadóttir OT-ADL
Neurobehavioral Evaluation
(A-ONE)

Name __Mr. H__   Date __05.01.1997__

Birthdate __03.04.1925__   Age __71__

Gender __Male__   Ethnicity __Caucasian__

Dominance __Right__   Profession __Retired, worked at an oil company__

Medical Diagnosis: Sustained Right-CVA 23.12.1996, resulting in left hemiparesis and left visual field defect. History of prior infarcts with apraxia. Also a 15 year history of Diabetes Mellitus.

Medication: Sotacor, Magnyl, Glucophage.

Social Situation: Lives with wife on the second floor in a condominium. Five grown up children. Worked in an oil company but retired at the age of 70. Wife is supportive. She does not work outside the home.

Summary of Independence:

Mr. H needs physical assistance with all the dressing tasks (putting on shirt, trousers, socks and fastenings) except for putting on shoes, because of sever spatial relations impairments as well as unilateral body neglect, bilateral motor apraxia and perseveration of movements and thoughts. Further, organization of activity steps is impaired and attention problems, such as field dependency, interfere with activity performance. Needs verbal assistance for grooming and hygiene activities and physical assistance with bating. In addition to the previously mentioned impairments, unilateral visual neglect interfered with grooming tasks. Needs verbal assistance for cutting, but is otherwise independent in feeding. Independent in transfers and mobility tasks except for tub transfers where physical assistance is needed. No communication problems were detected.

FUNCTIONAL INDEPENDENCE SCORE (optional)

FUNCTION	TOTAL SCORE	% SCORE
Dressing	1,1,1,2,1=6/20	
Grooming and hygiene	2,4,4,4,4,1=19/24	
Transfer and mobility	4,4,4,4,1,=17/20	
Feeding	4,4,4,2=14/16	
Communication	4,4,=8/8	

© 1988, Guðrún Árnadóttir

List of Neurobehavioral Impairments Observed:

SPECIFIC IMPAIRMENT	D	G	T	F	C
Motor Apraxia	3	1		2	
Ideational Apraxia					
Unilateral Body Neglect	3	2		2	
Somatoagnosia					
Spatial Relations	3	1		2	
Unilateral Spatial Neglect		1		1	
Abnormal Tone: Right					
Abnormal Tone: Left	1	1	1	1	
Perseveration	3	1			
Organization	2	2			
Topographical Disorientation					
Other					
Sensory Aphasia					
Jargon Aphasia					
Anomia					
Paraphasia					
Expressive Aphasia					

PERVASIVE IMPAIRMENT	ADL
Astereognosis	
Visual Object Agnosia	
Visual Spatial Agnosia	✓
Associative Visual Agnosia	
Anosognosia	
R/L discrimination	✓
Short–Term Memory	✓
Long–Term Memory	
Disorientation	
Confabulation	
Lability	
Euphoria	
Apathy	
Depression	
Aggressiveness	
Irritability	
Frustration	

PERVASIVE IMPAIRMENT	ADL
Restlessness	
Concrete Thinking	✓
Decreased Insight	✓
Impaired Judgment	✓
Confusion	
Impaired Alertness	
Impaired Attention	✓
Distractibility	✓
Impaired Initiative	
Impaired Motivation	
Performance Latency	
Absent mindedness	
Other	
Field dependency	✓

Use (√) for presence of specific impairments in different ADL domains (D = dressing, G = grooming, T = transfers, F = feeding, C = communication), and for presence of pervasive impairments detected during the ADL evaluation.

Summary of Neurobehavioral Impairments:

Mr. H had spatial relations impairments, bilateral motor apraxia and unilateral body inattention that interfered considerably with dressing performance, as well as grooming and hygiene performance and feeding. Premotor and prefrontal perseveration, field dependency and organization and sequencing problems regarding activity steps were also noted. Unilateral visual inattention was present as well as some lack of full strength in the left body side

Treatment Considerations:

Use of Functional Approach utilizing compensation and adaptation principles to improve independence in ADL. Activate the right hemisphere with non-verbal auditory stimuli and vestibular stimuli to affect general motivation, attention and neglect. This could be done by movement and music therapy groups where tactile and proprioceptive stimuli would also be incorporated. Avoid activating the left hemisphere by verbal stimuli during task performance, as it makes attention problems more apparent. Use feedback regarding errors in performance to increase insight into impairments, both direct feedback during performance as well as videotapes of performance with discussion. Use functional tasks such as washing and waxing car to improve strength, standing balance, endurance, and praxis. Also to affect organization of activity steps and improve spatial relations. Use of kitchen tasks and leisure tasks to establish new roles.

Occupational Therapist: Carol

A-ONE certification Number: ÍS-92 085

© 1988, Guðrún Árnadóttir

Appendix 10–1. Continues

A-ONE Part I
Functional Independence Scale and
Neurobehavioral Specific Impairment Subscale

Name Mr. H   Date   05.01.97

INDEPENDENCE SCORE (IP):

4 = Independent and able to transfer activity to other environmental situations.
3 = Independent with supervision.
2 = Needs verbal assistance.
1 = Needs demonstration or physical assistance.
0 = Unable to perform. Totally dependent on assistance.

NEUROBEHAVIORAL SCORE (NB):

0 = No neurobehavioral impairments observed.
1 = Patient is able to perform without additional information, but some neurobehavioral impairment is observed.
2 = Patient is able to perform with additional verbal assistance, but neurobehavioral impairment can be observed during performance.
3 = Patient is able to perform with demonstration or minimal to considerable physical assistance.
4 = Patient is unable to perform due to neurobehavioral impairment. Needs maximum physical assistance.

LIST HELPING AIDS USED:

-Prosthetic tooth brush for dentures

-Glasses for some ADL items

PRIMARY ADL ACTIVITY	SCORING	COMMENTS AND REASONING

DRESSING	IP SCORE	
Shirt (or dress)	4 3 2 ① 0	Px. assist with sleeve and neck hole.
Pants	4 3 2 ① 0	Re. how to turn clothes, and find holes.
Socks	4 3 2 ① 0	Re. heal turned wrong.
Shoes	4 3 ② 1 0	Incorrect right/left shoe
Fastenings	4 3 2 ① 0	Px for zipper, verbal for buckle on shoe.
Other		

NB IMPAIRMENT	NB SCORE	
Motor apraxia	0 1 2 ③ 4	Manipulating fastenings
Ideational apraxia	⓪ 1 2 3 4	
Unilateral body neglect	0 1 2 ③ 4	Shirt and trousers on left side.
Somatoagnosia	⓪ 1 2 3 4	
Spatial relations	0 1 2 ③ 4	Correct: arm, neck and leg holes.
Unilateral spatial neglect	⓪ 1 2 3 4	However, used items on R-side first.
Abnormal tone: Right	⓪ 1 2 3 4	
Abnormal tone: Left	0 ① 2 3 4	All movements present but a little weaker.
Perseveration	0 1 2 ③ 4	Gets stuck pulling on sock, sleeve.
Organization/Sequencing	0 1 ② 3 4	Shoes before trousers, fastenings.
Other Field dependency		Grabs whatever catches his attention.

Note: All definitions and scoring criteria for each deficit are in the Evaluation Manual.

© 1988, Guðrún Árnadóttir

Appendix 10–1. Continues

Functional Independence Scale and Neurobehavioral Specific Impairment Subscale cont.

PRIMARY ADL ACTIVITY	SCORING	COMMENTS AND REASONING

GROOMING AND HYGIENE — IP SCORE

GROOMING AND HYGIENE	IP SCORE					COMMENTS
Wash face and upper body	4	3	②	1	0	Reminded to: wash face, hands,
Comb hair	④	3	2	1	0	underarms, include soap and
Brush teeth	④	3	2	1	0	rinse soap off left side.
Shave/make up	④	3	2	1	0	
Continence/toilet	④	3	2	1	0	
Bath	4	3	2	①	0	
Other						

NB IMPAIRMENT	NB SCORE					
Motor apraxia	0	①	2	3	4	Bilateral clumsiness: brush teeth, hold comb.
Ideational apraxia	⓪	1	2	3	4	
Unilateral body neglect	0	1	②	3	4	Wash left side, use left hand.
Somatoagnosia	⓪	1	2	3	4	
Spatial relations	0	①	2	3	4	Many trials to turn teeth correctly.
Unilateral spatial neglect	0	①	2	3	4	Did not notice towel falling.
Abnormal tone: Right	⓪	1	2	3	4	Gathers all items in right visual field.
Abnormal tone: Left	0	①	2	3	4	
Perseveration	0	①	2	3	4	Washes face x 2, and combs x 3.
Organization/Sequencing	0	1	②	3	4	Include all activity steps. Rinse off soap.
Other Field dependency						Uses prosthetic brush for hands.

TRANSFERS AND MOBILITY	IP SCORE					
Sitting up in bed	④	3	2	1	0	
Transfers to/from bed (chair)	④	3	2	1	0	
Maneuver around	④	3	2	1	0	
Toilet transfers	④	3	2	1	0	
Tub transfers	4	3	2	①	0	
Other						

NB IMPAIRMENT	NB SCORE					
Motor apraxia	⓪	1	2	3	4	
Ideational apraxia	⓪	1	2	3	4	
Unilateral body neglect	⓪	1	2	3	4	
Spatial relations	0	①	2	3	4	Sometimes too far away from seat
Unilateral spatial neglect	⓪	1	2	3	4	for transferring.
Abnormal tone: Right	⓪	1	2	3	4	
Abnormal tone: Left	0	①	2	3	4	
Perseveration	⓪	1	2	3	4	
Organization/Sequencing	⓪	1	2	3	4	
Topographical disorientation	⓪	1	2	3	4	Knows his way around the Rehab.
Other						

© 1988, Guðrún Árnadóttir

Appendix 10–1. Continues

Functional Independence Scale and Neurobehavioral Specific Impairment Subscale cont.

PRIMARY ADL ACTIVITY	SCORING	COMMENTS AND REASONING

FEEDING	IP	SCORE				
Drink from a mug	④	3	2	1	0	
Use fingers/sandwich	④	3	2	1	0	
Use fork or spoon	④	3	2	1	0	
Use knife	4	3	②	1	0	
Other						

NB IMPAIRMENT	NB	SCORE				COMMENTS
Motor apraxia	0	1	②	3	4	Poor manipulation of knife.
Ideational apraxia	⓪	1	2	3	4	Requires bilateral hand use.
Unilateral body neglect	0	1	②	3	4	Reminded to include R-hand.
Spatial relations	0	1	②	3	4	Misjudges distances when buttering.
Unilateral spatial neglect	0	①	2	3	4	Does not notice some items
Abnormal tone: Right	⓪	1	2	3	4	in L-visual field.
Abnormal tone: Left	0	①	2	3	4	
Perseveration	⓪	1	2	3	4	
Organization/Sequencing	⓪	1	2	3	4	
Other						

COMMUNICATION	IP	SCORE			
Comprehension	④	3	2	1	0
Speech	④	3	2	1	0

NB IMPAIRMENT	NB	SCORE (0 = absent, 1 = present)			
Wernicke's aphasia / Sensory aphasia	⓪	1			
Jargon aphasia	⓪	1			
Anomia	⓪	1			
Paraphasia	⓪	1			
Perseveration	⓪	1			
Broca's Aphasia / Expressive aphasia	⓪	1			
Dysarthria	⓪	1			
Other	⓪	1			

Results from specific sensory and motor tests:

-Sensory tests including tactile location, proprioception and pain sensation are normal.

-Normal eye movements.

-Muscle strength Lower extremities: Left side: 4/5   Right side: 5/5

-Muscle strength upper extremities: Left side: 3^+-4/5   Right side: 5/5

   Isolated finger movements of all fingers on left side are present.

-Slightly increased tone on passive movements of left arm.

© 1988, Guðrún Árnadóttir

Appendix 10–1. Continues

A-ONE Part I
Neurobehavioral Pervasive
Impairment Subscale

Name <u>Mr. H</u>   Date <u>05.01.1997</u>

Scoring criteria: Circle one
0 = Impairment is absent
1 = Impairment is present

Pervasive signs may be observed or noted in any Activities of daily Living (ADL) domain, according to specific instructions in the manual.

NEUROBEHAVIORAL IMPAIRMENT	NB SCORE				COMMENTS AND REASONING
AGNOSIA					
1. Tactile/astereognosis: Right/Left side?	⓪	1			Able to recognize objects
2. Motor impersistence	⓪	1			Able to maintain positions
3. Visual object agnosia	⓪	1			
4. Visual spatial agnosia	0	①			Problems finding correct holes
5. Associative visual agnosia	⓪	1			on clothes. Misjudges distances.
6. Anosognosia	⓪	1			
BODY SCHEME DISTURBANCES					
1. Right/Left disorientation	0	①			Did not refer to the body sides
2. Body part identification	⓪	1			correctly as to R/L on command
EMOTIONAL/AFFECTIVE DISTURBANCES					
1. Lability	⓪	1			
2. Euphoria	⓪	1			
3. Apathy	⓪	1			
4. Depression	⓪	1			
5. Aggression	⓪	1			
6. Irritability	⓪	1			
7. Frustration	⓪	1			
8. Restlessness	⓪	1			
COGNITIVE DISTURBANCES					
1. Concrete thinking	0	①			Some trouble with simple calculations.
2. Decreased insight	0	①			Not aware of all impairments, nor how
3. Impaired judgment	0	①			they affect task performance
4. Confusion	⓪	1			Claimed it did not matter if clothes turned
OTHER DYSFUNCTIONS					incorrectly. Did not use feedback from ── errors appropriately.
1. Impaired alertness	⓪	1			
2. Impaired attention	0	①			Field dependent behavior. Distracted by
3. Distractibility	0	①			stimuli that were not relevant to particular
4. Impaired initiative	⓪	1			activity steps. Picks up irrelevant items.
5. Impaired motivation	⓪	1			
6. Performance latency	⓪	1			
7. Absentmindedness	⓪	1			
8.					

© 1988, Guðrún Árnadóttir

Appendix 10–1. Continues

Neurobehavioral Pervasive Impairment Subscale continued:

NEUROBEHAVIORAL IMPAIRMENT   NB SCORE   COMMENTS AND REASONING

MEMORY DISTURBANCES					
1. Short-term memory loss	0	(1)			Repeated instruction.
2. Long-term memory loss	(0)	1			
3. Disorientation	(0)	1			Only two days off the present date,
4. Confabulation	(0)	1			which is within normal limits.

Summary:

 Visual spatial agnosia (spatial relations impairment) interfered with all dressing tasks and manifested in difficulties finding correct holes of clothes. Problems with right-left discrimination manifested during dressing and upon confrontation.

 Cognitive impairments: Concrete thoughts manifested as difficulties with simple calculations, for example related to the time of retirement. Lack of insight into own condition was apparent as Mr.H was not able to identify any impairments as a result of the stroke except for the weakness. He also indicated that he could be discharged shortly and become an outpatient as he could drive in every day, not accounting for the severe spatial relations impairments that would certainly interfere with his driving performance. Lack of judgment manifested in comments such as "it does not matter if the clothes turn inside out", when that performance was pointed out to him. Did not use feedback from own errors even though they were indicated to him.

 Some short term memory problems were noted and instructions did at times have to be frequently repeated. Lack of attention probably affected short term memory as well. Specific visual stimuli that were not relevant for a particular activity frequently distracted him. Picked up irrelevant items, and at one point incorporated an item into performance of a previous activity indicating prefrontal perseveration and field dependency.

 Tactile discrimination was intact. Mr.H was well oriented towards time and place and his long term memory was intact. No affective or emotional disturbances were noted at the time of the evaluation

Use of Groups in the Rehabilitation of Persons with Head Injury: Reasoning Skills Used by the Group Facilitator

SHARAN SCHWARZBERG, EdD, OTR, FAOTA

- Climate Setting
- Closed Group
- Concrete Thinking
- Functional Group
- Open Group

- Patient-Oriented Style
- Peer-Facilitated Group
- Professionally Led Group
- Task-Oriented Style
- Unstable Affect

On completion of this chapter, the reader will be able to:

- Identify advantages of using various types of groups as a modality in cognitive and perceptual rehabilitation programs
- Understand differences between professionally led and peer-facilitated groups
- Identify practical concerns in forming a group
- Recognize the potential influence of cognitive and perceptual dysfunction on members' functioning in a group and the skills potentially enhanced by participating in a therapeutic or support group
- Understand the types of reasoning used by occupational therapists in facilitating group interventions for individuals with cognitive and perceptual dysfunction
- Successfully work through the Review Questions

≡ INTRODUCTION

The purpose of this chapter is to present the reasoning behind the use of groups in cognitive and perceptual rehabilitation. The chapter opens with a discussion of types of professionally led therapeutic groups and peer-led support groups. Therapist guidelines for facilitating a group for individuals with head injury are given. Clinical reasoning behind practice is explained and two case studies of a group's process are examined in detail.

≡ THE GROUP WORK MODEL

There are several advantages to the use of group treatment or intervention in cognitive perceptual rehabilitation. In addition to its cost-effectiveness (Duncombe & Howe, 1995; Trahey, 1991), the group format offers clients an opportunity to learn from actual experience in performance areas such as activities of daily living (ADLs); work and productive areas; play and leisure; and sensorimotor, cognitive, and psychosocial or psychological functional components and social skills. The performance context is easily adapted in groups and closely approximates natural settings. In addition, a group facilitator is able to modify the group format and process to accommodate the variety of problems that result from a brain injury.

The premise of group work is supported by Soderback and Ekholm's (1993) review of the literature on the use of occupational therapy in brain-damage rehabilitation. They found that many intervention programs used group sessions. The group activities included social club activities, bowling, cooking, and discussion with video feedback and were used as training media for individuals with traumatic brain injury, stroke, or dementia. Group process was also used to aid nonverbal communication and expression of feelings and included media such as ceramics, painting, drama, and music. They report: "The aims of the group process are to make the individuals aware of their own identity in relation to others and to master behavioral problems" (p. 344).

TYPES OF GROUPS

Groups can be broadly categorized as either professionally led or peer facilitated. The differences are mostly derived from the degree of structure and involvement from professional helpers and who initiates the group's formation. Group formats can range from minimal to no professional involvement, to trained leaders actively establishing and managing the group's agenda. Another form of groups, **functional groups,** bridges these two models. A comparison of professionally led occupational therapy groups versus peer-led groups is given in Table 11–1, and each is described in more detail in this chapter. Functional groups are then discussed.

Peer-Facilitated Groups

Peer-facilitated groups include self-help groups, advocacy groups, and support groups (Rootes & Aanes, 1992). Table 11–2 provides the types of peer-facilitated groups. For the purposes of this discussion, these groups

FEATURES	PROFESSIONALLY LED GROUP	PEER-LED GROUP
Focused, shared goals		X
Group-centered leadership		X
Leader centered	X	
Heterogeneous aims	X	
Monetary gain	X	
Self-supporting		X
Time and resource limited	X	
Open ended		X

Table 11–1. A comparison of professionally led and peer-led groups

are referred to as *peer-facilitated groups* and are not considered mutually exclusive. Riordan and Beggs (1988) believed that distinctions between self-help groups and peer-support groups stem from whether the group is begun by a professional organization or individual versus the members themselves. Self-help groups emphasize autonomy and the use of internal group resources rather than professional direction. Rootes and Aanes (1992) defined the self-help group using the following criteria. The group, as a self-governing structure:

1. is supportive and educational and formed for a single purpose that is focused on adaptation rather than personality change,
2. has leadership that comes from within the group,
3. is focused on a single major disruptive life event that is shared by the members,
4. is voluntary and, for personal growth with change, is the responsibility of the individual member,
5. has no monetary or profit orientation, and
6. has membership that is anonymous and participation that is confidential.

Professionally Led Groups

Therapy groups fall within the format of **professionally led groups**. These groups are typically focused on individual treatment goals. The groups are conducted by trained professionals, including occupational therapists, social workers, psychologists, doctors, rehabilitation counselors, and other health

Table 11–2. Types of peer-facilitated groups

FEATURES	SELF-HELP GROUP	ADVOCACY GROUP	SUPPORT GROUP
Initiated by members; nonprofit	X		
Initiated by professionals			X
Has a political agenda		X	
Emphasizes autonomy, self-governance, internal leadership	X		
Individual growth	X		
System change		X	
Shared major life disruption to self	X		
External life crisis			X
Information sharing and support	X		
Anonymity and confidentiality not central		X	X

personnel. In occupational therapy, there are several formats and conceptual models for group practice. The various types of occupational therapy groups include neurobehavioral, rehabilitatory, psychoeducational, developmental, task oriented, occupational behavioral, and functional. These categories mostly cover the variety of types of groups found in occupational therapy. The common feature of occupational therapy groups is the focus on functional goals or underlying skills (Table 11–3).

Functional Groups

The functional group model (Howe & Schwartzberg, 1995) is the vantage point of this chapter. This model is applied to both peer- and professionally guided groups. Using this perspective, the group leader capitalizes on the use of group structure (Howe & Schwartzberg, 1988) and the therapeutic use of the self to enhance the group process and individual function. Using purposeful activities, the leader structures tasks to maximally involve members by enhancing the sense of individual as well as group identity; creating an atmosphere that encourages spontaneous involvement, support, and feedback; and forming a match between the members' abilities and required task and personal interactions. The leadership skills used include:

Table 11–3. Sample of cognitive-perceptual skills enhanced by group work

SKILL	RATIONALE: REMEDIAL APPROACHES	RATIONALE: ADAPTIVE APPROACHES
Attention	• Leader can provide reinforcements for attention behaviors, such as tokens. • Leader can modify activities to require sustained attention, selective attention, alternating attention, and divided attention.	• Leader can provide verbal cues to focus members' attention on task. • Leader can state procedures.
Orientation	• Members can practice skills related to orientation to person, place, or time.	• Leader can provide verbal cues, external aids such as written cue cards and calendars, and opportunities for rehearsal using external aids.
Memory	• Members can rehearse and practice with memory retraining programs. • Leader can present information in several contexts with recall prompts.	• Leader can provide information at a level that is understood and establish routines in group to promote habits and create opportunities for routine rehearsal.
Generalization	• Leader can provide training in attention/concentration and abstract reasoning.	• Leader can suggest strategies for problem solving and memory storage, provide opportunities to practice strategies in multiple environments and situations, give feedback for reality orientation, and relate new knowledge that comes up in group to previously learned knowledge and skills.

Adapted from Neistadt, 1990, 1994c, 1995b; Quintana, 1995.

- Genuineness and empathy
- Modeling behavior
- Reality testing
- Communicating: listening and reflectively responding; giving feedback in a supportive manner; and using concrete language, confrontation, and self-disclosure (Howe & Schwartzberg, 1995)

Howe and Schwartzberg's approach is consistent with Tickle-Degnen and Rosenthal's (1990) finding that clients with brain damage appear to take more initiative when instructed in a "patient-oriented manner" versus a "task-oriented manner." In a **task-oriented style**, the therapist helps the patient complete a task by giving verbal directives with little attention paid to the patient's capabilities. In contrast, the **patient-oriented style** directs the therapist to help the patient complete tasks in a more nondirective manner by taking the perspective of the patient and offering guidance as appropriate (Tickle-Degnan & Rosenthal, 1990).

The functional approach is concerned with a person's adaptation to the environment and capitalizes on the individual's strengths and resources. This is similar to Neistadt's (1990) categorization of "adaptive" approaches in occupational therapy interventions for perceptual deficits in adults with brain injury. Building on the client's intact skills to offset residual disability, "therapists following the *adaptive approach* train clients in actual functional activities to help them regain function" (Neistadt, 1995b, p. 437). The functional group approach primarily provides opportunity for learning functional behavior in ADLs rather than focusing on the mediation of component skills. This approach includes community living skills programs because they tend to be driven by the context of the social setting (DePoy, 1987; Dikengil, King, & Monda, 1992; Giles & Shore, 1988; Meghji et al., 1995). Thus, it is different from "remedial" approaches (Neistadt, 1990), which attempt to nurture the recovery or reorganization of impaired central nervous system functions. "Therapists using the *remedial approach* train clients in the component skills that are necessary to do functional activities" (Neistadt, 1995b, p. 437).

In addition to adaptive approaches, some occupational therapy group settings for clients with cognitive and perceptual problems are organized for the primary purpose of singular skill development or remediation (Okkema, 1993; Lysaght & Bodenhamer, 1990; Johnson & Newton, 1987). It is also common to find group process formats that combine remedial and adaptive approaches (Hill & Carper, 1985; Lundgren & Persechino, 1986; Scheibel-Schmitt, 1992; Sladyk, 1992). It is speculated that, as in perceptual remedial retraining for adults with diffuse acquired brain injury (Neistadt, 1994c), repetition of functional group activities, with different tasks in different contexts, is more effective than remedial retraining approaches. Such interventions are particularly suitable for concrete thinkers and for those who have difficulty transferring learning to different situations. Neistadt (1994c) concluded that this may not be the case for individuals with localized lesions and preserved abstract reasoning who have been explicitly taught to transfer learning across a variety of treatment activities.

A group organized with the functional group perspective not only monitors and fosters the development or redevelopment of social skills but promotes the *social process* (M. H. Fleming, personal communication, January 28, 1997). Thus, this approach can potentially alter a process of intersubjective social reconstruction, making it a powerful tool. Functional groups are then quite different in focus from professionally led groups, either psychologically or specific-skills oriented (M. H. Fleming, personal communication, January 28, 1997).

≡ PRACTICAL GUIDELINES FOR FACILITATING A HEAD INJURY SUPPORT GROUP

For the purposes of this example, two types of group protocols are discussed. These are professionally organized groups and peer-organized groups. For both types of groups, the role of the leader, or facilitator, must be established. Second, the group goals are identified along with methods and procedures. This may include the sequence of the sessions; methods of recruiting members; whether the group will be an **open** or **closed group** (i.e., whether new members can join after the group has formed); and resources needed, such as guest speakers and written materials. When the group is initiated by professional staff, leaders can predetermine the group's composition and screen members for particular capabilities, such as attention span.

It is common for group facilitators to have a co-leader and work within interdisciplinary teams. This often occurs when the group is large, affiliated with a training program, or uses team approaches such as peer and professional facilitators and interdisciplinary treatment approaches. In addition, for several reasons, group membership may fluctuate from meeting to meeting. Usually new members join a group as others leave (or terminate). These reasons may be known or unknown to the participants and facilitator. Termination may occur because the member was not adequately prepared to be in a social setting. There may be situations such as the member's feeling unsafe, misunderstood, or confused by the process or content. Or in some circumstances, there are very concrete reasons, such as inadequate transportation.

Based on the importance of group cohesiveness, it is recommended that individuals with head injuries be treated in separate groups (Forssmann-Falck, Christian, & O'Shanick, 1989). Individuals with head injuries have been found to be more accepting of feedback and confrontation about appropriate behaviors from peers with head injuries rather than professional staff (Forssmann-Falck, Christian, & O'Shanick, 1989; Schwartzberg, 1994). It may be difficult for individuals with other neurological difficulties who have focal problems to identify with and understand the emotional trauma and diverse functional problems that may result from a head injury.

PEER-ORGANIZED GROUPS

In the case of a peer support group, it is suggested that whenever possible, the leader establish a contract with the group members before the group's formation. The agreement should delineate the facilitator's role, method of payment, group composition, and referral mechanisms as well as general group format and program activities.

PROFESSIONALLY ORGANIZED GROUPS

In a professionally led group, the group's goals are often established by an interdisciplinary team. The leader's role is complementary to the occupational therapy treatment goals. In all instances the leader must maintain flexibility to the degree of structure and support provided and in the complexity of activities. The leader must continually adjust responses on the basis of multiple verbal and nonverbal cues.

≡ CLINICAL REASONING BEHIND GROUP PRACTICE

Problems that present special challenges to clinical reasoning and effective practice are the influence of members' **concrete thinking** and **unstable affect**. A clinical example of each of these will be discussed from the perspective of Fleming's (1991) typology of three types of reasoning in occupational therapy: (1) procedural reasoning, (2) interactive reasoning, and (3) conditional reasoning. A brief review of clinical reasoning applied to group work is followed by the clinical examples.

REVIEW OF CLINICAL REASONING RELATED TO GROUP WORK

Whether in the treatment or the facilitator role, the therapist should attend to the members at the three levels described by Fleming (1991): "(a) the physical ailment, (b) the client as a person, and (c) the person as a social being in the context of family, environment, and culture" (p. 1007). The therapist pays attention to the members' physical needs, such as incoordination and cognitive-perceptual deficits in procedural reasoning. The leader adjusts the activity to the level of functional performance of individuals and the group as a whole. In interacting with individuals and perceiving the group as a whole, the therapist becomes acquainted with individual group members and attempts to understand the effects of the injury on the individual's self-image and maintenance of a sense of self through daily activities. This interactive reasoning helps the therapist understand the person better and employ conditional reasoning. In the latter form of reasoning, conditional reasoning, the therapist moves back and forth between images of what the person was like before the injury, who the person is now, and what the person's future life may become. In constructing these visions, the therapist is simultaneously imagining both the individuals and the life of the group itself. This is because the group, whether it is a closed or open group or a short- or a long-term group, has its own identity, history, and future. The functional group methodology is illustrated in the following description of facilitating a support group for head-injured individuals. Case examples are given to demonstrate the reasoning behind the therapist's actions.

GROUP EXAMPLE 1: THE INFLUENCE OF MEMBERS' CONCRETE THINKING

In the forming stage of a group, the facilitator explains the goals of the group and helps members get to know one another while promoting feelings of safety. In **climate setting**, the facilitator may ask members to go around and introduce themselves. Name tags are often used as memory aids. This may lead to misunderstandings about the group's purpose, facilitator role, and activity process as well as procedures.

An example of the former scenario follows. The group has been meeting on alternating weeks, for about 6 months, with a relatively stable membership. Table 11–4 provides an outline of the group events (numbered in the corresponding text of the following group discussion), type of clinical reasoning used (Mattingly & Fleming, 1994), and the therapist's underlying thought processes that relate to this example.

Facilitator: Why don't we have the older members introduce themselves and tell their stories and have other people have a chance to tell their story (1).
Ann (in an angry, dismissive voice): I'm not going first.

Table 11–4. The influence of members' concrete thinking: Clinical events and reasoning

GROUP EVENT	REASONING USED	UNDERLYING THOUGHT PROCESS
Facilitator invites name sharing (1)	PR, IR	• Orient group to structure, purpose, and people • Promote feelings of safety • Set climate
Facilitator scans group (2)	CR	• Identify group tone and mood states • Determine facilitator role
Facilitator makes inquiry (3)	IR	• Clarify meaning to enhance communication
Facilitator reorients group (4)	PR, IR	• Fulfill leader and group roles to reiterate purpose or group will founder

CR = conditional reasoning; IR = interactive reasoning; PR = procedural reasoning. Numbers refer to corresponding clients in Group Example 1.

Facilitator (visually scans the group circle) (2): Does everybody know everybody's name? That's probably what we should do first. Maybe we should just quickly go around and say our names (1).

Linda: I will go and get labels for everybody because that helps a lot.

Ann: I really don't like that.

Facilitator (in empathetic inquiring tone): What is that?

Ann: Because it really bothers me.

Facilitator: What bothers you? (3)

Ann: Labels.

Facilitator: You mean name tags? Why? (3)

Gail: Because it's distracting?

Ann: Because it is insulting.

Gail: Why?

Diane: For brain-injured people?

Judy (in flat tone): For anyone.

Diane: My ability before my brain injury was to remember everything about a person. Now I forget their names. But I remember everything about them. I guess.

Ralph: No. Because I can't remember people's names at all. But the things I remember, I remember their faces and their gestures and ... I don't know why.

Diane: But the people you met before your brain injury.
Ralph: I remember them.
Diane (in a lively voice): Yep. Yep.
Gail: Ann was saying that she objected, Linda, to name tags.
Linda: But why?
Facilitator: I think that we were just starting out talking. (4)
Ann: That was a very noncompassionate thing for me to say because I strengthen my memory by not having things like name tags so I can really work on remembering names. I have to be compassionate that there are people who have strength in other things that I have more trouble with and that name tags are necessary.
Judy: Since we're not together every day. If we were, we might remember.
Gail: So, Ann said she didn't want to be the first one to tell her story.
Facilitator: Linda? (4)

Review of Events

From this vignette we see the facilitator gathering cues and responding from (1) observing nonverbal behavior, (2) probing members for their concerns to clarify meanings, and (3) listening to what is said and not said. Although the group has been meeting for 6 months, it is in some respects in the formation stage because of functional problems, such as memory loss. In this stage, members are encouraged to establish goals and learn the routine of the group's process. The facilitator attempts to establish a foundation for trust through being consistent and clear about expectations, providing structure in the group format as needed, listening to all the members' needs, and then responding in a manner that promotes feelings of safety and self-esteem. The facilitator also responds in a manner that models role behaviors that will enable members to learn to support each other. As such, the aim of the facilitator is to foster group-centered leadership rather than leader-centered leadership.

The therapist is facilitating the discussion by simultaneously attending to the members' self-perceptions and to the limitations imposed on them by their clinical conditions. She is listening to the members' subjective experiences, not always verbalized or conscious, and to cues about performance concerns expected as a result of the brain injury. Special attention is given, for example, to expected memory loss, distractibility, heightened affect, loss of self-control, time-management problems, and effects of concrete thinking (e.g., the inability to prioritize or understand subtle meanings of language that is context driven). Furthermore, the therapist knows that members have differing experiences and responses to situations. These are based on a variety of things, such as prior experience and developmen-

BOX 11–1. THERAPIST REASONING AND REFLECTIONS—GROUP EXAMPLE 1

As group facilitator, I was concerned that Ann felt rejected. It also occurred to me that she may have concretely interpreted the meaning of "label" to mean "being labeled" rather than "name tag." I alternated between considering Ann's physical condition and Ann as person. In thinking about her physical condition, the head injury, I wondered about its resulting imposition on cognitive functioning. In reflecting upon Ann as a person, I wondered about her perception of me, the group, herself, and her disability. In constructing this image, I began to feel some anxiety. However, as I recognized these feelings, my strategy became immediately apparent.

My actions in the group (i.e., my intervention) was to be focused on promoting feelings of safety and acceptance. Ann was feeling labeled and "noncompassionate" about other members of the group, also head injured. I worried that she felt uncomfortable with a self-image of being disabled. It also concerned me that although Ann shared the same diagnosis, she might feel guilty for rejecting her peers because of their disability. These were signals that self-esteem was at risk, and my responses needed to be concrete and honest. They also genuinely reflected my interest and genuine wish to be in the group. I was willing to experience and tolerate the pain of the group.

tal stage as well as individual strengths, environmental supports, and the nature of the traumatic brain injury.

Fleming (1994a) observed that experienced therapists have tacit knowledge of the clinical condition. They can simultaneously move, as illustrated in the previous example, between the condition and the experience of the person. Their procedural skills grow immediately from this capability combined with the therapist's values and role perception. Therapist reasoning behind strategies and interventions with this group is provided in Box 11–1.

GROUP EXAMPLE 2: THE INFLUENCE OF MEMBERS' UNSTABLE AFFECT

It is common to find members confronting the facilitator and each other with strong affect that may rapidly fluctuate. This may involve tears and loud outbursts. The importance of establishing ground rules and clear expectations cannot be emphasized enough. Group members can help each other by setting limits and appropriate expectations as well as acting as

Table 11–5. The influence of members' unstable affect: Clinical events and reasoning

GROUP EVENT	REASONING USED	UNDERLYING THOUGHT PROCESS
Limit setting (1)	PR, IR, CR	• Substitute structure for safety to promote future image of adaptation • Without external controls, affect will escalate
Protect member safety (2)	PR, IR	• Substitute judgment
Reality testing (2, 3)	PR, IR	• Substitute judgment

CR = conditional reasoning; IR = interactive reasoning; PR = procedural reasoning. Numbers refer to corresponding clients in Group Example 2.

role models for each other. Nevertheless, it can be expected that whether consciously or unconsciously mobilized, these limits will be tested. Given the group perspective, the leader attempts to understand these reactions at the physiological, individual, and group-as-a-whole levels. In all instances, the facilitator must protect the safety of each individual and avoid a member's being used as a scapegoat. This calls on therapists to examine their own feelings, to understand the basis of the members' response, and to maintain appropriate therapeutic boundaries and positive relatedness. An example of such a situation is described below. Table 11–5 outlines the group events (numbered in corresponding text), type of clinical reasoning used (Mattingly & Fleming, 1994), and the therapist's underlying thought processes that relate to this example.

Facilitator (overhearing two members arguing loudly, voices growing more intense): One of our ground rules is no shouting (1).

June (in a loud and agitated voice): We are discussing. You don't understand because you are not head injured.

Ann: That's right.

Facilitator (in a calm and firm tone): In order for me to participate in the group, I cannot tolerate shouting (1). The words can be hurtful and regrettable (2). People cannot hear what each other means when there is shouting (3).

June: That is because you are not head injured.

Later that evening and the next day, several group members telephoned to explain to the facilitator that it was her misunderstanding. There was no problem in communication. The shouting was fine. Two members explained that it was the facilitator who could not understand because she was not head injured. Another member confirmed this perspective but also added that she was concerned about one of the members who was screaming. He had yelled at her the other day on the phone. She was afraid he might get violent when alone with her. The member, in a flat tone, added that she had to ask him to leave her house just the other day.

Review of Events

Fleming (1994a) explains that the term *conditional reasoning* refers to three types of therapist reasoning and is a "multidimensional" process. Conditional reasoning thereby includes:

1. Thinking about the person, illness, and meaning of the illness to the person and members of his or her social or cultural world—the whole condition,
2. Imagining a revised condition or how the condition could change, and
3. Remembering that client's participation in therapeutic activities is a necessary condition for achieving the desired outcome.

Therapist and client participate in the construction of the image of the possible outcome and work toward it together.

In this vignette we see the therapist gathering verbal and nonverbal cues. She holds an image of the group in the "here-and-now" while also en-

---

BOX 11–2. THERAPIST REASONING AND REFLECTIONS— GROUP EXAMPLE 2

As group facilitator, I recall feeling anxious about my ability to manage the group if members became physically out of control. My sense of competence as a professional relied on the members' remaining safe. In my heart, I did not really feel in any personal danger.

In thinking about the need for clear boundaries and rules, I decided to accept the "price" of exerting authority on the group. It was my decision— ultimate power as facilitator—to set the ground rules and enforce the rules regardless of criticism that was to be forthcoming. I believe a sense of trust was established by working with members, listening to their concerns, and allowing the issues and feelings to surface. Through this experience the foundation was laid for members to share intimate concerns about functional problems and to learn new strategies for adapting to a new and foreign world view as a person recovering from a head injury.

visioning the future interactions for individuals and the group as a whole. As noted by Fleming (1994a), "Conditional reasoning seems to relate to and guide the phenomenological aspects of practice" (p. 133). These illustrations show the therapist's attempts to evaluate and integrate the procedural and interactive modes through the use of conditional reasoning (Box 11–2).

SUMMARY

Group work is a viable modality in cognitive and perceptual rehabilitation. The format is flexible. It provides an opportunity for the therapist and members to establish goals and methods that are compatible with individual member goals for recovery and common group needs, such as peer support. It is demonstrated to be particularly suitable for neurological problems that influence function because group processes can be adapted for use within both remedial and compensatory intervention approaches.

≡ REVIEW QUESTIONS

1. For the purposes of continuing study, the two case studies presented in this chapter will be altered by three common occurrences. These are: (a) co-leadership, (b) a new member joins the group, and (c) vacations.
   A. In the former two case examples, the facilitator led the group alone. Imagine if the leader had a co-leader. Imagine if a new member was to join the group.

      ● How might this affect the group's process?
      ● Would you respond differently? If so, what would you say or do?
      ● What is your reasoning for employing a different approach or maintaining the same format and methodology?

   B. Leaders who facilitate open-ended groups are faced with managing groups during vacation periods. Imagine if there was no one to lead the group during the therapist's vacation period.

      ● How would you prepare the group members?
      ● What is your reasoning for employing this approach?

   C. Imagine if your co-leader was to lead the group alone or a temporary therapist was to fill in during your absence.

- What concerns would you expect to emerge in consideration of members' functional problems in the cognitive and perceptual domain as well as related psychological and social functioning?
- What strategies would you use to address these concerns?

2. In order to further your knowledge concerning the use of groups when working with clients who have cognitive and perceptual problems, review the following journal articles: Cole (1993), Jackson (1994), Kurasik (1967), Miller (1992), and Wilson (1979) and the book chapter Sohlberg and Mateer (1989). Provide a brief summary of each paper.

Glossary of Terms

Achromatopsia Difficulty with recognizing or matching colors or sorting different shades of the same color. All colors appear less bright. In severe cases of achromatopsia, the world may be viewed in shades of grey and white.

Activity Defined by Christiansen and Baum (1997) as the productive action required for development, maturation, and the use of cognitive, psychological, sensory, motor, and social functions. Activity is a way to acquire, maintain, or redevelop skills necessary to provide satisfaction and fulfill occupational roles. An activity does not need to yield an object.

Activity analysis A problem-solving strategy for examining activities that involves breaking down activities into their components in order to understand and evaluate them. In this way, the therapeutic potential activities can be analyzed.

Activity grading Any modifications made to an activity to ensure it is at the "just-right level" so that the client is optimally challenged. Activity grading is usually done before the client begins the task.

Adaptation Promoting quality of occupational performance by modifying the method used to accomplish a task, modifying the task itself, or changing the environment. Using the World Health Organization's classification of a health event (1980), adaptation is targeted at the level of disability.

Agnosia A failure of recognition of stimuli (e.g., visual, auditory, tactile) that is not due to sensory problems. See also prosopagnosia, astereognosis.

Alertness The capacity to maintain a state of wakefulness in which the person is ready and able to respond to events in the environment. The capacity to concentrate is dependent on a normal level of alertness.

Alexia Loss of the capacity to read or comprehend written language. Clients with this disorder do not usually have difficulty with oral (i.e., spoken) language.

Alternating concentration The capacity to move flexibly between tasks and respond appropriately to the demands of each task.

Anosognosia Presents as a denial of affected part of body as belonging to the person or lack of insight into or denial of paralysis or disability. Although anosognosia may be classified as a simple perceptual problem, many clinicians deal with this problem in relation to body scheme disorders.

Anterograde amnesia The inability to acquire and retain new information. Amnesia for events subsequent to the episode that precipitated the disorder.

Aphasia Difficulties comprehending the spoken word or with speech expression, including grammatical errors and errors in word choice.

Apraxia Difficulties executing skilled learned movements not caused by any primary motor or sensory deficit or attributable to lack of comprehension, attention, or willingness to perform the movement. Generally two forms are discussed in the literature, ideomotor and ideational.

Astereognosis Tactile agnosia, the inability to recognize objects by touch alone (with vision occluded) despite intact sensory abilities. Astereognosis involves impaired perception of shape, texture, temperature, weight, density, and therefore identity (Bradshaw & Mattingley, 1995). It is important to distinguish between tactile anomia (i.e., inability to name an object by touch despite recognizing what the object is) and tactile agnosia (i.e., inability to recognize an object by touch).

Attention Refer to concentration and unilateral neglect.

Auditory agnosia The inability to distinguish between sounds or to recognize familiar sounds despite intact hearing.

Behavioral goal A statement (sometimes referred to as a *long-term goal*) about what the client will achieve over a relatively long space of time, such as the duration of the therapy program or several weeks. Behavioral goals are written using the who, given what, does what, how well, by when method.

Behavioral objective A statement (sometimes referred to as a *short-term goal*) about the things a client will achieve in a relatively short space of time, such as a therapy session or a week. Behavioral objectives are written using the who, given what, does what, how well, by when method.

Body scheme An individual's capacity to perceive his or her own postural model. Body scheme disorders are defective perception of body position, including and involving the relation of body parts to each other. Body scheme disorders include somatoagnosia, difficulty with right–left discrimination, finger agnosia, unilateral body neglect, and anosognosia.

Buccofacial apraxia The same kind of disorder as ideomotor apraxia but relates to the execution of purposeful movements of the face and lips for language production and emotional expression.

Capacity The opposite of impairment (using the World Health Organization's definitions of disease, impairment, disability, and handicap). Possessing normal psychological, physiological, or anatomical structure or function.

Climate setting The practice of a group facilitator of creating an environment for the group. An example of this is to invite members to introduce themselves.

Clinical reasoning The ongoing thinking or cognitive processes and decision-making that therapists use to guide their work. The main forms of clinical reasoning discussed in occupational therapy are scientific, pragmatic, procedural, interactive, and conditional reasoning.

Closed group A group that new members cannot join after it has formed.

Cognition The capacities that enable us to think, which include the capacity to concentrate (i.e., pay attention), remember, and learn. The conscious thought processes that include knowing and understanding (see also higher-order cognition).

Collaborative consultation A method of building on the collaborative relationships necessary to foster the success of therapeutic interventions using principles of therapeutic rapport (Tickle-Degnen, 1995) to foster openness and trust. Collaborative consultation is similar to therapeutic rapport because they are both based on mutual and collaborative relationships among equals.

Color agnosia An inability to associate objects with particular colors, although color vision is intact. For example, a client with color agnosia is unable to name a color shown or point to a color named by the examiner, but correct color associations can be made.

Compensation The goal of achieving a "correct" performance by limiting the effects of the deficit and using other intact skills. The emphasis is on skills training and reinforcement of successful responses to resolve a problem or complete a task. Compensation involves altering the way the client performs the task or the task itself. Compensation strategies and adaptive approaches may be adopted to facilitate a client's successful return to community living.

Concentration Purposefully and voluntarily directing one's thoughts and actions toward a stimulus or stimuli (Stringer, 1996). The ability to focus on relevant features according to the task, past experiences, or needs and to inhibit focus on distracting stimuli.

Concrete thinking A lack of abstract thought that often includes misinterpretation and difficulties in understanding the subtle meanings of language.

Conditional reasoning Conditional reasoning is not always conscious and is therefore difficult to define. Clinicians use this form of reasoning when they try to understand what is meaningful to the client in his or her world by imagining what his or her life was like before the illness or disability and what it could be like in the future. Conditional reasoning takes the whole of the client's condition into account as the therapist considers the client's temporal contexts (i.e., past, present, and future) and their personal, cultural, and social contexts. Therapists use conditional reasoning to integrate procedural and interactive reasoning to create an image of the client's future. In addition, conditional reasoning calls for an understanding of the ways the condition has affected the individual's work, social situation and leisure, and his or her view of self.

Constructional abilities The capacity to reproduce designs in two or three dimensions

Contextual interference Potential distractors that are normally found in an environment. An environment with contextual interference is complex, requires higher processing demands, and is usually designed to make a goal more difficult to achieve in order to strengthen a learning pattern.

Contextual congruence A simple environment that requires minimal processing demands is said to posses contextual congruence. A congruent environment is designed to match the task with the goal.

Contralesional The side of the person or hemispace opposite the side of their brain lesion.

Cue Subjective or objective information or data provided or received. For example, in cue acquisition the therapist gathers information about the client and his or her difficulties. During a treatment session, a therapist may provide the client with verbal (i.e., spoken or sung by therapist or voice recording) or visual (i.e., pictures or written instructions) cues to aid activity completion.

Decision making The process of making choices about preferred courses of action.

Depth perception The capacity to perceive the correct depth or distance of an object or body part.

Diagnostic reasoning The component of procedural reasoning that involves the evaluation and identification of a client's problems from an occupational therapist's viewpoint.

Distraction or distractibility Anything that diverts a person's concentration away from the task they are engaged in.

Divided concentration The capacity to respond simultaneously to two or more tasks. This is required when more than one response is required or more than one stimuli needs to be monitored.

Dysarthria The impairment of speech after damage to or loss of control of peripheral speech structures. This results in a mechanical speech problem, such as slurring.

Effective performance The capacity for quality control, including the capacity to self-monitor and self-correct one's behavior. Because effective self-monitoring and self-correction are the primary features of the performance of persons with problems with effective performance, clients may not even perceive their mistakes, but others may identify them but take no action to correct them (Lezak, 1995).

Executive abilities The behavioral manifestations of executive functions in the context of daily life task performances, including personal or instrumental activities of daily living.

Executive functions A group of capacities and mental processes that occur within the brain. Executive functions are considered higher level cortical capacities. Disorders of executive functions can be considered impairments within the World Health Organization classification of impairment, disability, and handicap (World Health Organization, 1980).

Expert therapist A therapist who does not need to rely on rules and guidelines to take appropriate action but rather has an intuitive grasp of the situation. Experts often find it difficult to explain this intuition.

Extinction This is evident in situations when the client can attend to isolated stimuli coming from either the contralesional or the ipsilesional side. However, when presented with double or simultaneous stimuli (i.e., stimuli from both sides), the client may respond to the ipsilesional stimuli only, thus "extinguishing" the concurrent, contralesional stimuli. Motor extinction is particularly evident in bilateral tasks (particularly if the client has good motor control of the affected side). In motor extinction, the client typically fails to use the limb normally in bilateral tasks such as holding a cup or catching a ball.

Figure/ground discrimination The capacity to isolate a shape or an object from its background. Also described as the capacity to differentiate the foreground from the background.

Finger agnosia Impaired capacity to identify the fingers on one's own hand or the hand of another person. Difficulty with naming fingers on command or knowing which finger has been touched.

Focused (selective) concentration The capacity to concentrate on an occupation despite environmental visual or auditory stimuli. Difficulty with focused concentration is often referred to as *distractibility*.

Form discrimination The capacity to perceive a familiar shape or object as the same even though it might be observed in a variety of conditions (e.g., distance, orientation, location, or lighting).

Functional group Group that includes the group leader's capitalizing on the use of group structure and therapeutic use of self to enhance the group process and individual function. Using purposeful activities, the leader structures a task to maximally involve members; enhance the sense of individual as well as group identity; create an atmosphere that encourages spontaneous involvement, support, and feedback; and form a match between the member's abilities and the required action.

Generalization The capacity to use a newly learned strategy or skill in different situations.

Hemianesthesia Sensory loss on either the right or left side of the body.

Hemianopia Refer to homonymous hemianopia.

Hemiplegia Muscle weakness on one side of the body.

Higher-order cognition Complex cognitive functions such as the capacity to plan, manipulate information, initiate and terminate activities, and recognize errors.

Homonymous hemianopia or hemianopsia A visual field defect of either the left or right half of the visual field.

Hypothesis testing A nonstandardized approach to assessment in which the therapist selects a functional activity to undertake with the client and then generates one or a number of hypotheses that are tested by manipulating variables and observing change in client performance. Hypothesis testing has many similarities to the four-stage model of problem solving outlined by Elstein, Shulman, and Sprafka (1978) and the dynamic interaction approach to assessment developed by Toglia (1989) (see Chapter 3).

Hypoxia, cerebral Extreme deficiency of oxygen to the brain.

Ideational apraxia An incapacity to formulate a plan of action successfully because of a loss of the mental representation of what is to be done. It can occur when a person is carrying out automatic actions or when performing on command.

Ideomotor apraxia Although understanding what is to be done, a person with ideomotor apraxia is unable to implement the required action successfully. However, an individual may carry out the action automatically (i.e,. when they are not considering the movement consciously).

Impairment The abnormality or loss of physiological, anatomical, or psychological function or structure.

Intention tremor A jerky movement that is absent when the limbs are inactive but becomes more prominent as action continues and fine adjustment of the movement is demanded.

Information processing The mental capacity to perceive and react to the environment.

Insight Awareness of a person's whole self: one's own condition and resulting impairments and disabilities.

Instrumental activities of daily living Domestic and community activities of daily living, such as cleaning, shopping, and driving.

Interactive reasoning The type of reasoning that occurs as a clinician engages in therapy with a client and therefore takes place during face-to-face encounters between clinicians and their clients. Therapist are using this form of reasoning when verifying information, asking clients about themselves, and sharing information with clients.

Ipsilateral On the same side.

Ipsilesional The same side of the body as the side of the brain lesion.

Judgment The capacity to make realistic decisions based on environmental information.

Learning A relatively permanent change in the capacity for responding that results from practice and experience, persists with time, resists environmental changes, and can be generalized in response to new tasks and situations (Schmidt, 1988). It allows an individual to cope with the ever-changing demands of the environment (Farber & Abreu, 1993).

Macro perspective In the quadraphonic approach to therapy, two orientations in the area of cognitive retraining are described. One of these is reductionistic in character, employing a micro perspective, and the other is holistic or humanistic and proceeds through a macro perspective (Abreu, 1994). Macro perspectives have also been described as adaptive, functional, and top down (see Chapter 1) (Abreu, 1994). The macro orientation is guided by four characteristics unique to each client (refer to Chapter 5 for complete description).

Markers Temporal, social, or task-related cues that inform a person that a performance error has occurred. More specifically, ". . . a marker is basically a message that some future behavior or event should not be treated as routine and instead, some particular aspect of the situation should be viewed as especially relevant for action" (Shallice & Burgess, 1991, p. 737).

Memory The capacity to store experiences (including concepts and tasks) and perceptions for recall and recognition. At the neurocellular level, it is a functional property of any nervous system component that aids in retaining information.

Metacognition A complex cognitive function that includes an understanding of one's own cognition. This is sometimes describes as "knowing about knowing." Metacognition includes an awareness of the self and executive functions.

Metamemory An individual's subjective knowledge about his or her capacity to acquire, retain, and recall information.

Micro perspective An orientation in the area of cognitive retraining that is reductionistic in character. Micro perspectives have also been called restorative or bottom-up (as described in Chapter 1). In the quadraphonic approach, the micro orientation is guided by four theories: information processing, teaching-learning, neurodevelopmental, and biomechanical (Abreu, 1990).

Motivation The desire to reach a goal and demonstrate actual follow-through.

Narrative reasoning The use of story making and storytelling to assist the therapist in reaching an understanding.

Neglect Refer to unilateral neglect.

Neuropsychology The study of the relationships between the brain and behavior.

Novice therapist The opposite of expert. Novices don't have experience of the situations they will be involved in. A novice therapist is usually rigid in the application of rules, principles, and theories to clinical situations.

Open group A type of group in which new members can join after the group has formed.

Orientation An awareness of one's environment, situation, or both and the capacity to use this information appropriately in a functional setting.

Patient-oriented style or client-oriented style Style that directs a therapist to help a client complete tasks in a more nondirective manner by taking the perspective of the client and offering guidance as appropriate (Tickle-Degnan & Rosenthal, 1990).

Peer-facilitated group Group that is facilitated by members or run by persons on an equal basis. Peer-facilitated groups can be defined to include self-help groups, advocacy groups, and support groups (Rootes & Aanes, 1992).

Perception The capacity to transform information from the senses (i.e., touch, hearing, vision, smell, taste, and kinaesthesia) and use this to interact appropriately with the environment. It is a selective, integrative, and dynamic process using mental capacities and physical sensations through which the individual integrates what he currently experiences and his past experiences to interact appropriately with the environment.

Perceptual anchor A technique used to "pattern" attention to the unattended side with clients who experience unilateral neglect (this is usually the left side). This involves teaching the client to begin scanning to the left by first locating an anchor on the left side of the task such as the left arm or table edge, thus using the arm or table edge as a "perceptual anchor" (Robertson, North, & Geggie, 1992).

Performance areas Daily living activities, work or productivity, and leisure.

Performance components The capacities that are required for successful engagement in performance areas, including cognition and perception and sensorimotor, motor, psychosocial, and psychological skills.

Performance contexts The temporal or environmental factors that influence an individual's participation in a performance area.

Phenomenology Concerned with the ways meanings are made and how they are embodied in everyday habits and activities. Taking a phenomenological perspective means attempting to understand a person from his or her own point of view and to see people as they see themselves and their lives, families, and environments.

Planning The capacity to logically and systematically outline what is to be done. It involves the capacity to look ahead and conceptualize change, conceive of alternatives, and weigh and make choices (Lezak, 1995).

Post-traumatic amnesia A period of confusion and disorientation that generally follows traumatic brain injury during which a person does not have the capacity to form new memories. The duration of post-traumatic amnesia is often used as a measure of head-injury severity.

Pragmatic reasoning The reasoning processes associated with a clinician's practice setting and personal context. Pragmatic reasoning includes consideration of organizational, political, and economic constraints and opportunities and incorporates personal motivation, values, and beliefs (Schell & Cervero, 1993).

Praxis The execution of skilled, purposeful movement.

Problem solving The capacity to analyze information related to a given situation and generate appropriate responses.

Procedural reasoning The kind of thinking used when determining what a client's problems are and how to reduce their effects. Therapists use procedural forms of reasoning when they think about which assessments or approaches they will use to identify a client's functional problems, set goals, and plan treatment.

Professionally led group A therapy group. These groups are focused on treatment goals and are conducted by trained professionals, including occupational therapists, social workers, psychologists, doctors, rehabilitation counselors, and other health care personnel.

Prompt A brief cue (usually provided by the therapist but can be environmental) used to assist a client during an activity in which they need guidance to continue. A prompt can be provided verbally or nonverbally.

Prosopagnosia An inability to recognize familiar faces despite intact sensory capacities. Clients with this condition know that faces are different but cannot tell who the person is.

Purposive action Capacities for productivity and self-regulation (including the capacity to structure an effective and fluent course of action by initiating, maintaining, switching, and stopping complex action sequences in an orderly manner) to realize a goal.

Quadraphonic approach A treatment model based on creating a confluent environment designed to empower the client to increase the opportunity and the capacity for action, achieve goals, and increase life satisfaction. This approach is a holistic rehabilitation method that incorporates the reductionist orientation necessary for effective cognitive retraining with the holistic orientation necessary to produce an effective evaluation model.

Rehabilitation The process of working with a disabled client to develop maximum independence and promote a sense of well-being.

Reliability The precision, consistency, and stability of a test or a method used for measurement.

Remediation To improve or restore lost or damaged performance components or capacities. Using the World Health Organization's classification of a health event (1980), remediation is targeted at the level of impairments.

Residual Left behind or remaining.

Retrograde amnesia The inability to use information acquired before an injury, illness, or the onset of amnesia. Amnesia for events before the episode that precipitated the disorder.

Right/left discrimination The capacity to discriminate between right and left in terms of one's own body and the external environment.

Scanning The capacity to review the environment visually, usually achieved by planned eye movements from side to side.

Scientific reasoning The process of hypothesis generation and testing that is generally referred to as *hypothetico-deductive reasoning*. This form of reasoning is most often used when making a diagnosis of a client's medical condition. Scientific reasoning assists the clinician in thinking about the medical aspects of the client's condition and its implications.

Simultanagnosia Difficulty in recognizing the elements of a visual array. Although the elements of such an array may be correctly perceived, clients with this form of agnosia have difficulty in recognizing the meaning of the total picture.

Somatoagnosia An unawareness of body structure and a failure to recognize one's own body parts and their relationship to each other. This problem is also referred to as *autopagnosia* or, simply, *body agnosia*.

Spatial relations The capacity to relate objects to each other and to one's self.

Standardized assessment An assessment that has a uniform procedure for administration and scoring and possesses normative data. The manual of a standardized assessment contains information concerning reliability and validity, which are essential for correct interpretation of assessment results.

Sustained concentration The capacity to consistently concentrate on relevant information during a continuous activity. Also referred to as *concentration span*.

Tacit knowledge Information that a person has that is difficult to describe with language. Tacit knowledge is understood or implied without being stated.

Tactile agnosia See astereognosis.

Task-oriented style A therapist's technique of helping a client complete a task by giving directives.

Taxonomy An approach to classification usually according to a set of principles.

Theoretical reasoning Form of reasoning concerned with generalities, or what we can reliably predict or hold to be true. We can learn theoretical reasoning from textbooks.

Temporal organization Within the context of the Assessment of Motor and Process Skills (Fisher, 1997a), the ability to initiate, continue, sequence, and terminate the actions or steps of an activity or the activity itself.

Topographical orientation The capacity to recall the spatial arrangements of familiar surroundings and therefore find one's way around and learn new routes.

Unilateral neglect A lateralized disorder affecting the ability to attend and interact with objects, the self, or space. The inability to report or to orientate to stimuli on the side of extrapersonal space or the body contralateral to a lesion, which is not due to a primary motor or sensory loss. A client with a unilateral neglect due to a right lesion may neglect the left hemispace, or body.

Unstable affect Emotional reactions or moods that fluctuate rapidly.

Validity The degree to which a test actually measures the characteristics it reports to measure.

Visual object agnosia The inability to recognize familiar objects and forms by looking at them despite intact vision. Cases of pure visual object agnosia are rare; they are usually seen in conjunction with other forms of agnosia.

Visuospatial disorders A collection of disorders including defective judgment of depth and distance, difficulties with spatial relations, topographical disorientation, and unilateral spatial neglect.

Visualization The creation of a picture in one's mind of what is being discussed.

Volition The capacity to determine what one needs and wants to do and the capacity to conceptualize a future realization of one's needs and wants. Volition requires the capacity to formulate a goal or an intention and then to initiate task performance.

References

Abreu, B. C. (1981). Interdisciplinary approach to the adult visual perceptual function: dysfunction continuum. In B. C. Abreu (Ed.), *Physical disabilities manual* (pp. 51–181). New York: Raven.

Abreu, B. C. (1990). *The quadraphonic approach: Management of cognitive and postural dysfunction.* New York: Therapeutic Service Systems.

Abreu, B. C. (1992). The quadraphonic approach: Management of cognitive-perceptual and postural control dysfunction. *Occupational Therapy Practice, 3,* 12–29.

Abreu, B. C. (1994). Perceptual motor skills: Assessment and intervention strategies. In C. B. Royeen (Ed.), *AOTA Self-study series: Cognitive rehabilitation* (pp. 6–48). Rockville, MD: American Occupational Therapy Association.

Abreu, B. C. (1995). The effect of environmental regulations on postural control after stroke. *American Journal of Occupational Therapy, 49,* 517–525.

Abreu, B. C. (1998a). The quadraphonic approach: Holistic rehabilitation for brain injury. In N. Katz (Ed.), *Cognition and occupation in rehabilitation* (pp. 51–97). Rockville, MD: American Occupational Therapy Association.

Abreu, B. C. (1998b). Additional uses for data. In J. Hinojosa & P. Kramer (Eds.), *Occupational therapy evaluation: obtaining and interpreting data* (pp. 213–234). Bethesda, MD: American Occupational Therapy Association, Inc.

Abreu, B. C., Duval, M., Gerber, D., & Wood, W. (1994). Occupational performance and the functional approach. In C. B. Royeen (Ed.), *AOTA Self-study series: Cognitive rehabilitation* (pp. 1–36). Rockville, MD: American Occupational Therapy Association.

Abreu, B. C., & Hinojosa, J. (1992). The process approach for cognitive-perceptual and postural control for adults with brain injuries. In N. Katz (Ed.), *Cognitive rehabilitation: Models for intervention in occupational therapy* (pp. 167–194). Boston: Andover Medical.

Abreu, B. C., Seale, G., Podlesak, J., & Hartley, L. (1996). Development of critical paths for postacute brain injury rehabilitation: Lessons learned. *American Journal of Occupational Therapy, 50,* 417–427.

Abreu, B. C., & Toglia, J. P. (1987). Cognitive rehabilitation: An occupational therapy model. *American Journal of Occupational Therapy, 41,* 439–448.

Affolter, F., & Bichøfberger, W. (1996). *Behandling af Perceptionsforstyrrelser.* Copenhagen: Munksgaard.

Agency for Health Care Policy and Research (1995). *Post Stroke Rehabilitation Guidelines. No. 95–0662.* Washington, DC: Author.

Agostoni, E., Coletti, A., Orlando, G., & Tredici, G. (1983). Apraxia in deep cerebral lesions. *Journal of Neurology, Neurosurgery and Psychiatry, 46,* 804–808.

Aja, D., Jacobs, K., & Hermenau, D. (1992). *Americans with Disabilities Act Work Site Assessment.* Boston: Author.

Alexander, M., Baker, E., Naeser, M., et al. (1992). Neuropsychological and neuroanatomical dimensions of ideomotor apraxia. *Brain, 115,* 87–107.

Allen, C. K. (1982). Independence through activity: The practice of occupational therapy (psychiatry). *American Journal of Occupational Therapy, 36,* 731–739.

485

Allen, C. K. (1985). *Occupational therapy for psychiatric diseases: measurement and management of cognitive disabilities.* Boston: Little, Brown & Co.

Allen, C. K. (1990). *Allen cognitive level test manual.* Colchester, CT: S & S/ Worldwide.

Allen, C. K. (1992). Cognitive disabilities. In N. Katz (Ed.), *Cognitive rehabilitation: Models for intervention in occupational therapy* (pp. 1–21). Boston: Andover Medical.

Allen, C. K., Earhart, C. A., & Blue, T. (1992). *Occupational therapy treatment goals for the physically and cognitively disabled.* Rockville, MD: American Occupational Therapy Association.

Allen, C. K., Kehrberg, K., & Burns, T. (1992). Evaluation instruments. In C. K. Allen, C. A. Earhart, & T. Blue (Eds.), *Occupational therapy treatment goals for the physically and cognitively disabled (pp. 31–84).* Rockville, MD: American Occupational Therapy Association.

Almli, C. R., & Finger, S. (1992). Brain injury and recovery of function: Theories and mechanisms of functional reorganization. *Journal of Head Trauma Rehabilitation, 7,* 70–77.

Alnervik, A., & Sviden, G. (1996). On clinical reasoning: Patterns of reflection on practice. *Occupational Therapy Journal of Research, 16,* 98–110.

Aloisio, L. (1998). Visual dysfunction. In G. Gillen & A. Burkhardt (Eds.), *Occupational therapy management of the CVA patient* (pp. 267–284). St. Louis, MO: C. V. Mosby.

American Heart Association (1991). *Heart and stroke facts.* Dallas, TX: Author.

American Occupational Therapy Association. (1990). *1990 Member Data Survey Summary Report.* Rockville, MD: Author.

American Occupational Therapy Association. (1994a). Uniform terminology for occupational therapy—third edition. *American Journal of Occupational Therapy, 48,* 1047–1054.

American Occupational Therapy Association. (1994b). Uniform terminology— third edition: Application to practice. *American Journal of Occupational Therapy, 48,* 1055–1059.

Anastasi, A. (1988). *Psychological testing* (6th ed.). New York: Macmillan Publishing Co.

Archibald, Y. (1987). Persisting apraxia in two left handed, aphasic patients with right hemisphere lesions. *Brain and Cognition, 6,* 412–428.

Árnadóttir, G. (1990). *The brain and behavior: Assessing cortical dysfunction through activities of daily living.* St. Louis, MO: C. V. Mosby.

Árnadóttir, G. (1996). *Árnadóttir OT-ADL Neurobehavioral Evaluation (A-ONE) course notes.* Unpublished manuscript, Reykjavik, Iceland.

Árnadóttir, G. (1998). Impact of neurobehavioral deficits on ADL. In G. Gillen & A. Burkhardt (Eds.), *Occupational therapy management of the CVA patient* (pp. 285–333). St. Louis, MO: C. V. Mosby.

Atkinson, R. C., & Shiffrin, R. M. (1968). Human memory: A proposed system and its control processes. In K. W. Spence (Ed.), *The psychology of learning and motivation: Advances in research and theory, 2* (pp. 189–195). New York: Academic Press.

Australian Association of Occupational Therapists (1991). *1991 Member Census.* Melbourne: Author.

Averbuch, S., & Katz, N. (1992). Cognitive rehabilitation: A retraining approach for brain-injured adults. In N. Katz (Ed.), *Cognitive rehabilitation: Models for intervention in occupational therapy* (pp. 219–239). Boston: Andover Medical.

Ayres, A. J. (1972). *Southern California sensory integration tests.* Los Angeles: Western Psychological Services.

Ayres, A. J. (1985). *Developmental dyspraxia and adult-onset apraxia.* Torrance, CA: Sensory Integration International.

Ayres, A. J. (1989). *Sensory integration and praxis tests.* Los Angeles: Western Psychological Services.

Baddeley, A. (1992). Is working memory working? The Fifteenth Bartlett Lecture. *The Quarterly Journal of Experimental Psychology, 44A,* 1–31.

Banich, M. T. (1997). *Neuropsychology: The neural bases of mental function.* Boston: Houghton Mifflin.

Barlow, D. H., & Hersen, M. (1984). *Single case experimental designs: Strategies for studying behavior change* (2nd ed.). Oxford: Pergamon Press.

Baron, K., & Curtin, C. (1990). *A manual for use with the Self Assessment of Occupational Functioning.* Unpublished manuscript, Department of Occupational Therapy, University of Illinois at Chicago.

Barton, S. (1994). Chaos, self-organization, and psychology. *American Psychologist,* 5–14.

Basso, A., Luzzatti, C., & Spinnler, H. (1980). Is ideomotor apraxia the outcome of damage to well-defined regions of the left hemisphere? *Journal of Neurology, Neurosurgery and Psychiatry, 43,* 118–126.

Bauer, R. M., & Rubens, A. B. (1993). Agnosia. In K. M. Heilman & E. Valenstein (Eds.), *Clinical neuropsychology* (3rd ed., pp. 215–278). Oxford: Oxford University Press.

Baum, C. M., & Edwards, D. F. (1993). Cognitive performance in senile dementia of the Alzheimer's type: the Kitchen Task Assessment. *American Journal of Occupational Therapy, 47,* 431–436.

Bear, M. F., Connors, B. W., & Paradiso, M. A. (1996). *Neuroscience: Exploring the brain.* Baltimore: Williams & Wilkins.

Benardi-Coletta, B., Dominowski, R. L., Buyer, L. S., & Rellinger, E. R. (1995). Metacognition and problem solving: A process-oriented approach. *Journal of Experimental Psychology: Learning, Memory, and Cognition, 21,* 205–223.

Benner, P. (1984). *From novice to expert: Excellence and power in clinical nursing practice.* Menlo Park, CA: Addison-Wesley Publishing Company.

Benner, P., & Tanner, C. (1987). Clinical judgment: How expert nurses use intuition. *American Journal of Nursing, 87,* 23–31.

Benton, A. L. (1993). Visuoperceptual, visuospatial, and visuoconstructive disorders. In K. M. Heilman & E. Valenstein (Eds.), *Clinical neuropsychology* (3rd ed., pp. 165–214). Oxford: Oxford University Press.

Benton, A. L., des Hamsher, K., Varney, N. R., & Otfried, S. (1983). *Contributions to neuropsychological assessment.* New York: Oxford University Press.

Benton, A., & Sivan, A. B. (1993). Disturbances of the body schema. In K. M. Heilman & E. Valenstein (Eds.), *Clinical neuropsychology* (3rd ed., pp. 123–140). New York: Oxford University Press.

Benton, A., & Tranel, D. (1993). Visuoperceptual, visuospatial, and visuoconstructive disorders. In K. M. Heilman & E. Valenstein (Eds.), *Clinical neuropsychology* (3rd ed., pp. 165–213). New York: Oxford University Press.

Benton, A. L., & Van Allen, M. W. (1968). Impairment of facial recognition in patients with cerebral disease. *Cortex, 4,* 344–358.

Berg Rice, V. (Ed.). (1998). Ergonomics in health care and rehabilitation. Newton, MA: Butterworth Heinemann.

Berlyne, D. E. (1969). Laughter, humor, and play. In G. Lindzert & E. Aronson (Eds.), *The handbook of social psychology*. Reading, MA: Addison-Wesley.

Bernspång, B., & Fisher, A. G. (1995a). Differences between persons with right or left CVA on the Assessment of Motor and Process Skills. *Archives of Physical Medicine and Rehabilitation, 76,* 1144–1151.

Bernspång, B., & Fisher, A. G. (1995b). Validation of the Assessment of Motor and Process Skills for use in Sweden. *Scandinavian Journal of Occupational Therapy, 2,* 3–9.

Bernstein, N. (1967). *The coordination and regulation of movements.* London: Pergamon.

Berthier, M., Starkstein, S., & Leiguarda, R. (1987). Behavioural effects of damage to the right insula and surrounding regions. *Cortex, 23,* 673–678.

Bhavnani, G., Cockburn, J., Whiting, S., Lincoln, N. (1983). The reliability of the Rivermead Perceptual Assessment. *British Journal of Occupational Therapy, 46,* 17–19.

Bisiach, E., & Luzzatti, C. (1978). Unilateral neglect of representational space. *Cortex, 14,* 129–133.

Bjork, R. A. (1994). Memory and metamemory: Considerations in the training of human beings. In J. Metcalfe & A. P. Shimamura (Eds.), *Metacognition: Knowing about knowing* (pp. 185–206). Cambridge, MA: The Massachusetts Institute of Technology Press.

Blackmer, E. R., & Mitton, J. L. (1991). Theories of monitoring and the timing of repairs in spontaneous speech. *Cognition, 39,* 173–194.

Boys, M., Fisher, P., Holzberg, C., & Reid, D. W. (1988). The OSOT Perceptual Evaluation: a research perspective. *American Journal of Occupational Therapy, 42,* 92–98.

Bradburn, S. L. (1992). *Psychiatric occupational therapists' strategies for engaging patients in treatment during the initial interview.* Unpublished master's thesis. Tufts University, Medford, MA.

Bradshaw, J. L., & Mattingley, J. B. (1995). *Clinical neuropsychology: Behavioral and brain science.* San Diego: Academic Press.

Breines, E. B. (1995). *Occupational therapy: Activities from clay to computers.* Philadelphia: F. A. Davis.

Broadbent, D. (1958). *Perception and Communication.* Oxford: Pergamon.

Brockmann-Rubio, K. (1998). Treatment of neurobehavioral deficits: A function based approach. In G. Gillen & A. Burkhardt (Eds.), *Occupational therapy management of the CVA patient* (pp. 334–352). St. Louis, MO: C. V. Mosby.

Brooke, M. M., Questad, K. A., Patterson, D. R., & Vallois, T. A. (1992). Driving evaluation after traumatic brain injury. *The American Journal of Physical Medicine and Rehabilitation, 71,* 177–182.

Brown, A. (1987). Metacognition, executive control, self-regulation, and other more mysterious mechanisms. In F. E. Weinert & R. H. Kluwe (Eds.), *Metacognition, motivation, and understanding* (pp. 65–116). Hillsdale, NJ: Lawrence Erlbaum Associates.

Butler, J. A. (1996a). Does sensory input influence recovery in ideomotor apraxia? *Brain Research Association Abstracts, 13,* 66.

Butler, J. A. (1996b). Intervention in a case of ideomotor apraxia. *Proceeds of the British Psychological Society, 4,* 55.

Buxbaum, L. J., Schwartz, M. F., Coslett, H. B., & Carew, T. G. (1995). Naturalistic action and praxis in callosal apraxia. *Neurocase, 1,* 3–17.

Campione, J. C. (1987). Metacognitive components of instructional research with problem learners. In F. E. Weinert & R. H. Kluwe (Eds.), *Metacognition, motivation, and understanding* (pp. 117–141). Hillsdale, NJ: Lawrence Erlbaum Associates.

Campione, J. C., Brown, A. L., & Bryant, N. R. (1985). Individual differences in learning and memory. In R. J. Sternberg (Ed.), *Human abilities: an information-processing approach* (pp. 103–126). New York: W. H. Freeman and Company.

Canadian Association of Occupational Therapists. (1991). Guidelines for the client-centered practice of occupational therapy. Toronto: CAOT Publications ACE.

Cavanaugh, J. C., & Perlmutter, M. (1982). Metamemory: A critical examination. *Child Development, 53,* 11–28.

Cermak, S. A., & Hausser, J. (1989). The Behavioural Inattention Test for unilateral visual neglect: A critical review. *Physical and Occupational Therapy in Geriatrics, 7,* 43–53.

Cermak, S. A., Katz, N., McGuire, E., et al. (1995). Performance of Americans and Israelis with cerebrovascular accident on the Loewenstein Occupational Therapy Cognitive Assessment (LOTCA). *American Journal of Occupational Therapy, 49,* 500–506.

Chi, M. T. H., Feltovich, P. J., & Glaser, R. (1979). Categorization and representation of physics problems by experts and novices. *Cognitive Science, 5,* 121–152.

Chi, M. T. H., Leeuw, N. D., Chi, M. H., & LaVancher, C. (1994). Eliciting self-explanations improves understanding. *Cognitive Science, 18,* 439–477.

Christiansen, C. (1993). Continuing challenges of functional assessment in rehabilitation: Recommended changes. *American Journal of Occupational Therapy, 47,* 258–59

Christiansen, C. H., & Baum, C. M. (1997). *Occupational therapy: Enabling performance and well being* (2nd ed.). Thorofare, NJ: Slack Inc.

Churchland, P. M. (Ed.). (1995). *The engine of reason, the seat of the soul.* Cambridge, MA: The Massachusetts Institute of Technology Press.

Cicerone, K. D. (1996). Attention deficits and dual task demands after mild traumatic brain injury. *Brain injury, 10,* 79–89.

Cicerone, K. D., & Tupper, D. E. (1991). Neuropsychological rehabilitation: Treatment of errors in everyday functioning. In D. E. Tupper & K. D. Cicerone (Eds.), *The neuropsychology of everyday life: Issues in development and rehabilitation* (pp. 271–292). London: Kluwer Academic.

Classen, J., Kunesch, E., Binkofski, F., et al. (1995). Subcortical origin of visuomotor apraxia. *Brain, 118,* 1365–1374.

Cockburn, J., Bhavnani, G., Whiting, S., Lincoln, N. (1982). Normal performance on some tests of perception in adults. *British Journal of Occupational Therapy, 45,* 67–68.

Cockburn, J., Wilson, B. A., & Baddeley, A. D. (1990). Assessing everyday memory in patients with perceptual deficits. *Clinical Rehabilitation, 4,* 129–135.

Cohen, E. S. (1989). Fieldwork education: Shaping a foundation for clinical reasoning. *American Journal of Occupational Therapy, 43,* 240–244.

Cohen, E. S. (1991). Nationally speaking. Clinical Reasoning: Explicating complexity. *American Journal of Occupational Therapy, 45,* 969–971.

Cohen, G. (1991). *Memory in the real world.* Hillsdale, NJ: Lawrence Erlbaum Associates.

Cohen, N. J., & Eichenbaum, H. (1994). *Memory, amnesia, and the hippocampal system.* Cambridge, MA: The Massachusetts Institute of Technology Press.

Cohen, R. F., & Mapou, R. L. (1988). Neuropsychological assessment for treatment planning: A hypothesis-testing approach. *Journal of Head Trauma Rehabilitation, 3,* 12–23.

Cole, M. B. (1993). *Group dynamics in occupational therapy: The theoretical basis and practice application of group treatment.* Thorofare, NJ: Slack.

Collins, L. F., & Affeldt, J. (1996). Bridging the clinical reasoning gap. *OT Practice, 1,* 33–35.

Cooper, B., Rigby, P., & Letts, L. (1995). Evaluation of access to home, community, and workplace. In C. Trombly (Ed.), *Occupational therapy for physical dysfunction* (4th ed., pp. 55–72). Baltimore: Williams & Wilkins.

Cornoldi, C., & De Beni, R. (1996). Mnemonics and metacognition. In D. Herrmann, C. McEvoy, C. Hertzog, P., et al. (Eds.), *Basic and applied memory research: Practical Applications* (vol. 2, pp. 237–253). Mahwah, NJ: Lawrence Erlbaum Associates, Publishers.

Crepeau, E. B. (1991). Achieving intersubjective understanding: Examples from an occupational therapy treatment session. *American Journal of Occupational Therapy, 45,* 1016–1025.

Croce, R. (1993). A review of the neural basis of apractic disorders with implications for remediation. *Adapted Physical Activity Quarterly, 10,* 173–215.

Cromwell, F. S. (1976). *Occupational therapist's manual for basic skill assessment: Primary prevocational evaluation.* Altadena, CA: Fair Oaks Printing.

Csikszentmihalyi, M. (1975). Play and intrinsic rewards. *Humanistic Psychology, 15,* 41–63.

Cubie, S. H., & Kaplan, K. (1982). A case analysis method for the model of human occupation. *American Journal of Occupational Therapy, 36,* 645–656.

Cummins, J. L. (1995). Anatomic and behavioral aspects of frontal-subcortical circuits. In J. Grafman, K. J. Holyoak, & F. Boller (Eds.), *Annals of the New York Academy of Sciences (Structure and function of the human prefrontal cortex)* (vol. 769, pp. 1–13). New York: New York Academy of Sciences.

Cytowic, R. E. (Ed.). (1996). *The neurological side of neuropsychology.* Cambridge, MA: The Massachusetts Institute of Technology Press.

Dackis, C. A., & Gold, M. S. (1990). Medical, endocrinological, and pharmacological aspects of cocaine addiction. In N. D. Volkow & A. C. Swann (Eds.), *Cocaine in the brain* (pp. 135–154). New Brunswick, NJ: Rutgers University Press.

Damasio, H., & Damasio, A. R. (1989). *Lesion analysis in neuropsychology.* New York: Oxford University Press.

Darragh, A., Sample, P. L., & Fisher, A. G. (in press). The effect of the environment on functional task performance: Use of the Assessment of Motor and Process Skills with adults with acquired brain injury. *Archives of Physical Medicine and Rehabilitation.*

de Clive-Lowe, S. (1996). Outcome measurement, cost-effectiveness and clinical audit: The importance of standardised assessment to occupational therapists in meeting these new demands. *British Journal of Occupational Therapy, 59,* 357–362.

Demeurisse, G., Hublet, C., Paternot, J., Colson, C., & Serniclaes, W. (1997). Pathogenesis of subcortical visuo-spatial neglect. A HMPAO SPECT study. *Neuropsychologia, 35,* 731–735.

Demore-Taber, M. (1995). Job analysis during employer site visit. In K. Jacobs & C. Bettencourt (Eds.), *Ergonomics for therapists* (pp. 237–244). Boston: Butterworth-Heinemann.

DePoy, E. (1987). Community-based occupational therapy with a head-injured adult. *American Journal of Occupational Therapy, 41,* 461–464.

DePoy, E., & Burke, J. P. (1992). Viewing cognition through the lens of the Model of Human Occupation. In N. Katz (Ed.), *Cognitive rehabilitation: Models for intervention in occupational therapy* (pp. 240–257). Boston: Andover Medical.

De Renzi, E., Fabrizia, M., & Nichelli, P. (1980). Imitating gestures. A quantitative approach to ideomotor apraxia. *Archives of Neurology, 37,* 6–10.

De Renzi, E., & Lucchelli, F. (1988). Ideational apraxia. *Brain, 111,* 1173–1185.

Diamant, J. J., & Hakkaart, P. J. W. (1989). Cognitive rehabilitation in an information-processing perspective. *Cognitive Rehabilitation, 7,* 22–28.

Dickerson, A. E., & Fisher, A. G. (1993). Age differences in functional performance. *American Journal of Occupational Therapy, 47,* 686–692.

Dickerson, A. E., & Fisher, A. G. (1995). Culture-relevant functional performance assessment of the Hispanic elderly. *Occupational Therapy Journal of Research, 15,* 50–68.

Dickerson, A. E., & Fisher, A. G. (1997). The effects of familiarity of task and choice on the functional performance of young and old adults. *Psychology and Aging, 12,* 247–254.

Dickoff, J., James, P., & Wiedenbach, E. (1968). Theory in a practice discipline. Part I: Practice oriented theory. *Nursing Research, 17,* 415–435.

Dikengil, A., King, C., & Monda, D. (1992). Communication functional skills group: An integrated group therapy approach to head injury rehabilitation. *Journal of Cognitive Rehabilitation, 10,* 28–31.

Doble, S. E., Fisk, J. D., Fisher, A. G., et al. (1994). Functional competence of community-dwelling persons with multiple sclerosis using the Assessment of Motor and Process Skills. *Archives of Physical Medicine and Rehabilitation, 75,* 843–851.

Doble, S. E., Fisk, J. D., MacPherson, K. M., et al. (1997). Measuring functional competence in older persons with Alzheimer's disease. *International Psychogeriatrics, 9,* 25–38.

Dowie, J., & Elstein, A. (1988). *Professional judgment: A reader in clinical decision-making.* Cambridge: Cambridge University Press.

Dreyfus, S. E., & Dreyfus, H. L. (1980). *A five-stage model of the mental activities involved in directed skill acquisition.* Unpublished report supported by the Air Force Office of Scientific Research (AFSC), USAF (Contract F49620-79-C-0063), University of California at Berkeley.

Dreyfus, H. L., & Dreyfus, S. E. (1986). *Mind over machine: The power of human intuition and expertise in the era of the computer.* New York: Free Press.

Driver, J., & Halligan, P. W. (1991). Can visual neglect operate in object-centred co-ordinates? An affirmative single-case study. *Cognitive Neuropsychology, 8,* 475–496.

Duchek, J. M., & Abreu, B. C. (1997). Meeting the challenges of cognitive disabilities. In C. Christiansen & C. Baum (Eds.), *Occupational therapy: Enabling function and well-being* (2nd ed., pp. 288–311). Thorofare, NJ: Slack.

Duncombe, L. W., & Howe, M. C. (1995). Group treatment: Goals, tasks, and economic implications. *American Journal of Occupational Therapy, 49,* 199–205.

Duran, L., & Fisher, A. G. (1996). Male and female performance on the Assessment of Motor and Process Skills. *Archives of Physical Medicine and Rehabilitation, 77,* 1019–1024.

Dutton, R. (1995). *Clinical reasoning in physical disabilities.* Baltimore: Williams & Wilkins.

Earhart, C. A., & Allen, C. K. (1992). *Cognitive disabilities: Expanded activity analysis.* Colchester, CT: S & S/Worldwide.

Eichenbaum, H. (1996). Olfactory perception and memory. In R. Llinás & P. S. Churchland (Eds.), *The mind-brain continuum: Sensory processes,* (pp. 173–201). Cambridge, MA: The Massachusetts Institute of Technology Press.

Ellenberg, D. B. (1996). Outcomes research: The history, debate, and implications for the field of occupational therapy. *American Journal of Occupational Therapy, 50,* 435–441.

Ellis, A. W., & Young, A. W. (1988). *Human Cognitive Neuropsychology.* Hillsdale, NJ: Lawrence Erlbaum Associates.

Ellwanger, J., Rosenfeld, J. P., Sweet, J. J., & Bhatt, M. (1996). Detecting simulated amnesia for autobiographical and recently learned information using the P300 event-related potential. *International Journal of Psychophysiology, 23,* 9–23.

Elstein, A. S., Shulman, L. S., & Sprafka, S. A. (1978). *Medical problem solving: An analysis of clinical reasoning.* Massachusetts: Harvard University Press.

Faglioni, P., & Basso, A. (1985). Historical perspectives on neuroanatomical correlates of limb apraxia. In E. A. Roy (Ed.), *Neuropsychological studies of apraxia and related disorders* (pp. 3–44). Oxford: North-Holland.

Farber, S. D. (1982). *Neurorehabilitation: A multisensory approach.* Philadelphia: W. B. Saunders Company.

Farber, S. D., & Abreu, B. A. (1993). Understanding the brain and learning theories related to cognitive function and rehabilitation. In C. B. Royeen (Ed.), *AOTA Self-study series: Cognitive rehabilitation* (pp. 1–28). Rockville, MD: American Occupational Therapy Association.

Fidler, G., & Fidler, J. (1963). *Occupational therapy: A communication process in psychiatry.* New York: Macmillan.

Fisher, A. G. (in press). Uniting practice and theory in an occupational framework: 1998 Eleanor Clark Slagle Lectureship. *American Journal of Occupational Therapy, 52.*

Fisher, A. G (1993). The assessment of IADL motor skills: An application of many-faceted Rasch analysis. *American Journal of Occupational Therapy, 47,* 319–329.

Fisher, A. G. (1994). Functional assessment and occupation: Critical issues for occupational therapy. *New Zealand Journal of Occupational Therapy, 45,* 13–19.

Fisher, A. G. (1995). *The Assessment of Motor and Process Skills: A sensitive and powerful tool for the occupational therapist.* Unpublished manual, Colorado State University, Colorado.

Fisher, A. G. (1997a). *Assessment of Motor and Process Skills* (2nd ed.). Fort Collins, CO: Three Star Press.

Fisher, A. G. (1997b). An expanded rehabilitative model of practice. In A. G. Fisher (Ed.), *Assessment of Motor and Process Skills* (2nd ed., pp. 73–85). Fort Collins, CO: Three Star Press.

Fisher, A. G., Liu, Y., Velozo, C. A., & Pan, A. W. (1992). Cross-cultural assessment of process skills. *American Journal of Occupational Therapy, 46,* 876–885.

Fisher, A. G., & Kielhofner, G. (1995). Mind-brain-body performance subsystem. In G. Kielhofner (Ed.), *The model of human occupation* (2nd ed., pp. 83–90). Baltimore: Williams & Wilkins.

Fisher, A. G., & Short de Graf, M. (1993). Improving functional assessment in occupational therapy: Recommendations and philosophy for change. *American Journal of Occupational Therapy, 47,* 199–201.

Flavell, J. H. (1979). Metacognition and cognitive monitoring: A new area of cognitive development inquiry. *American Psychologist, 34,* 906–911.

Fleming, M. H. (1989). The therapist with the three-track mind. *The APTA Practice Symposium Program Guide.* Rockville, MD: American Occupational Therapy Association.

Fleming, M. H. (Ed.). (1990). Proceedings of the institute on clinical reasoning for occupational therapy. *Educators.* Medford, MA: Clinical Reasoning Institute, Tufts University.

Fleming, M. H. (1991). The therapist with the three-track mind. *American Journal of Occupational Therapy, 45,* 1007–1014.

Fleming, M. H. (1994a). The therapist with the three-track mind. In C. Mattingly & M. H. Fleming (Eds.), *Clinical reasoning: Forms of inquiry in a therapeutic practice.* Philadelphia: F. A. Davis.

Fleming, M. H. (1994b). Procedural reasoning. Addressing functional limitations. In C. Mattingly & M. H. Fleming (Eds.), *Clinical reasoning: Forms of inquiry in a therapeutic practice.* Philadelphia: F. A. Davis.

Fleming, M. H. (1994c). Conditional reasoning. Creating meaningful experiences. In C. Mattingly & M. H. Fleming (Eds.), *Clinical reasoning: Forms of inquiry in a therapeutic practice.* Philadelphia: F. A. Davis.

Fogel, M. L. (1967). Picture description and interpretation in brain-damaged patients. *Cortex, 3,* 433–448

Forssmann-Falck, R., Christian, F. M., & O'Shanick, G. (1989). Group therapy with moderately neurologically damaged patients. *Health and Social Work, 14,* 235–243.

Foto, M. (1996). Nationally speaking: Outcome studies: The what, why, how, and when. *American Journal of Occupational Therapy, 50,* 87–88.

Freeman, W. J. (1991). The physiology of perception. *Scientific American, February,* 78–85.

Friedman, R. B., Ween, J. E., & Albert, M. L. (1993). Alexia. In K. M. Heilman & E. Valenstein (Eds.), *Clinical neuropsychology* (3rd ed., pp. 37–62). Oxford: Oxford University Press.

Fuster, J. M. (1993). Frontal lobes. *Current Opinion in Neurobiology, 3,* 160–165.

Fuster, J. M. (1995). *Memory in the cerebral cortex: An empirical approach to neural networks in the human and nonhuman primate.* Cambridge, MA: The Massachusetts Institute of Technology Press.

Gainotti, G. (1994). The dilemma of unilateral spatial neglect. *Neuropsychological Rehabilitation, 4,* 127–132.

Gainotti, G., D'Erme, P., & Bartolomeo, P. (1991). Early orientation of attention toward the half space ipsilateral to the lesion in patients with unilateral brain damage. *Journal of Neurology, Neurosurgery and Psychiatry, 54,* 1082–1089.

Galaski, T., Bruno, R., & Ehle, H. (1993). Prediction of behind the wheel driving performance in patients with cerebral brain damage function analysis. *American Journal of Occupational Therapy, 47,* 391–396.

Gasquoine, P. G., & Gibbons, T. A. (1994). Lack of awareness of impairment in institutionalized, severely and chronically disabled survivors of traumatic brain injury. *Journal of Head Trauma Rehabilitation, 9,* 16–24.

Gauggel, S., & Niemann, T. (1996). Evaluation of a short-term computer-assisted training programme for the remediation of attentional deficits after brain injury: A preliminary study. *International Journal of Rehabilitation Research, 19,* 229–239.

Gazzaniga, M. S., & LeDoux, J. E. (1981). *The integrated mind.* New York: Plenum Press.

Gentile, A. M. (1987). Skill acquisition: Action, movement, and neuromotor processes. In J. H. Carr, R. B. Shepherd, J. Gordon, et al. (Eds.), *Movement science foundations for physical therapy in rehabilitation,* (pp. 93–154). Rockville, MD: Aspen Publishers.

Geschwind, N. (1975). The apraxias: Neural mechanisms of disorders of learned movement. *American Scientist, 63,* 188–195.

Gianutsos, R. (1994). Driving advisement with the Elementary Driving Simulator (EDS). *Behavioral Research Methods, 26,* 183–186.

Gianutsos, R., & Klitzner, C. (1981). *Computer programs for cognitive rehabilitation.* Bayport: Life Science Associates.

Giles, G. M. (1992). A neurofunctional approach to rehabilitation following severe brain injury. In N. Katz (Ed.), *Cognitive rehabilitation: Models for intervention in occupational therapy* (pp. 195–218). Boston: Andover Medical.

Giles, G. M., & Wilson, J. C. (1992). *Occupational therapy for the brain injured adult: A neurofunctional approach.* London: Chapman and Hall.

Giles, G. M., & Shore, M. (1988). The role of the transitional living center in rehabilitation after brain injury. *Cognitive Rehabilitation, 6,* 26–31.

Glaser, R. (1990a). The reemergence of learning theory within instructional research. *American Psychologist, 45,* 29–39.

Glaser, R. (1990b). Expert knowledge and the thinking process. *Chemtech, 20,* 394–397.

Glaser, R. (1990c). Toward new models for assessment. *International Journal of Educational Research, 14,* 475–483.

Glaser, R., & Chi, M. T. H. (1988). Overview. In M. T. H. Chi, R. Glaser & M. J. Farr (Eds.), *The nature of expertise* (pp. xv–xviii). Hillsdale, NJ: Lawrence Erlbaum Associates.

Glosser, G., & Goodglass, H. (1990). Disorders of executive control functions among aphasic and other brain-damaged patients. *Journal of Clinical and Experimental Neuropsychology, 12*, 485–501.

Gobbo, C., & Chi, M. (1986). How knowledge is structured and used by expert and novice children. *Cognitive Development, 1*, 221–237.

Golding, E. (1989). *Middlesex Elderly Assessment of Mental State*. Suffolk: Thames Test Valley.

Goldman, S. L., & Fisher, A. G. (1997). Cross-cultural validation of the Assessment of Motor and Process Skills (AMPS). *British Journal of Occupational Therapy, 60*, 77–85.

Goldstein, M. (1990). Traumatic brain injury: A silent epidemic. *Annals of Neurology, 27*, 327.

Goodgold-Edwards, S., & Cermak, S. (1990). Integrating motor control and motor learning concepts with neuropsychological perspectives on apraxia and developmental dyspraxia. *American Journal of Occupational Therapy, 44*, 431–439.

Goto, S., Fisher, A. G., & Mayberry, W. L. (1996). AMPS applied cross-culturally to the Japanese. *American Journal of Occupational Therapy, 50*, 798–806.

Graff-Radford, N., Welsh, K., & Godersky, J. (1987). Callosal apraxia. *Neurology, 37*, 100–105.

Gray, J. M. (1990). The remediation of attentional disorders following brain injury of acute onset. In R. L. Wood & I. Fussey (Eds.). *Cognitive rehabilitation in perspective* (pp. 29–47). London: Taylor & Francis.

Gray, J. J., Kennedy, B. L., & Zemke, R. (1996). Application of dynamic systems theory to occupation. In R. Zemke & F. Clark (Eds.), *Occupational science: The evolving discipline* (pp. 309–324). Philadelphia: F. A. Davis.

Grieve, J. (1993). *Neuropsychology for occupational therapists: Assessment of perception and cognition*. Oxford: Blackwell Scientific Publications.

Gronwall, D. (1977). Paced Auditory Serial Addition Task: A measure of recovery from concussion. *Perceptual and Motor Skills, 44*, 367–373.

Guide for the Uniform Data Set for Medical Rehabilitation (Adult FIM[SM]), (1993). Version 4.0. Buffalo, NY: State University of New York at Buffalo.

Haenggi, D., & Perfetti, C. A. (1994). Processing components of college-level reading comprehension. *Discourse Processes, 17*, 83–104.

Hagedorn, R. (1996). Clinical decision making in familiar cases: A model of the process and implications for practice. *British Journal of Occupational Therapy, 59*, 217–222.

Halligan, P. W., & Marshall, J. C. (1988). How long is a piece of string? A study of bisection in a case of visual neglect. *Cortex, 24*, 321–328.

Halligan, P. W., & Marshall, J. C. (1993). The history and clinical presentation of neglect. In I. H. Robertson & J. C. Marshall (Eds.), *Unilateral neglect: Clinical and experimental studies* (pp. 3–25). Hove, England: Lawrence Erlbaum Associates Ltd.

Halligan, P. W., Marshall, J. C., & Wade, D. T. (1989). Visuospatial neglect: Underlying factors and test sensitivity. *The Lancet, Oct*, 908–910.

Halligan, P. W., Marshall, J. C., & Wade, D. T. (1992). Left on right: Allochiria in a case of left visuo-spatial neglect. *Journal of Neurology, Neurosurgery and Psychiatry, 55*, 717–719.

Halsband, U., Ito, N., Tanji, J., & Freund, H. (1993). The role of the pre-motor and the supplementary motor area in the temporal control of movement in man. *Brain, 116*, 243–266.

Hammond, K. R. (1988). Judgment and decision-making in dynamic tasks. *Information and decision-making technologies, 14*, 3–14.

Hart, T., & Jacobs, H. E. (1993). Rehabilitation and management of behavioral disturbances following frontal lobe injury. *Journal of Head Trauma Rehabilitation, 8*, 1–12.

Hartley, L. L. (1995). *Cognitive communicative abilities following brain injury. A functional approach.* San Diego: Singular Publishing Group, Inc.

Hattrup, R. A., & Bickel, W. E. (1993). Teacher-researcher collaborations: Resolving the tensions. *Educational Leadership, 50*, 38–40.

Heilman, K. M., & Gonzalez-Rothi, L. J. (1993). Apraxia. In K. M. Heilman & E. Valenstein (Eds.), *Clinical neuropsychology* (3rd ed., pp. 141–163). New York: Oxford University Press Inc.

Heilman, K. M., & Valenstein, E. (Eds.). (1993). *Clinical neuropsychology* (3rd ed.). New York: Oxford University Press.

Heilman, K. M., & Van Den Abell, T. (1980). Right hemisphere dominance for attention: The mechanism underlying hemispheric asymmetries of inattention (neglect). *Neurology, 30*, 327–330.

Heilman, K. M., & Watson, M. T. (1978). Changes in the symptoms of neglect induced by changing task strategy. *Archives of Neurology, 35*, 47–49.

Heilman, K. M., Watson, R. T., & Valenstein, E. (1993). Neglect and related disorders. In K. M. Heilman & E. Valenstein (Eds.), *Clinical neuropsychology* (3rd ed., pp. 279–336). New York: Oxford University Press Inc.

Hermsdorfer, J., Mai, N., Spatt, J., et al. (1996). Kinematic analysis of movement imitation in apraxia. *Brain, 119*, 1575–1586.

Hertel, P. T. (1996). Practical aspects of emotion and memory. In D. Herrman, C. McEnvoy, C. Hertzog, P., et al. (Eds.), *Basic and applied memory research therapy in context* (vol. 1, pp. 317–336). Mahwah, NJ: Lawrence Erlbaum Associates, Publishers.

Higgs, J. (1992). Developing clinical reasoning competencies. *Physiotherapy, 78*, 575–581.

Hill, J., & Carper, M. (1985). Greenery: Group therapeutic approaches with the head injured. *Cognitive Rehabilitation, 3*, 18–29.

Hobson, J. A. (1996). How the brain goes out of its mind. *Endeavour, 20*, 86–89.

Hodges, J. R., & McCarthy, R. A. (1995). Loss of remote memory: A cognitive neuropsychological perspective. *Current Opinion in Neurobiology, 5*, 178–183.

Holm, M. B., & Rogers, J. C. (1989). The therapists thinking behind functional assessment II. In C. B. Royeen (Ed.), *AOTA Self-study series: Assessing function* (pp. 1–30). Rockville, MD: American Occupational Therapy Association Inc.

Holstein, J. A., & Gubrium, J. F. (1995). *The active interview: Qualitative research methods series 37.* Thousand Oaks, CA: Sage Publications.

Hong, E. (1995). A structural comparison between state and trait self-regulation models. *Applied Cognitive Psychology, 9*, 333–349.

Hooper, H. E. (1983). *Hooper visual organization test*. Los Angeles: Western Psychological Services.

Hopkins, H. L., & Smith, H. D. (Eds.). (1993). *Willard and Spackman's Occupational Therapy* (8th ed.). Philadelphia: J. B. Lippincott.

Horn, L. J., & Zasler, N. D. (Eds.). (1996). *Medical rehabilitation of traumatic brain injury*. Philadelphia: Hanley and Belfus, Inc.

Howe, M. C., & Schwartzberg, S. L. (1988). Structure and process in designing a functional group. *Occupational Therapy in Mental Health, 8*, 1–8.

Howe, M. C., & Schwartzberg, S. L. (1995). *A functional approach to group work in occupational therapy* (2nd ed.). Philadelphia: J. B. Lippincott.

Humphreys, G. W., & Riddoch, M. J. (1987). *To see but not to see: A case study of visual agnosia*. London: Lawrence Erlbaum Associates.

Itzkovich, M., Elazar, B., Averbuch, S., & Katz, N. (1990). *The Loewenstein Occupational Therapy Assessment (LOTCA) manual*. Pequanock, NJ: Maddak Inc.

Jackson, J. D. (1994). After rehabilitation: Meeting the long-term needs of persons with traumatic brain injury. *American Journal of Occupational Therapy, 48*, 251–255.

Jacobs, K. (1991). *Occupational therapy: Work-related programs and assessments*. Boston: Little, Brown & Co.

Jacobs, K. (1995). Preparing for return to work. In C. Trombly (Ed.), *Occupational therapy for physical dysfunction* (4th ed., pp. 329–349). Baltimore: Williams & Wilkins.

Jacobs, K., & Bettencourt, C. (Eds.). (1994). *Ergonomics for therapists*. Newton, MA: Butterworth-Heinemann.

Jesshope, H. J., Clarke, M. S., & Smith, D. S. (1991). The RPAB: Its application to stroke-patients and relationship with function. *Clinical Rehabilitation, 5*, 115–122.

Johnson, D. A., & Newton, A. (1987). HIPSIG: A basis for social adjustment after head injury: Head injured persons social interaction group. *British Journal of Occupational Therapy, 50*, 47–52.

Johnstone, B., & Frank, R. G. (1995). Neuropsychological assessment in rehabilitation: Current limitations and applications. *NeuroRehabilitation, 5*, 75–86.

Jongbloed, L. E., Stacey, S., & Brighton, C. (1989). Stroke rehabilitation: Sensorimotor integrative treatment versus functional treatment. *American Journal of Occupational Therapy, 43*, 391–397.

Josman, N., & Katz, N. (1991). Problem solving version of the Allen Cognitive Level Test. *American Journal of Occupational Therapy, 45*, 331–338.

Josselson, R., & Lieblich, A. (Eds.). (1995). *Interpreting experience: The narrative study of lives* (vol. 3). Thousand Oaks, CA: Sage Publications, Inc.

Kandel, E. R. (1976). *Cellular basis of behavior: An introduction to behavioral neurobiology*. San Francisco: W. H. Freeman & Company.

Kandel, E. R. (1985). Processing of form and movement in the visual system. In E. R. Kandel & J. H. Schwartz (Eds.), *Principles of neural science* (2nd ed., pp. 366–383). New York: Elsevier.

Kanehura & Company (1977). *The Ishihara Color Plates*. Tokyo: Author.

Kaplan, S. (1996). Critical evaluation of standardized tests. *Occupational Therapy in Health Care, 10*, 3–14.

Kaplan, E., et al. (1991). *WAIS-R NI Manual: WAIS-R as a neuropsychological instrument*. San Antonio, TX: The Psychological Corporation.

Katz, N. (Ed.). (1992). *Cognitive rehabilitation: Models for intervention in occupational therapy*. Boston: Andover Medical.

Katz, N., & Hartman-Maeir, A. (1997). Occupational performance and metacognition. *Canadian Journal of Occupational Therapy, 64*, 53–62.

Katz, N., Hefner, D., & Reuben, R. (1990). Measuring clinical change in cognitive rehabilitation of patients with brain damage: Two cases, traumatic brain injury and cerebral vascular accident. *Occupational Therapy in Health Care, 7*, 23–43.

Katz, N., & Heimann, N. (1990). Review of research conducted in Israel on cognitive disability instrumentation. *Occupational Therapy in Mental Health, 10*, 1–15.

Katz, N., Itzkovich, M., Averbuch, S., & Elazar, B. (1989). Loewenstein occupational therapy cognitive assessment (LOTCA), battery for brain injured patients: Reliability and validity. *American Journal of Occupational Therapy, 43*, 184–192.

Keh-chung, L. (1996). Right hemisphere activation approaches to neglect rehabilitation poststroke. *American Journal of Occupational Therapy, 50*, 504–515.

Kehrberg, K. (1993). *The Larger Allen Cognitive Level Test*. Colchester, CT: S & S/Worldwide.

Kelly-Hayes, M., Wolf, P. A., Kase, C. S., et al. (1989). Time course of functional recovery after stroke. The Framingham study. *Journal of Neurological Rehabilitation, 3*, 65–70.

Kelso, J. A. S., & Tuller, B. H. (1981). Towards a theory of apractic syndromes. *Brain and Language, 12*, 224–245.

Kertesz, A., & Ferro, J. M. (1984). Lesion size and location in ideomotor apraxia. *Brain, 107*, 921–933.

Kielhofner, G. (1992). *Conceptual foundations of occupational therapy*. Philadelphia: F. A. Davis.

Kielhofner, G. (1995a). *A model of human occupation: Theory and application* (2nd ed.). Baltimore: Williams & Wilkins.

Kielhofner, G. (1995b). Habituation subsystem. In G. Kielhofner (Ed.), *A model of human occupation: Theory and application* (2nd ed., pp. 63–81). Baltimore: Williams & Wilkins.

Kielhofner, G. (1997). *Conceptual foundations of occupational therapy* (2nd ed.). Philadelphia: F. A. Davis.

Kielhofner, G, Borell, L., Burke, J., et al. (1995). Volition subsystem. In G. Kielhofner (Ed.), *A model of human occupation: Theory and application* (2nd ed., pp. 39–62). Baltimore: Williams & Wilkins.

Kielhofner, G., & Burke, J. P. (1980). A model of human occupation, part 1. Conceptual framework and content. *American Journal of Occupational Therapy, 34*, 572–581.

Kielhofner, G., & Neville, A. (1983). *The modified interest checklist*. Unpublished manuscript, Department of Occupational Therapy, University of Illinois at Chicago.

Kinsbourne, M. (1993). Orientational bias model of unilateral neglect: Evidence from attentional gradients within hemispace. In I. H. Robertson & J. C. Marshall (Eds.), *Unilateral neglect: Clinical and experimental studies* (pp. 27–39). Hillsdale, NJ: Lawrence Erlbaum Associates.

Kinsbourne, M., & Warrington, E. (1962). A disorder of simultaneous form perception. *Brain, 85*, 461–486.

Kintsch, W. (1994). Text comprehension, memory, and learning. *American Psychologist, 49*, 294–303.

Kirshner, H. (1991). The apraxias. In W. Bradley, R. Daroff, G. Fenichel, & C. Marsden (Eds.), *Neurology in clinical practice: Principles of diagnosis and management* (vol. 1, pp. 117–122). London: Butterworth-Heinmann.

Klatzy, K. (1980). *Human memory: Structure and processes.* San Francisco: W. H. Freeman.

Klopfer, L. E. (1986). The coming generation of tutoring software. *The Science Teacher, 56*, 34–37.

Koriat, A. (1994). Memory's knowledge of its own knowledge: The accessibility account of the feeling of knowing. In J. Metcalfe & A. P. Shimamura (Eds.), *Metacognition: Knowing about knowing* (pp. 115–135). Cambridge, MA: The Massachusetts Institute of Technology Press.

Konow, A., & Pribram, K. H. (1970). Error recognition and utilization produced by injury to the frontal cortex in man. *Neuropsychologia, 8*, 489–491.

Kortleing, J. E., & Kaptein, M. A. (1996). Neuropsychological driving fitness tests for brain-damaged subjects. *Archives of Physical Medicine and Rehabilitation, 77*, 138–146.

Kottorp, A., Bernspång, B., Fisher, A. G., & Bryze, K. (1995). IADL ability measured with the AMPS: Relation to two classification systems of mental retardation. *Scandinavian Journal of Occupational Therapy, 2*, 121–128.

Kurasik, S. (1967). Group dynamics in rehabilitation of hemiplegic patients. *Journal of the American Geriatric Society, 15*, 852–855.

Lamport, N. K., Coffey, M. S., & Hersch, G. I. (1993). *Activity analysis handbook* (2nd ed.). Thorofare, NJ: Slack Inc.

Langthaler, M. (1990). *The components of a therapeutic relationship in occupational therapy.* Unpublished master's thesis. Tufts University, Medford, MA.

Laver, A. J. (1990). Test Review: The Rivermead Perceptual Assessment Battery. In J. R. Beech & L. Harding. *Assessment of the Elderly* (pp. 134–138). Windsor: NFER Nelson.

Laver, A. J. (1991). Test Review: The Functional Performance Record. *The British Journal of Occupational Therapy, 54*, 22–23.

Laver, A. J. (1994a). The structured observational test of function. *Gerontology Special Interest Section Newsletter, 17*, 1–2.

Laver, A. J. (1994b). *The Development of the Structured Observational Test of Function (SOTOF).* Unpublished doctoral dissertation. University of Surrey, Guildford, England.

Laver, A. J. (1996). The Occupational Therapy Intervention Process. Section I Occupational Therapy Assessment and Evaluation of Older Clients. In K. O. Larson, R. G. Stevens-Ratchford, L. W. Pedretti, & J. L. Crabtree (Eds.), *ROTE: The Role of Occupational Therapy with the Elderly–A Self-Paced Clinical Course* (pp. 503–533). Bethesda, MD: American Occupational Therapy Association.

Laver, A. J., & Huchison, S. (1994). The performance of normal elderly people on the Chessington Occupational Therapy Neurological Assessment Battery (COTNAB). *British Journal of Occupational Therapy, 57*, 137–142.

Laver, A. J., & Powell, G. E. (1995). *The Structured Observational Test of Function (SOTOF).* Windsor: NFER-NELSON.

Law, M. (1987). Measurement in occupational therapy: Scientific criteria for evaluation. *Canadian Journal of Occupational Therapy, 54,* 133–138.

Law, M., Baptiste, S., Carswell, A., et al. (1994). *The Canadian Occupational Performance Measure.* Toronto: Canadian Association of Occupational Therapy.

Leinhardt, G. (1990). Capturing craft knowledge in teaching. *Educational Researcher, 19,* 18–25.

Leinhardt, G., & Ohlsson, S. (1990). Tutorials on the structure of tutoring from teachers. *Journal of Artificial Intelligence in Education, 2,* 21–46.

Leinhardt, G., Weidman, C., & Hammond, K. M. (1987). Introduction and integration of classroom routines by expert teachers. *Curriculum Inquiry, 17,* 135–176.

Lennon, S. (1994). Task specific effects in the rehabilitation of unilateral neglect. In M. J. Riddoch & G. W. Humpreys (Eds.), *Cognitive Neuropsychology and Cognitive Rehabilitation* (pp. 187–203). Hove: Lawrence Erlbaum Associates.

Leon-Carrion, J. (Ed.). (1997). *Neuropsychological rehabilitation: Fundamentals, innovations and directions.* Delray Beach, FL: GR/St. Lucie Press.

Leonesio, R. J., & Nelson, T. O. (1992). Do different metamemory judgments tap the same underlying aspects of memory? In T. O. Nelson (Ed.), *Metacognition core readings* (pp. 159–170). Needham Heights, MA: Allyn & Brown–Simon & Schuster, Inc.

Levine, R. E., & Brayley, C. R. (1991). Occupation as a therapeutic medium. In C. Christiansen & C. Baum (Eds.), *Occupational Therapy: Overcoming human performance deficits* (pp. 590–631). Thorofare, NJ: SLACK Inc.

Levinson, R. (1995). A computer model of prefrontal cortex function. In J. Grafman, K. J. Holyoak, & F. Boller (Eds.), *Annals of the New York Academy of Sciences (Structure and function of the human prefrontal cortex)* (vol. 769, pp. 381–388). New York: New York Academy of Sciences.

Levitt, J. J., O'Donnell, B. F., McCarley, R. W., et al. (1996). Correlations of premorbid adjustment in schizophrenia with auditory event-related potential and neuropsychological abnormalities. *American Journal of Psychiatry, 153,* 1347–1349.

Levy, L. L. (1992). The use of the cognitive disability frame of reference in rehabilitation of cognitively disabled older adults. In N. Katz (Ed.), *Cognitive rehabilitation: Models for intervention in occupational therapy* (pp. 22–50). Boston: Andover Medical.

Lezak, M. D. (1993). Newer contributions to the neuropsychological assessment of executive functions. *Journal of Head Trauma Rehabilitation, 8,* 24–31.

Lezak, M. D. (1995). *Neuropsychological assessment* (3rd ed.). New York: Oxford University Press.

Lhermitte, F. (1986). Human anatomy and the frontal lobes. Part II: Patient behavior in complex and social situations: The "environmental dependency syndrome." *Annals of Neurology, 19,* 335–343.

Light, K. E. (1990). Information processing for motor performance in aging adults. *Physical Therapy, 10,* 820–826.

Lincoln, N. B., & Edmans, J. A. (1989). A shortened version of the Rivermead Perceptual Assessment Battery. *Clinical Rehabilitation, 3,* 199–204.

Llinás, R., & Churchland, P. S. (Eds.). (1996). *The mind-brain continuum: Sensory processes.* Cambridge, MA: The Massachusetts Institute of Technology Press.

Llorens, L. A. (1986). Activity analysis: Agreement among factors in a sensory processing model. *American Journal of Occupational Therapy, 40,* 103–110.

Loxterman, J. A., Beck, I. L., & McKeown, M. G. (1994). The effects of thinking aloud during reading on students' comprehension of more or less coherent test. *Reading Research Quarterly, 29,* 353–368.

Lundgren, C. C., & Persechino, E. L. (1986). Cognitive group: A treatment program for head injured adults. *American Journal of Occupational Therapy, 40,* 397–401.

Luria, A. R. (1963). *Restoration of function after brain injury.* New York: Basic Books.

Luria, A. R. (1966). *Higher cortical functions in man.* New York: Basic Books.

Luria, A. R. (1973). *The working brain: An introduction to neuropsychology.* New York: Basic Books.

Lysaght, R., & Bodenhamer, E. (1990). The use of relaxation training to enhance functional outcomes in adults with traumatic head injuries. *American Journal of Occupational Therapy, 44,* 797–802.

Magalhães, L., Fisher, A. G., Bernspång, B., & Linacre, J. M. (1996). Cross-cultural assessment of functional ability. *Occupational Therapy Journal of Research, 16,* 45–63.

Mahoney, F., & Barthel, D. (1965). Functional evaluation: The Barthel Index. *Maryland State Medical Journal, 14,* 61–65.

Malec, J. F., Zweber, B., & DePompolo, R. (1990). The Rivermead Behavioural Memory Test, laboratory neurocognitive measure, and everyday functioning. *Journal of Head Trauma Rehabilitation, 5,* 60–68.

Mapou, R. L., & Spector, J. (Eds.). (1995). *Clinical neurospychological assessment: A cognitive approach.* New York: Plenum Press.

Matchar, D. B., McCrory, D. C., Barnett, H. J. M., & Feussner, J. R. (1994). Medical treatment for stroke prevention. *Annals of Internal Medicine, 121,* 41–53.

Mateer, C. A. (1997). Rehabilitation of individuals with frontal lobe impairment. In J. Leon-Carrion (Ed.), *Neuropsychological rehabilitation: Fundamentals, Innovations and Directions.* Delray Beach, FL: GR/St. Lucie Press.

Mateer, C. A., Kerns, K. A., & Eso, K. L. (1996). Management of attention and memory disorders following traumatic brain injury. *Journal of Learning Disabilities, 29,* 618–632.

Mateer, C. A., Sohlberg, M. M., & Youngman, P. K. (1990). The management of acquired attention and memory deficits. In R. L. Wood & I. Fussey (Eds.), *Cognitive rehabilitation in perspective* (pp. 68–95). London: Taylor & Francis.

Mathiowetz, V. (1993). Role of physical performance component evaluations in occupational therapy functional assessment. *American Journal of Occupational Therapy, 47,* 225–230.

Mathiowetz, V., Volland, G., Kashman, N., & Weber, K. (1985). Adult norms for the box and block test of manual dexterity. *American Journal of Occupational Therapy, 39,* 386–91.

Matsatsuyu, J. S. (1969). The Interest Check List. *American Journal of Occupational Therapy, 23,* 323 –327.

Matthey, S., Donnelly, S. M., & Hextell, D. L. (1993). The clinical usefulness of the Rivermead Perceptual Assessment Battery. *British Journal of Occupational Therapy, 56,* 365–370.

Mattingly, C. (1989). *Thinking with stories: Stories and experience in a clinical practice.* Unpublished doctoral dissertation. Massachusetts Institute of technology, Cambridge, MA.

Mattingly, C. (1991). What is clinical reasoning? *American Journal of Occupational Therapy, 45,* 979–986.

Mattingly, C. (1994a). Occupational therapy as a two-body practice: The body as Machine. In C. Mattingly & M. H. Fleming (Eds.), *Clinical reasoning: Forms of inquiry in a therapeutic practice* (pp. 37–63). Philadelphia: F. A. Davis.

Mattingly, C. (1994b). The narrative nature of clinical reasoning. In C. Mattingly & M. H. Fleming (Eds.), *Clinical reasoning: Forms of inquiry in a therapeutic practice* (pp. 239–269). Philadelphia: F. A. Davis.

Mattingly, C. (1994c). Clinical revision: Changing the therapeutic story in midstream. In C. Mattingly & M. H. Fleming (Eds.), *Clinical reasoning: Forms of inquiry in a therapeutic practice* (pp. 270–291). Philadelphia: F. A. Davis.

Mattingly, C., & Fleming, M. H. (1994). *Clinical reasoning: Forms of inquiry in a therapeutic practice.* Philadelphia, F. A. Davis.

Mattingly, C., & Gillette, N. (1991). Anthropology, occupational therapy, and action research. *American Journal of Occupational Therapy, 45,* 972–978.

Mayer, M. A. (1988). Analysis of information processing and cognitive disability theory. *American Journal of Occupational Therapy, 42,* 176–183.

Mayer, N. H., Reed E., Schwartz M. F., et al. (1990). Buttering a hot cup of coffee: An approach to the study of errors of action in patients with brain damage. In D. E. Tupper & K. D. Cicerone (Eds.), *The neuropsychology of everyday life: Assessment and basic competencies* (pp. 259–284). London: Kluwer Academic Publishers.

Mayes, A. R., Downes, J. J., McDonald, C., et al. (1994). Two tests for assessing remote public knowledge: A tool for assessing retrograde amnesia, *Memory, 2,* 183–210.

McAdams, S. (1996). Audition: Cognitive Psychology of Music. In R. Llinás & P. S. Churchland (Eds.), *The mind-brain continuum: Sensory processes* (pp. 251–279). Cambridge, MA: The Massachusetts Institute of Technology Press.

McKeehan, K. M. (1981). Conceptual framework for discharge planning. In K. M. McKeehan (Ed.), *Continuing care: A multidisciplinary approach to discharge planning* (pp. 3–17). Toronto: C. V. Mosby.

Meadows, J. C. (1974). Disturbed perception of colors associated with localized cerebral lesions. *Brain, 97,* 615–632.

Meghji, C., Lonneberg, E., Bridgman, E., et al. (1995). Practice makes perfect: An interdisciplinary community living skills group for persons with brain injury. *Journal of Cognitive Rehabilitation, 13,* 4–14.

Mesulam, M. (1981). A cortical network for directed attention and unilateral neglect. *Annals of Neurology, 10,* 309–325.

Mesulam, M. (1985). *Principles of behavioral neurology.* Philadelphia: F. A. Davis.

Meier, M. J., Strauman, S., & Thompson, W. G. (1987). Individual differences in neuropsychological recovery: An overview. In M. Meier, A. Benton, & L. Diller (Eds.), *Neuropsychological rehabilitation* (pp. 71–110). New York: Guilford.

Merriam-Webster's collegiate dictionary (10th Ed.). (1995). Springfield, MA: Merriam-Webster, Inc.

Metcalfe, J. (1993). Novelty monitoring, metacognition, and control in a composite holographic associative recall model: Implications for Korsakoff amnesia. *Psychological Review, 100,* 3–22.

Miller, W. G., & Gil, E. B. (1994). Neuropsychological assessment of the traumatic head-injured patient. In S. Touyz, D. Byrne, & A. Gilandas (Eds.), *Neuropsychology in clinical practice* (pp. 79–106). Sydney: Academic Press.

Miller, L. (1992). When the best help is self-help, or, everything you always wanted to know about brain injury support groups. *Journal of Cognitive Rehabilitation, 10,* 14–17.

Milner, B. (1971). Interhemispheric differences in the localization of psychological processes in man. *British Medical Bulletin, 27,* 272–277.

Molloy, M. P. (1994). Computer-enhanced rehabilitation in the private practice setting. In S. Touyz, D. Byrne, & A. Gilandas (Eds.), *Neuropsychology in clinical practice* (pp. 359–370). Sydney: Academic Press.

Monnier, M. (1975). *Functions of the nervous system.* New York: American Elsevier Publishing Company, Inc.

Moore, J. C. (1993). *Brain atlas & functional systems.* Rockville, MD: American Occupational Therapy Association, Inc.

Mosey, A. C. (1993). Working taxonomies. In C. B. Royeen (Ed.), *AOTA Self-study series: Cognitive rehabilitation* (pp. 23–34). Rockville, MD: American Occupational Therapy Association.

Mosey, A. C. (1986). *Psychosocial components of occupational therapy.* New York: Raven Press.

Mozaz, M. J. (1992). Ideational and ideomotor apraxia: A qualitative analysis. *Behavioural Neurology, 5,* 11–17.

Mozaz, M., Marti, J., Carrera, E., & de la Puente, E. (1990). Apraxia in a patient with lesion located in right sub-cortical area: Analysis of errors. *Cortex, 26,* 651–655.

Narens, L., Graf, A., & Nelson, T. D. (1996). Metacognitive aspects of implicit/explicit memory. In L. M. Reder (Ed.), *Implicit memory and metacognition* (pp. 137–170). Mahwah, NJ: Lawrence Erlbaum Associates.

Neistadt, M. E. (1987). Classroom as clinic: A model of teaching clinical reasoning in occupational therapy education. *American Journal of Occupational Therapy, 41,* 631–637.

Neistadt, M. E. (1988). Occupational therapy for adults with perceptual deficits. *American Journal of Occupational Therapy, 42,* 434–440.

Neistadt, M. E. (1990). A critical analysis of occupational therapy approaches for perceptual deficits for adults with brain injury. *American Journal of Occupational Therapy, 44,* 299–304.

Neistadt, M. E. (1992a). The classroom as clinic: Applications for a method of teaching clinical reasoning. *American Journal of Occupational Therapy, 46,* 814–819.

Neistadt, M. E. (1992b). The Rabideau kitchen evaluation-revised: An assessment of meal preparation skill. *Occupational Therapy Journal of Research, 12,* 242–255.

Neistadt, M. E. (1994a). The neurobiology of learning: Implications for treatment of adults with brain injury. *American Journal of Occupational Therapy, 48,* 421–430.

Neistadt, M. E. (1994b). A meal preparation treatment protocol for adults with brain injury. *American Journal of Occupational Therapy, 48,* 431–438.

Neistadt, M. E. (1994c). Perceptual retraining for adults with diffuse brain injury. *American Journal of Occupational Therapy, 48,* 225–233.

Neistadt, M. E. (1995a). Assessing learning capabilities during cognitive and perceptual evaluations for adults with traumatic brain injury. *Occupational Therapy in Health care, 9,* 3–16.

Neistadt, M. E. (1995b). Treatment activity preferences of occupational therapists in adult physical dysfunction settings. *American Journal of Occupational Therapy, 49,* 437–443.

Neistadt, M. E. (1996). Teaching strategies for the development of clinical reasoning. *American Journal of Occupational Therapy, 50,* 676–684.

Neistadt, M. E., & Atkins, A. (1996). Analysis of the orthopedic content in an occupational therapy curriculum from a clinical reasoning perspective. *American Journal of Occupational Therapy, 50,* 669–675.

Nelson, T. O., & Narens, L. (1992). Metamemory: A theoretical framework and new findings. In T. O. Nelson (Ed.), *Metacognition core readings* (pp. 117–129). Needham Heights, MA: Allyn & Bacon.

Norman, D. A., & Shallice, T. (1986). Attention to action: Willed and automatic control of behavior. In R. J. Davidson, G. E. Schwartz, & D. Shapiro (Eds.), *Consciousness and self-regulation: Advances in research and theory* (vol. 4, pp. 1–18). New York: Plenum Press.

Nyberg, L., McIntosh, A. R., Cabeza, R., et al. (1996). Network analysis of positron emission tomography regional cerebral blood flow data: Ensemble inhibition during episodic memory retrieval. *The Journal of Neuroscience, 16,* 3753–3759.

Nygård, L., Bernspång, B., Fisher, A. G., & Winblad, B. (1994). Comparing motor and process ability of persons with suspected dementia in home and clinic settings. *American Journal of Occupational Therapy, 48,* 689–696.

Oakley, F., Kielhofner, G., & Barris, R. (1985). An occupational therapy approach to assessing psychiatric patients' adaptive functioning. *American Journal of Occupational Therapy, 39,* 147–154.

Oakley, F., Kielhofner, G., Barris, R., & Reichler, R. K. (1986). The Role Checklist: Development and Empirical Assessment of Reliability. *Occupational Therapy Journal of Research, 6,* 157 –170.

Oakley, F., & Sunderland, T. (1997). The Assessment of Motor and Process Skills as a measure of IADL functioning in pharmacologic studies of people with Alzheimer's disease: A pilot study. *International Psychogeriatrics, 9,* 197–206.

Okkema, K. (1993). *Cognition and perception in the stroke patient: A guide to functional outcomes in occupational therapy.* Gaithersburg, MD: Aspen Publishers.

Omahoney, D., Coffey, J., Murphy, J., et al. (1996). Event-related potential prolongation in Alzheimer's disease signifies frontal lobe impairment: Evidence from SPECT imaging. *Journals of Gerontology Series A–Biological Sciences and Medical Sciences, 51,* M102–M107.

Pan, A. W., & Fisher, A. G. (1994). The Assessment of Motor and Process Skills of persons with psychiatric disorders. *American Journal of Occupational Therapy, 48,* 775–780.

Palmer, S. E. (1975). The effect of contextual scenes of the identification of objects. *Memory & Cognition, 3,* 519–526.

Papagno, C., Della Salla, S., & Basso, A. (1993). Ideomotor apraxia without aphasia and aphasia without apraxia: The anatomical support for a double dissociation. *Journal of Neurology, Neurosurgery and Psychiatry, 56,* 286–289.

Papanicolaou, A. C. (1987). Electrophysiological methods for the study of attentional deficits in head injury. In H. S. Levin, J. Grafman, & H. M. Eisenberg (Eds.), *Neurobehavioral Recovery from Head Injury* (pp. 379–389). New York: Oxford University Press.

Parham, L. D. (1987). Toward professionalism: The reflective therapist. *American Journal of Occupational Therapy, 41,* 555–561.

Paris, S. G., & Winograd, P. (1990). How metacognition can promote academic learning and instruction. In B. F. Jones & L. Idol (Eds.), *Dimensions of Thinking and Cognitive Instruction* (pp. 15–51). Hillsdale, NJ: Lawrence Erlbaum.

Park, S., Duran, L., & Fisher, A. G. (1997). Evaluation and intervention planning: Enhancing ADL performance. In A. G. Fisher (Ed.), *Assessment of Motor and Process Skills* (2nd ed., pp. 87–117). Fort Collins, CO: Three Star Press.

Park, S., Fisher, A. G., & Velozo, C. A. (1994). Using the Assessment of Motor and Process Skills to compare occupational performance between clinic and home settings. *American Journal of Occupational Therapy, 48,* 697–709.

Parker, R. S. (1990). *Traumatic brain injury and neuropsychological impairment.* New York: Springer-Verlag.

Parkin, A. J., Bell, W. P., & Leng, N. R. C. (1988). A study of metamemory in amnesic and normal adults. *Cortex, 24,* 143–148.

Pedretti, L. R. (Ed.). (1985). *Occupational therapy: Practice skills for physical dysfunction* (3rd ed.). St. Louis: C. V. Mosby.

Pedretti, L. R. (Ed.). (1996). *Occupational therapy: Practice skills for physical dysfunction* (4th ed.). St. Louis: C. V. Mosby.

Pelland, M. J. (1987). A conceptual model for the instruction and supervision of treatment planning. *American Journal of Occupational Therapy, 41,* 351–359.

Peloquin, S. M. (1996). Using the arts to enhance confluent learning. *American Journal of Occupational Therapy, 50,* 148–151.

Pierce, S. (1996). A roadmap for driver rehabilitation. *OT Practice, 1,* 30–38.

Phillips, M. E., & Wolters, S. (1996). Assessment in practice: Common tools and methods. In C. B. Royeen (Ed.), *AOTA Self-study series: Stroke: Strategies, treatment, rehabilitation, outcomes, knowledge, and evaluation* (pp. 1–30). Bethesda, MD: American Occupational Therapy Association.

Pilgrim, E. J., & Humphreys G. W. (1994). Rehabilitating ideomotor apraxia. In J. Riddock & G. W. Humphreys (Eds.), *Cognitive Neuropsychology and Cognitive Rehabilitation* (pp. 271–285). Hove: Laurence Erlbaum Associates Ltd.

Perfetti, C. A. (1995). Cognitive research can inform reading education. *Journal of Research in Reading, 18,* 106–115.

Poeck, K. (1986). The clinical examination of apraxia. *Neuropsychologia, 24,* 129–134.

Poizner, H., Mack, L., Verfaellie, M., et al. (1990). Three dimensional computergraphic analysis of apraxia: Neural representations of learned movement. *Brain, 113,* 85–101.

Ponsford, J. (1990). The use of computers in the rehabilitation of attentional disorders. In R. L. Wood & I. Fussey (Eds.), *Cognitive rehabilitation in perspective* (pp. 48–67). London: Taylor & Francis.

Ponsford, J. L., & Kinsella, G. (1988). Evaluation of a remedial programme for attentional deficits following closed head injury. *Journal of Clinical and Experimental Neuropsychology, 10,* 693–708.

Ponsford, J. L., & Kinsella, G. (1991). The use of a rating scale of attentional behaviour. *Neuropsychological Rehabilitation, 1,* 241–257.

Ponsford, J. L., & Kinsella, G. (1992). Attentional deficits following closed head injury. *Journal of Clinical and Experimental Neuropsychology, 14,* 822–838.

Ponsford, J., Sloan, S., & Snow, P. (1995). *Traumatic brain injury: Rehabilitation for everyday adaptive living.* Hove: Lawrence Erlbaum.

Posner, M. I. (1988). Introduction: What is it to be an expert? In M. T. H. Chi, R. Glaser, & M. J. Farr (Eds.), *The Nature of Expertise* (pp. xxix–xxxvi). Hillsdale, NJ: Lawrence Erlbaum Associates.

Posner, M. I., & Peterson, S. E. (1990). The attention system of the human brain. *Annual Review of Neuroscience, 13,* 25–42.

Prichard, D., & Bernard, E. (1995). Making group work work. In M. A. Chamberlain, V. Neumann, & A. Tennant (Eds.), *Traumatic brain injury rehabilitation: Services, treatments and outcomes* (pp. 180–192). London: Chapman and Hall.

Quintana, L. A. (1995). Remediating cognitive impairments. In C. A. Trombly (Ed.), *Occupational therapy for physical dysfunction* (4th ed., pp. 539–548). Baltimore: Williams & Wilkins.

Raade, A. S., Gonzalez Rothi, L. J., & Heilman, K. M. (1991). The relationship between buccofacial and limb apraxia. *Brain and Cognition, 16,* 130–146.

Rafal, R. (1994). Neglect. *Current Opinion in Neurobiology, 4,* 321–326.

Rappaport, M. (1986). Brain evoked potentials in coma and the vegetative state. *Head Trauma Rehabilitation, 1,* 15–29.

Reder, L. M. (Ed.). (1996). *Implicit memory and metacognition.* Mahwah, NJ: Lawrence Erlbaum Associates, Inc.

Reed, E. S. (1989a). Changing theories of postural development. In M. H. Wollacott & A. Shumway-Cook (Eds.), *Development of posture and gait across the life span,* (pp. 3–24). Colombia, SC: University of South Carolina Press.

Reed, E. S. (1989b). Neural regulation of adaptive behavior. *Ecological Psychology, 1,* 97–118.

Riordan, R. J., & Beggs, M. S. (1988). Some critical differences between self-help and therapy groups. *Journal for Specialists in Group Work, 13,* 24–29.

Riddock, M J., Humphreys, G. W., & Price, C. (1989). Routes to action: Evidence from apraxia. *Cognitive Neuropsychology, 6,* 437–454.

Rizzolatti, G., & Berti, A. (1993). Neural mechanisms of spatial neglect. In I. H. Robertson & J. C. Marshall (Eds.), *Unilateral neglect: Clinical and experimental studies* (pp. 87–105). Hove: Lawrence Erlbaum Associates Ltd.

Robertson, I. H. (1994). The rehabilitation of attentional and hemi-inattentional disorders. In M. J. Riddoch & G. W. Humphreys (Eds.), *Cognitive Neuropsychology and Cognitive Rehabilitation* (pp. 173–186). Hove: Lawrence Erlbaum Associates.

Robertson, L. J. (1996). Clinical reasoning, Part 2: Novice/expert differences. *British Journal of Occupational Therapy, 59,* 212–216.

Robertson, L. C., & Eglin, M. (1993). Attentional search in unilateral visual neglect. In I. H. Robertson & J. C. Marshall (Eds.), *Unilateral neglect: Clinical and experimental studies* (pp. 169–192). Hove: Lawrence Erlbaum Associates.

Robertson, I. H., & North, N. T. (1993). Active and passive activation of left limbs: Influence on visual and sensory neglect. *Neuropsychologia, 31,* 293–300.

Robertson, I. H., North, N. T., & Geggie, C. (1992). Spatio-motor cueing in unilateral left neglect: Three case studies of its therapeutic effects. *Journal of Neurology, Neurosurgery and Psychiatry, 55,* 799–805.

Robertson, I. H., Tegnér, R., Goodrich, S. J., & Wilson, C. (1994). Walking trajectory and hand movements in unilateral left neglect: A vestibular hypothesis. *Neuropsychologia, 32,* 1495–1502.

Robertson, I. H., Tegnér, R., Than, K., et al. (1995). Sustained attention training for unilateral neglect: Theoretical and rehabilitation implications. *Journal of Neurology, Neurosurgery & Psychiatry, 17,* 416–430.

Robertson, I., Ward, T., Ridgeway, Y., & Nimmo-Smith, I. (1994). *The test of everyday attention.* Bury St. Edwards: Thames Valley Test Co.

Robinson, B. C. (1983). Validation of a Caregiver Strain Index. *Journal of Gerontology, 38,* 344–348.

Rogers, J. C. (1983). Eleanor Clarke Slagle Lectureship–1993: Clinical reasoning: The ethics, science and art. *American Journal of Occupational Therapy, 37,* 601–616.

Rogers, J. C., & Holm, M. B. (1989). The therapists thinking behind functional assessment I. In Royeen C. B. (Ed.), *AOTA Self-study series: Assessing function* (pp. 1–30). Rockville, MD: American Occupational Therapy Association.

Rogers, J. C., & Holm, M. B. (1991). Occupational therapy diagnostic reasoning: A component of clinical reasoning. *American Journal of Occupational Therapy, 45,* 1045–1053.

Rogers, J. C., & Holm, M. B. (1994). Accepting the challenge of outcome research: Examining the effectiveness of occupational therapy practice. *American Journal of Occupational Therapy, 48,* 871–876.

Rogers, J. C., & Holm, M. B. (1997). Diagnostic reasoning: The process of problem identification. In C. Christiansen & C. Baum (Eds.), *Occupational therapy: Enabling function and well being* (2nd ed., pp. 137–156). Thorofare, NJ: SLACK Incorporated.

Rogers, J. C., & Masagatani, G. (1982). Clinical reasoning of occupational therapists during the initial assessment of physically disabled patients. *Occupational Therapy Journal of Research, 2,* 195–219.

Roland, P. E. (1982). Cortical regulation of selective attention in man. A regional cerebral blood flow study. *Journal of Neurophysiology, 48,* 1059–1078.

Rootes, L. E., & Aanes, D. L. (1992). A conceptual framework for understanding self-help groups. *Hospital and Community Psychiatry, 43,* 379–381.

Royeen, C. B. (Ed.). (1993). *AOTA Self-study series: Cognitive rehabilitation.* Rockville, MD: American Association of Occupational Therapy.

Rubio, K. B., & Van Deusen, J. (1995). Relation of perceptual and body image dysfunction to activities of daily living of persons after stroke. *American Journal of Occupational Therapy, 49,* 551–559.

Ryerson, S., & Levit, K. (1997). *Functional movement reeducation: A contemporary model for stroke rehabilitation.* New York, Churchill Livingstone.

Salamy, M., Simon, S., & Kielhofner, G. (1993). *The Assessment of Communication and Interaction Skills (Research Version).* Unpublished manuscript, Department of Occupational Therapy, University of Illinois at Chicago.

Selnes, O., Pestronk, A., Hart, J., & Gordan, B. (1991). Limb apraxia without aphasia from a left sided lesion in a right handed patient. *Journal of Neurology, Neurosurgery and Psychiatry, 54,* 734–737.

Schacter, D. L. (1996). *Searching for memory.* New York: Basic Books.

Schacter, D. L., & Tulving, E. (Eds.). (1994). *Memory systems 1994.* Cambridge, MA: The Massachusetts Institute of Technology Press.

Scheibel-Schmitt, C. (1992, July 9). Stroke treatment: Meeting individual goals together. *OT Week,* pp. 16–17.

Scheiman, M. (Ed.). (1996). *Understanding and managing vision deficits: A guide for occupational therapists.* Thorofare, NJ: Slack Inc.

Schell, B. A., & Cervero, R. M. (1993). Clinical reasoning in occupational therapy: An integrative review. *American Journal of Occupational Therapy, 47,* 605–610.

Schmidt, R. A. (1988). *Motor control and learning: A behavioral emphasis* (2nd ed.). Champaign, IL: Human Kinetics.

Schmidt, R. A., & Bjork, R. A. (1992). New conceptualizations of practice. Common principles in three paradigms suggest new concepts for training. *Psychological Science, 3,* 207–217.

Schneider, W. (1993). Varieties of working memory as seen in biology and in connectionist/control architectures. *Memory and Cognition, 21,* 184–192.

Schneider, W., Casey, B. J., & Noll, D. (1994). Functional MRI mapping of stimulus rate effects across visual processing stages. *Human Brain Mapping, 1,* 117–133.

Schneider, W., & Graham, D. J. (1992). Introduction to connectionist modeling in education. *Educational Psychologist, 27,* 513–530.

Schneider, W., Noll, D., & Cohen, J. (1993). Functional topographic mapping of the cortical ribbon in human vision with conventional MRI scanners. *Nature, 365,* 150–153.

Schnider, A., Gutbrod, K., Hess, C., & Schroth, G. (1996). Memory without context: Amnesia with confabulations after infarction of the right capsular genu. *Journal of Neurology, Neurosurgery and Psychiatry, 61,* 186–193.

Schön, D. A. (1983). *The reflective practitioner: How professionals think in action.* New York: Basic Books Inc.

Schön, D. A. (1988). *Educating the reflective practitioner.* San Francisco: Jossey-Bass Publishers.

Schwartz, R. K. (1985). *Therapy as learning.* Dubuque, IA: Kendall Publishing Company.

Schwartz, R. K. (1991). Education and training strategies: Therapy as learning. In C. Christiansen & C. Braun (Eds.), *Occupational Therapy: Overcoming Human Performance Deficits* (pp. 664–698). Thorofare, NJ: Slack.

Schwartz, M. F. (1995). Re-examining the role of executive functions in routine action production. In J. Grafman, K. J. Holyoak, & F. Boller (Eds.), *Annals of the New York Academy of Sciences (Structure and function of the human prefrontal cortex)* (vol. 769, pp. 321–335). New York: New York Academy of Sciences.

Schwartz, M. F., Mayer, N. H., Fitzpatrick-DeSalme, E .J., & Montgomery, M. W. (1993). Cognitive theory and the study of everyday action disorders after brain damage. *Journal of Head Trauma Rehabilitation, 8*, 59–72.

Schwartzberg, S. L. (1994). Helping factors in a peer-developed support group for persons with head injury, Part 1: Participant observer perspective. *American Journal of Occupational Therapy, 48*, 297–304.

Seil, F. J. (Ed.). (1997). *Neuronal Regeneration, reorganization, and repair.* Philadelphia: Lippincott-Raven.

Shallice, T. (1982). Specific impairments of planning. *Philosophical Transactions of the Royal Society of London, B298,* 199–209

Shallice, T., & Burgess, P. W. (1991). Deficits in strategy application following frontal lobe damage in man. *Brain, 114,* 727–741.

Sharrott, G. W. (1985/6). An analysis of occupational therapy theoretical approaches for mental health: Are the profession's major treatment approaches truly occupational therapy? *Occupational Therapy in Mental Health, 5,* 1–16.

Shriffin, R. M., & Schneider, W. (1977). Controlled and automatic human information processing: II. Perceptual learning, automatic attending, and a general theory. *Psychological Review, 84,* 127–190.

Shute, V. J., & Glaser, R. (1990). A large-scale evaluation of an intelligent discovery world: Smithtown. *Interactive Learning Environments, 1,* 51–77.

Siegler, C. C. (1987). *Functions of humor in occupational therapy.* Unpublished master's thesis. Tufts University, Medford, MA.

Simmons, W., & Resnick, L. (1993). Assessment as the catalyst of school reform. *Educational Leadership, 50,* 11–15.

Skarda, C. A., & Freeman W. J. (1987). How brains make chaos in order to make sense of the world. *Behavioral and Brain Sciences, 10,* 161–195.

Sladyk, K. (1992). Traumatic brain injury, behavioral disorder, and group treatment. *American Journal of Occupational Therapy, 46,* 267–270.

Slife, B., Weiss, J., & Bell, T. (1985). Separability of metacognition and cognition: Problem solving in learning disabled and regular students. *Journal of Educational Psychology, 77,* 437–445.

Sloan, R. L., Downie, C., Hornby, J., & Pentland, B. (1991). Routine screening of brain damaged patients: A comparison of the Rivermead Perceptual Assessment Battery and the Chessington Occupational Therapy Neurological Assessment Battery. *Clinical Rehabilitation, 5,* 265–272.

Smith, A. (1982). *Symbol Digit Modalities Test Manual.* Los Angeles: Western Psychological Services.

Söderback, I., Bengtsson, I., Ginsburg, E., & Eckholm, J. (1992). Video feedback in occupational therapy: Its effect in patients with neglect syndrome. *Archives of Physical Medicine and Rehabilitation, 73,* 1140–46.

Söderback, I., & Ekholm, J. (1993). Occupational therapy in brain damage rehabilitation. *Critical Reviews in Physical and Rehabilitation Medicine, 5,* 315–355.

Sohlberg, M. M., & Mateer, C. A. (1989). *Introduction to cognitive rehabilitation: Theory and practice.* New York: The Guilford Press.

Solet, J. M. (1974). *Solet test for apraxia.* Unpublished master's thesis. Boston University, Boston, MA.

Sörensen, L. (1978). *Cognitive test.* Gentofte, Denmark: Tranehaven.

Spreen, O., & Benton, A. L. (1969). *Embedded figure test.* Neuropsychology Laboratory, University of Victoria, Victoria, BC, Canada.

Spreen, O., & Strauss, E. (1991). *A compendium of neurospychological tests.* New York: Oxford University Press.

Springer, S. P., & Deutsch, G. (1989). *Left brain, right brain* (3rd ed.). New York: W. H. Freeman.

Squire, L. R. (1987). *Memory and Brain.* New York: Oxford University Press.

Squire, L., & Alvarez, P. (1995). Retrograde amnesia and memory consolidation: A neurobiological perspective. *Current Opinion in Neurobiology, 5,* 169–177.

Squire, L. R., Ojemann, J. G., Miezin, F. M., et al. (1992). Activation of the hippocampus in normal humans: A functional anatomical study of memory. *Proceedings of the National Academy of Sciences, USA, 89,* 1837–1841.

Squire, L. R., & Zola-Morgan, S. (1991). The medial temporal lobe memory system. *Science, 253,* 1380–1386.

Stanley, M., Sutterfield, J., Bowden, S., & Williams, C. (1995). Chessington Occupational Therapy Neurological Assessment Battery: Comparison of performance of people aged 50–65 years with people aged 66 and over. *Australian Occupational Therapy Journal, 42,* 55–65.

Starkstein, S. E., & Robinson, R. G. (1994). Neuropsychiatric aspects of stroke. In C. E. Coffey & J. L. Cummings (Eds.), *Textbook of geriatric neuropsychiatry* (pp. 455–475). Washington, DC: American Psychiatric Press, Inc.

Stone, E. L. (1992). The use of the cognitive disability frame of reference in a short-stay private psychiatric hospital. In N. Katz (Ed.), *Cognitive rehabilitation: Models for intervention in occupational therapy* (pp. 51–76). Boston: Andover Medical.

Strayer, D. L., & Kramer, A. F. (1994). Aging and skill acquisition: Learning-Performance distinctions. *Psychology and Aging, 9,* 589–605.

Stringer, A. Y. (1996). *A guide to adult neurological diagnosis.* Philadelphia: F. A. Davis.

Strong, J., Gilbert, J., Cassidy, S., & Bennett, S. (1995). Expert clinicians' and students' views on clinical reasoning in occupational therapy. *British Journal of Occupational Therapy, 58,* 119–122.

Stroop, J. R. (1935). Studies of inference in serial verbal reactions. *Journal of Experimental Psychology, 18,* 643–662.

Strub, R. L., & Black, F. W. (1985). *The mental status examination in neurology.* (2nd ed.). Philadelphia: F. A. Davis.

Stuss, D. T. (1991). Disturbance of self-awareness after frontal system damage. In G. P. Prigatano & D. L. Schacter (Eds.), *Awareness of Deficit After Brain Injury: Clinical and Theoretical Issues* (pp. 63–83). New York: Oxford University Press.

Stuss, D. T. (1992). Biological and physiological development of executive functions. *Brain and Cognition, 20,* 8–23.

Swiderek, B. (1996). Metacognition. *Journal of Adolescent and Adult Literacy, 39,* 418–419.

Tate, R., & McDonald, S. (1995). What is apraxia? The clinician's dilemma. *Neuropsychological Rehabilitation, 5,* 273–297.

Thelen, E. (1995). Motor development: A new synthesis. *American Psychologist, 50,* 79–95.

Thomas, C. (1997). *Taber's Cyclopedic Medical Dictionary.* 18th Edition. Philadelphia: F. A. Davis.

Tickle-Degnen, L. (1995). Therapeutic rapport. In C. A. Trombly (Ed.), *Occupational therapy for physical dysfunction* (4th ed., pp. 277–285). Baltimore: Williams & Wilkins.

Tickle-Degnen, L., & Rosenthal, R. (1990). The behavioral and cognitive response of brain-damaged patients to therapist instructional style. *Occupational Therapy Journal of Research, 10,* 345–359.

Tiffin, J. (1968). *Purdue Pegboard: Examiner manual.* Chicago: Science Research Associates.

Toglia, J. P. (1989a). Approaches to cognitive assessment of the brain injured adult: Traditional methods and dynamic investigation. *Occupational Therapy Practice, 1,* 36–55.

Toglia, J. P. (1989b). Visual perception of objects: an approach to assessment and intervention. *American Journal of Occupational Therapy, 43,* 587–595.

Toglia, J. (1991). Generalization of treatment: A multicontext approach to cognitive perceptual impairment in adults with brain injury. *American Journal of Occupational Therapy, 45,* 505–516.

Toglia, J. P. (1992a). *Cognitive perceptual rehabilitation: a dynamic interactional approach.* Unpublished workshop manual, Cornell University Medical Center, New York.

Toglia, J. P. (1992b). A dynamic interactional approach to cognitive retraining. In N. Katz (Ed.), *Cognitive rehabilitation: Models for intervention in occupational therapy* (pp. 104–143). Boston: Andover Medical Publishers.

Toglia, J. P. (1993a). *The contextual memory test manual.* Tucson, AZ: Therapy Skills Builders.

Toglia, J. (1993b). Attention and memory. In C. B. Royeen (Ed.), *AOTA Self study series: Cognitive rehabilitation* (pp. 1–72). Rockville, MD: American Occupational Therapy Association.

Trahey, P. J. (1991). A comparison of the cost-effectiveness of two types of occupational therapy services. *American Journal of Occupational Therapy, 45,* 397–400.

Tranel, D., Anderson, S. W., & Benton, A. (1994). Development of the concept of "executive function" and its relationship to the frontal lobes. In F. Boller & J. Grafman (Eds.), *Handbook of neuropsychology* (vol. 9, pp. 125–148). Amsterdam: Elsevier Science B. V.

Trexler, L. (1987). Neuropsychological rehabilitation in the United States. In M. Meier, A. Benton, & L. Diller (Eds.), *Neuropsychological Rehabilitation* (pp. 437–460). New York: Guilford Press.

Trombly, C. A. (Ed.), (1989). *Occupational therapy for physical dysfunction* (3rd ed.). Baltimore: Williams & Wilkins.

Trombly, C. (1993). The issue is anticipating the future: Assessment of occupational function. *American Journal of Occupational Therapy, 47,* 253–257.

Trombly, C. A. (Ed.), (1995a). *Occupational therapy for physical dysfunction* (4th ed.). Baltimore: Williams & Wilkins.

Trombly, C. A. (1995b). Planning, guiding and documenting therapy. In C. A. Trombly (Ed.), *Occupational therapy for physical dysfunction* (4th ed., pp. 29–40). Baltimore: Williams & Wilkins.

Trombly, C. A. (1995c). Theoretical foundations for practice. In C. A. Trombly (Ed.), *Occupational therapy for physical dysfunction* (4th ed., pp. 15–27). Baltimore: Williams & Wilkins.

Trombly, C. A. (1995d). Retraining basic and instrumental activities of daily living. In C. A. Trombly (Ed.), *Occupational therapy for physical dysfunction* (4th ed., pp. 289–318). Baltimore: Williams & Wilkins.

Tulving, E., & Schacter, D. L. (1990). Priming and human memory systems. *Science, 24,* 301–305.

Tyerman, R., Tyerman, A., Howard, P., & Hadfield, C. (1986). *COTNAB— Chessington Occupational Therapy Neurological Assessment Battery introductory manual.* Nottingham: Nottingham Rehab Limited.

Unsworth, C. A. (1996). Clients' perceptions of discharge housing decisions following stroke rehabilitation. *American Journal of Occupational Therapy, 50,* 207–216.

Unsworth, C. A. (1997). Team decision making in rehabilitation. *American Journal of Physical Medicine and Rehabilitation, 75,* 483–484.

Unsworth, C. A. (1998). Ergonomics for one: Cognitive disabilities. In V. Berg Rice (Ed.), *Ergonomics in health care and rehabilitation* (pp. 79–110). Newton MA: Butterworth Heinemann.

Unsworth, C. A., & Thomas, S. A. (1993). Information use in discharge accommodation recommendations for stroke patients. *Clinical Rehabilitation, 7,* 181–188.

Unsworth, C. A., Thomas, S. A., & Greenwood, K. M. (1995). Rehabilitation team decisions concerning discharge housing for stroke patients. *Archives of Physical Medicine and Rehabilitation, 76,* 331–340.

U. S. Army (1944). *Army Individual Test Battery. Manual of directions and scoring.* Adjutant General's Office.

Uzzell, B. P. (1997). Neuropsychological rehabilitation models. In J. Leon-Carrion (Ed.), *Neuropsychological rehabilitation: Fundamentals, innovations and directions* (pp. 41–46). Delray Beach, FL: GR/St. Lucie Press.

Vallar, G. (1993). The anatomical basis of spatial hemineglect in humans. In I. H. Robertson & J. C. Marshall (Eds.), *Unilateral neglect: Clinical and experimental studies* (pp. 27–59). Hove: Lawrence Erlbaum Associates Ltd.

Valli, L. (Ed.). (1992). *Reflective teacher education: Cases and critiques.* Albany, NY: State University of New York Press.

Van Deusen, J. (1988). Unilateral neglect: Suggestions for research by occupational therapists. *American Journal of Occupational Therapy, 42,* 441–448.

Van Deusen, J. (1993). *Body image and perceptual dysfunction in adults.* Philadelphia: W. B. Saunders.

van Zomeren, A. H., & Brouwer, W. H. (1994). *The clinical neuropsychology of attention.* New York: Oxford University Press.

von Bertalanffy, L. (1968). *General systems theory: Foundations, development, applications.* New York: George Braziller Inc.

Wang, P. I., & Ennis, K. E. (1986). Competency assessment in clinical populations: an introduction to the Cognitive Competency Test. In B. Uzzell & E. Gross (Eds.). *Clinical neuropsychology of intervention.* Boston: Martinus Nijhoff Publishing.

Walsh, K. (1994). *Neuropsychology: A clinical approach* (3rd ed.). London: Churchill Livingstone.

Warren, M. (1993a). A hierarchical model for evaluation and treatment of visual perceptual dysfunction in adult acquired brain injury: Part I. *American Journal of Occupational Therapy, 47*, 42–53.

Warren, M. (1993b). A hierarchical model for evaluation and treatment of visual perceptual dysfunction in adult acquired brain injury: Part II. *American Journal of Occupational Therapy, 47*, 55–66.

Warren, M. (1994). Visuospatial skills: Assessment and intervention strategies. In C. B. Royeen (Ed.), *AOTA Self-study series: Cognitive rehabilitation* (pp. 1–76). Rockville, MD: American Occupational Therapy Association.

Warren, M. (1996). Evaluation and treatment of visual deficits. In L. W. Pedretti (Ed.), *Occupational therapy practice skills for physical dysfunction* (4th ed., pp. 193–212). St. Louis, MO: C. V. Mosby.

Warrington, E. K. (1984). *Recognition Memory Test.* Windsor, UK: NFER-Nelson.

Weber, A. M. (1990). A practical clinical approach to understanding and treating attentional problems. *Journal of Head Trauma Rehabilitation, 5*, 73–85.

Weinberg, J., Diller, L., Gordon, W. A., et al. (1977). Visual scanning training affect on reading related tasks in acquired right brain damage. *Archives of Physical Medicine and Rehabilitation, 58*, 479–486.

Weinberger, D. R. (1988). Schizophrenia and the frontal lobe. *Trends in Neurosciences, 11*, 367–370.

Wertsch, J. V. (1985). Adult-child interaction as a source of self-regulation in children. In S. R. Yussen (Ed.), *The Growth of Reflection in Children* (pp. 69–97). Orlando, FL: Academic Press, Inc.

Whalley Hammell, K. R. (1994). Establishing objectives in occupational therapy practice, Part 2. *British Journal of Occupational Therapy, 57*, 45–48.

Whiting, S., Lincoln, N., Bhavnani, G., & Cockburn, J. (1985). *RPAB—Rivermead Perceptual Assessment Battery.* Windsor: NFER-NELSON.

Wickelgren, W. A. (1977). *Learning and memory.* Englewood Cliffs, NJ: Prentice-Hall, Inc.

Williams, J. H., Drinka, T. J. K., Greenberg, J. R., et al. (1991). Development and testing of the assessment of living skills and resources (ALSAR) in elderly community dwelling veterans. *The Gerontologist, 31*, 84–91.

Wilson, B. A. (1987). *Rehabilitation of memory.* New York: Guilford Press.

Wilson, B. (1988). Remediation of apraxia following an anaesthetic accident. In J. West & P. Spinks (Eds.), *Case studies in clinical psychology* (pp. 178–183). Bristol: John Wright & Sons Ltd.

Wilson, L. G. (1979). The use of a stroke group treatment program on an extended care unit. *Canadian Journal of Occupational Therapy, 46*, 19–20.

Wilson, P., & Calder, R. V. (1990). *Housing choices for older Australians.* Melbourne: The Australian Council on the Aging.

Wilson, B., Cockburn, J., & Baddely, A. (1991). *RBMT—The Rivermead Behavioural Memory Test.* Bury St. Edmunds, London: Thames Valley Test Company.

Wilson, B., Cockburn, J., Baddely, A., & Hiorns, R. (1989). Development and validation of a test battery for detecting and monitoring everyday memory problems. *Journal of Clinical and Experimental Neuropsychology, 11*, 885–870.

Wilson, B., Cockburn, J., & Halligan, P. W. (1987a). *Behavioural Inattention Test.* Bury St. Edmunds, England: Thames Valley Test Company.

Wilson, B., Cockburn, J., & Halligan, P. W. (1987b). Development of a behavioural test of visuospatial neglect. *Archives of Physical Medicine and Rehabilitation, 68*, 98–102.

Wilson, T. D., Lisle, D. J., Schooler, J. W., et al. (1993). Introspecting about reasons can reduce post-choice satisfaction. *Personality and Social Psychology Bulletin, 19*, 331–339.

Winegardner, J. (1993). Executive functions. In H. Cohen (Ed.), *Neuroscience for rehabilitation* (pp. 346–353). Philadelphia: Lippincott.

Winkler, P. A. (1995). Head injury. In D. A. Umphred (Ed.), *Neurological rehabilitation* (pp. 421–453). St. Louis: Mosby.

Winne, P. H. (1995). Inherent details in self-regulated learning. *Educational Psychologist, 30*, 173–187.

Witherell, C., & Noddings, N. (Eds.). (1991). *Stories lives tell: Narratives and dialogue in education.* New York: Teachers College Press.

Wood, R. L. (1987). *Brain injury rehabilitation: A neurobehavioral approach.* London: Croon Helm.

Wood, W., Abreu, B., Duval, M., & Gerber, D. (1994). Occupational performance and the functional approach. In C. B. Royeen (Ed.), *AOTA Self-study series: Cognitive rehabilitation* (pp. 1–50). Rockville, MD: American Occupational Therapy Association.

World Health Organization (1980). *International classification of impairments, disabilities and handicaps.* Geneva: Author.

Worthington, A. D. (1996). Cueing strategies in neglect dyslexia. *Neuropsychological rehabilitation, 6*, 1–17.

Young, G. (1996). Evaluating questions used to assess cognitive orientation for very old adults. *Psychological Reports, 78*, 827–833.

York Haaland, K., & Flaherty, D. (1984). The different types of limb apraxia errors made by patients with left vs. right hemisphere damage. *Brain and Cognition, 3*, 370–384.

Yuen, H. K. (1994). Neurofunctional approach to improve self-care skills in adults with brain damage. *Occupational Therapy in Mental Health, 12*, 31–45.

Zarit, S. H., Orr, N. K., & Zarit, J. M. (1985). *The hidden victims of Alzheimer's disease: Families under stress.* New York: New York University Press.

Zarit, S. H., Reever, K. E., & Bach-Peterson, J. (1980). Relatives of the impaired elderly, correlates of feeling of burden. *Gerontologist, 20*, 649–655.

Zarit, S. H., Todd, P. A., & Zarit, J. M. (1986). Relatives of the impaired elderly, correlates of feeling of burden. *Gerontologist, 26*, 260–266.

Zarit, S. H., & Zarit, J. M. (1983). Cognitive impairment. In P. M. Lewinsohn & L. Teri (Eds.), *Clinical Geropsychology: New directions in assessment and treatment.* New York: Pergamon Press.

Zemke, R. (1994). Task skills, problem solving and social interaction. In C. B. Royeen (Ed.), *AOTA Self-study series: Cognitive rehabilitation* (pp. 1–44). Rockville, MD: American Occupational Therapy Association.

Zoltan, B. (1996). *Vision, perception and cognition: A manual for the evaluation and treatment of the neurologically impaired adult* (3rd ed.). Thorofare. NJ: Slack Inc.

Zoltan, B., Jabri, J., Panikoff, L., & Ryckman, D. (1983). *Perceptual motor evaluation for head injured and other neurologically impaired adults.* San Jose, CA: Santa Clara Valley Medical Center.

Index

Page numbers followed by "f" indicate figures; page numbers followed by "t" indicate tables.